# Medicare Made Easy

# DATE DUE

| AP 30'98 | | | |
|---|---|---|---|
| AP 16'01 | | | |
| DE | | | |
| | | | |
| | | | |
| | | | |
| | | | |
| | | | |
| | | | |
| | | | |
| | | | |
| | | | |
| | | | |
| | | | |
| | | | |
| | | | |
| | | | |
| | | | |

# MEDICARE · MADE · EASY

## REVISED AND UPDATED EDITION

### Charles B. Inlander
President, People's Medical Society

### Michael A. Donio

**≡People's Medical Society®**

Allentown, Pennsylvania

The People's Medical Society is a nonprofit consumer health organization dedicated to the principles of better, more responsive, and less expensive medical care. Organized in 1983, the People's Medical Society puts previously unavailable medical information into the hands of consumers so that they can make informed decisions about their own health care.

Cover design by Hannus Design Associates
Text design by Joyce C. Weston

*Library of Congress Cataloging-in-Publication Data*

Inlander, Charles B.
     Medicare made easy. — Rev. and updated ed. / Charles B. Inlander, Michael A. Donio
         p.   cm.
     Includes bibliographical references and index.
     ISBN 1-882606-67-1 (pbk.)
     1. Medicare.   2. Medicare—Claims administration.   I. Donio, Michael A.   II. Title.
     HD7102.U4I56   1997
     368.4′2′0973—dc20                                           96-43924
                                                                          CIP

1 2 3 4 5 6 7 8 9 0

# Acknowledgments

No book can be written by the authors alone. In this case, many hard-working and dedicated people assisted. We would like to thank the dedicated employees of the Health Care Financing Administration (HCFA), the people who administer the Medicare program. Especially we thank Frank Sokolik, director, Division of Beneficiary Relations; Dick Getrost, Anne Hoffnar, and Carol Sampson, all HCFA public affairs specialists; and many other fine people at the Baltimore headquarters who helped us launch this project.

We also thank Margaret Jefferson, health insurance specialist with HCFA, for her assistance on Social Security and Medicare eligibility criteria.

From the People's Medical Society, we thank Linda Hager who managed the editorial revisions for this edition. We also thank Karla Morales, People's Medical Society vice president, for serving as the general editor and overall coordinator of the book; Jennifer Hay and Janet Worsley Norwood for editorial assistance; Karen Kemmerer, who handled all aspects of production; and Linda Swank for manuscript entry.

# Contents

# Introduction

Since 1983, when we created the People's Medical Society, I have traveled over two million miles listening and talking to people about medicine and health care. I have heard tales of horror and stories of inspiration. I have met victims of the medical system and persons alive today because of it.

And we get mail, as well. In fact, on average, the People's Medical Society receives tens of thousands of pieces of correspondence each year. And just as I find when on the road, the stories and questions cover the entire medical/health gamut.

By meeting and corresponding with hundreds of thousands of people, I have reached the following conclusions:

- Medical consumers want to be more involved in and in charge of their health care.
- The majority want reliable information about the quality of the services available so they can make informed medical decisions.
- Nobody can figure out Medicare!

This year thirty-eight million Americans will be covered by the program. More than $200 billion will be paid annually by Medicare to doctors and hospitals for services to elderly and to certain disabled citizens. That's almost 3 percent of the gross domestic product.

But that's only part of the story. Over $50 billion more is paid out each year from either the pockets of Medicare beneficiaries or their private supplemental insurers to pay for services Medicare did not cover entirely or at all.

Yet, despite the enormity of the program — Medicare is the costliest government entitlement program in the world — virtually no Medicare recipient really understands how it works or how it can work for him or her. In fact, many people deny themselves medical care, pay out-of-pocket for services Medicare will cover, refuse to appeal a denial of coverage, or allow themselves to be bullied or buffaloed by a doctor's receptionist, hospital accounting clerk, or insurance carrier's telephone representative simply because they do not understand Medicare.

People who are under the age of 65, are not disabled, or have not directly assisted a senior or disabled citizen in traversing the Medicare maze find it hard to believe that Medicare is such a complicated program. What could be so hard, they ask? You hit 65 or have a disability, you head down to the Social Security office and sign up for the program, and the rest is a smooth sail down an idyllic, albeit costly, medical stream.

Little do they know. In fact, a very alert 92-year-old woman once confided in me that she could not wait until the next year when her 64-year-old son would become eligible for Medicare. Her reason — now he would not think she was suffering from senile dementia every time she complained about her problems with Medicare.

Why is Medicare so complicated? Why can't reasonably intelligent people — the majority of whom are able to wend their way through the Internal Revenue Service's long income tax form without getting audited and incarcerated — make heads or tails out of Medicare?

The answer is simple. There has not been a single publication printed by the government (or anyone else, for that matter) that explains fully and clearly how to use the program, what it does and does not cover, how to appeal individual rulings and decisions, and most important, how to make Medicare work for the consumer.

Wait a minute. Doesn't Medicare itself publish a variety of publications that explain it all? The answer is both yes and no.

Yes, it does publish many publications. All are useful to some extent or another. In fact, the primary publication, *Your Medicare Handbook* — the one everyone gets after signing up — is a straightforward booklet that gives the basic information one needs. But, and this is a big, qualified but, it does nothing more than give a basic description of services.

The other Medicare publications are also helpful — most are single-topic brochures covering a specific issue or situation. Most people do not even know these publications exist, however.

The major gap in Medicare's own publications is what they do not say and, in some instances, what they cannot say.

Because Medicare is a government program, initiated by Congress, administered by a governmental bureaucracy, and partially operated by contracted insurance companies and paying private doctors, hospitals, and health maintenance organizations, the publications it produces must go through layer upon layer of review not only to ensure accuracy but also to avoid opening any of the parties involved to problems.

For example, the Medicare laws and regulations do not require doctors to accept assignment. Assignment is government talk for accepting what Medicare pays as full payment for services rendered.

Medicare's publications explain that. But what they do not tell you is the following:

- Some doctors do not accept assignment 100 percent of the time.
- You can negotiate with any doctor who does not accept assignment and possibly, in your case, get him or her to do so.

These are two glaring omissions. They are also extremely important bits of information for you, the beneficiary.

In other words, Medicare's publications are like the instructions you get with your federal income tax forms each year — they give you basic information, tell you what form you need, when and where to file, and so on. But they do not tell you how to get the maximum benefits, tactics and techniques you can use to save money, or how to make the most of the program.

That is why we have written *Medicare Made Easy*. It is essential for the Medicare beneficiary to have not only the basic information but all of the information needed to use and get the maximum benefit from the program.

We also wrote this book to help the reader cut through the bureaucratic red tape that envelops Medicare.

*Medicare Made Easy* goes beyond what Medicare tells its beneficiaries. We show readers what they need to know to get their benefits on the very first day eligible. We describe how one consumer can pay less for doctor and hospital services than a friend or neighbor who has the exact same coverage. We help beneficiaries in their selection of a Medicare supplemental insurance program (something Medicare itself cannot even talk about).

As the nation's largest consumer health advocacy organization, the People's Medical Society has no ax to grind, no insurance to sell, and no conflicts of interest. We exist for one purpose: to help medical consumers get the most from the health care system.

This book is designed to fulfill that goal. Everything in it is meant to help you.

Medicare is going through a period of major change. The increasing number of citizens enrolling in the program each year and the increase in the life span of all Americans has put the program under severe financial pressure. But this pressure is not new. The program has always been, and always will be, a fiscal challenge. And each time the program has shown signs of financial weakness, Congress has devised ways to meet the need.

No one can predict how long people will live and what their state of health will be. No one can foresee, with accuracy, the new medical technologies that emerge each year and what their fiscal impact will be. But one thing is certain, even with all the juggling and jiggling of the program, Medicare is here to stay. It is one of the most popular programs ever devised by the federal government and it is the cornerstone of every senior citizen's health program.

Even though Medicare will not vanish, it will change. The financial state of the nation, the ever-changing health care system, new and unique ways of delivering health care, and the political climate at any given time are all factors that force modifications to the program. That is why it is essential that you and your family fully understand the program.

Remember, Medicare is your health insurance plan. You pay for it; you elect people who have the oversight responsibility for it. In our democracy, you are the chairperson of the board. And just like any chief executive, make sure you are treated with the respect, dignity, and service you deserve.

CHARLES B. INLANDER
PRESIDENT, PEOPLE'S MEDICAL SOCIETY
ALLENTOWN, PENNSYLVANIA

In this chapter you will learn: How Medicare began  ▪  The role of the Social Security Administration  ▪  The role of the Health Care Financing Administration  ▪  The role of Medicare Carriers and Intermediaries  ▪  The role of the Peer Review Organizations

# 1. Understanding Medicare

Medicare is probably the largest and the most expensive single program that the federal government runs. It is also one of the most complex, because passage of the Medicare law in 1965 required a good deal of horse-trading, especially with the American Medical Association (AMA) and various health insurers. If at times Medicare seems not to make sense to you, keep in mind that it was never supposed to. The current law is the result of a long series of political deals that had to satisfy diverse interests in order for there to be any law at all.

You won't think too much about Medicare until you have occasion to file a claim. Assume that your health problems are simple and uncomplicated. Assume that all the care you need is within the bounds of what the program pays for. Assume that you have enough income to pay the Medicare Part B (doctor insurance) premium, the catastrophic insurance premium, and the premium for a good supplemental policy easily. Assume that you have selected a good Medicare supplemental insurance policy. Assume that everything each of your doctors does is clearly medically necessary. Assume that you get well or die quickly. If all of these assumptions are met, Medicare will appear benign and friendly. You will wonder why anyone ever has problems with it.

If Medicare is your only source of payment for health care, you can't afford supplemental insurance or pick a poor policy, and you require care in a nursing home, you are likely to have a nightmare. You will wonder how anyone could have designed a monstrosity that does to people what Medicare may well do to you. What you know can determine what kind of experience you will have with Medicare.

We have tried to keep this book short, simple, and to the point. Our goal is to put *you* in the driver's seat when you, as a Medicare beneficiary, deal with doctors, hospitals, the assorted Medicare carriers and intermediaries, and the needlessly large amount of paperwork involved. When we depart from the goal of KISS — Keep It Short and Simple — it is to provide you with background that you need to deal effectively with Medicare.

Medicare has been reformed almost continuously since it began, but it has been reformed piecemeal, with layers of controls being added atop one another. To avoid cluttering up the text with definitions and footnotes that the subject almost seems to demand, and to help you break the code language of Medicare and medicine, we've chosen to print special words in **boldface** the first few times they occur in the book (or in a chapter) as a clue that they are defined in the glossary at the back of the book. Points that we want to emphasize are in *italics*.

The American health care system embodies even more deals between the various parties involved than Medicare itself. They aren't public deals. Those who pay for health care in both the private and public sectors still don't feel as involved as they would like to be. Patients, consumers of medical services — you — have been involved in an effective way only in the last decade or so. Only in the last ten years have really effective health care consumer organizations emerged.

The impetus for Medicare arose in the early 1960s as part of the wave of New Frontier and Great Society programs started by President John F. Kennedy and continued by President Lyndon Johnson. A repeatedly quoted figure was that the elderly, at the time the law was passed, spent about 15 percent of their incomes on health care — a figure that was thought to be intolerable, as Senator Hubert Humphrey proclaimed with tears streaming down his face, arguing for passage of the law on the floor of the Senate. That was in 1965.

Yet today the elderly again spend more than 15 percent of their income on health care, even with Medicare. Does this mean that Medicare is a failure? Not really, if we measure it by other standards. Without it, the elderly and the disabled would spend far more than 15 percent of their incomes on health care, many would have to do without it, and the American people would have even less control over doctors and hospitals than they do today. And Medicare has helped to establish the idea that those who pay the bills in health care should make at least some of the rules.

Medicare has established, through the **Peer Review Organization** programs and their predecessors, that the medical profession and the hospital industry cannot really be trusted to guarantee quality care on their own. The peer review organizations are groups of doctors who make judgments about the medical necessity of what Medicare pays for. But they do it under contract with Medicare and aim at targets set by Medicare. They are constantly producing evidence that doctors need professional checkups as much as their patients need medical ones. (A list of the Peer Review Organizations is provided in appendix J.)

The **Diagnosis-Related Groups (DRG) system**, which we explain later, has shown that hospitals can give adequate care even if they are not rewarded with an endless shower of money. But Medicare has *not* relieved the elderly of the burden of paying for health care. It has only lightened it — and the elderly are paying more now, as a percentage of income, than when the law was passed.

Medicare does not pay for some of the services you may need the most. A common misconception, for example, is that Medicare pays for nursing home care. This misconception may have tragic consequences. Medicare will pay if you need short-term care in a **Skilled Nursing Facility** to assist in your recovery following a hospital stay. But no other nursing home care is paid for. "Custodial" care — care that you need because you can no longer function with complete independence — is *not* covered.

Medicare requires cost-sharing for most services. The average annual income from Social Security for a retired individual is $8,640; the average income for a retired couple is $14,580. This does not leave much room to pay more than 15 percent for health care, a burden that this program was supposed to alleviate.

Medicare imposes this burden on you because it is committed to the principle of cost-sharing. This is, in theory, a good idea. In practice, it has meant the loss of the original goals — somewhat equal access to health care and elimination of the threat of impoverishment because of illness — for many Americans. The amounts that you must pay for the Part B premiums (the part of Medicare that pays for doctor bills), for hospital care, and for doctors' services are raised automatically as the result of a formula, without regard for your ability to pay.

Medicare has established a national fee schedule for compensating doctors, called the **Resources-Based Relative Value Scale (RBRVS)**. Every procedure performed by doctors (primary care and specialists) is assigned a five-digit code along with a weighted value determined by the RBRVS. Medicare calculates the fee according to a formula that considers the resources needed to deliver the service. This new system not only makes Medicare fees more attractive to doctors, but it enables Medicare to more effectively manage expenditures on physician services. Another benefit is that more doctors might be encouraged to accept assignment. Only in Massachusetts, Pennsylvania, and Rhode Island are doctors required to accept what Medicare pays.

A national pay scale had been nearly unthinkable in part because doctors are not required to treat Medicare beneficiaries. Ensuring access to health care for older Americans without such a requirement is a chicken-and-egg problem. Older Americans need money to pay for health care. They also need doctors who will see them for the amounts that they can afford. Contrary to the image of the sainted doctor tending all the sick, the American Medical Association has maintained in its recent codes of ethics that a doctor has no obligation to treat any individual. (Stopping treatment against a patient's wishes is different, and it's considered unethical. It's called "abandonment" — but watch how fast you get abandoned if you can't pay your bill.) The AMA lobbied hard to ensure that no provision requiring doctors to treat beneficiaries went into the Medicare bill.

However, this hasn't stopped physicians and other practitioners from treating Medicare beneficiaries and participating in the Medicare program. More than three-quarters of physicians and other limited-license practitioners now participate in Medicare. As a result, some 90 percent of Medicare-allowed charges are now billed by participating providers. Participating providers include medical doctors (M.D.s), osteopathic doctors (D.O.s), chiropractors (D.C.s), nurse-practitioners (N.P.s), and physical therapists (P.T.s).

There are, of course, Medicare supplemental insurance plans that claim to cover the costs that Medicare doesn't cover. Some of them do a decent job, but others don't; nearly all of them fail to provide coverage for long-term care, which imposes the greatest risk of financial ruin on the elderly. (Relatively few of the elderly run up hospital bills that are enormous compared to others, and Medicare still picks up most of the tab for the usual length of hospital stay. It is long-term care, which about 5 percent of the over-65 population are using at any one time, that poses the real financial threat.) In this book, we show how to pick an affordable Medicare supplemental plan that fits your needs.

Medicare — and medicine — involve many special terms. Some

have the purpose of efficiently substituting one special word for several plain English ones. (Example: "assignment" instead of "the doctor's agreeing to take what Medicare determines is the fair price, handling the paperwork with Medicare for the patient, getting a check for 80 percent of the price directly from Medicare, and charging the patient or the patient's insurer only 20 percent," which could get cumbersome.) Others are just medical or bureaucratic jargon, having the effect of giving the laity less control over the process by introducing what can amount to the secret language of a club.

## Who Dealt This Mess, Anyway?

Who really runs Medicare? The answers may surprise you.

*The Law*

Medicare, as it currently exists, is a compromise between politicians' desire to provide what they thought was good-quality medical care to the elderly and their fear of what it would cost. It's between doctors and hospitals who fear loss of control over patients and medicine in general and their desire for federal dollars. It's between the public's notion that health care is a right and the reality that even the federal government cannot enforce such rights throughout fifty states and four territories. Add the desire of large health insurers, such as Blue Cross and Blue Shield, not to be locked out of the picture. Like the camel, it is a horse put together by a committee. And Medicaid — another federal health insurance program primarily for the nonelderly poor, which even the most starry-eyed legislators had not expected to see passed — was tacked on at the last second.

Like other benefits provided by the federal government to the middle class, the current form of Medicare has become something of a sacred cow. Legislators and the public fear changing it, because they fear losing what has been gained.

This means that, in contrast to some other federal programs, much of the driving force for change comes from the small professional bureaucracy that runs it and from the small segments of the other parts of government and the public that have learned to deal with them. Some of them toil on the staffs of congressional committees. Some work in the domestic policy section of the **Office of Management and Budget (OMB)**. Others work in the **Congressional Budget Office**. Some are in universities. The inner workings of the Medicare program are almost as far removed from public scrutiny as those of the Department of Defense.

Congress could never adjourn if all the details of federal program management were worked out on the floor of the House and Senate. Laws passed by Congress broadly authorize the programs; appropriations passed as part of the federal budget each year provide money for them. Everything else is left to the various **executive departments,** which write regulations for them that "have the force of law." This means that they are just like laws passed by Congress, but Congress never passed them, and most congresspersons never see them. Except in very special situations, all of them are published in the *Federal Register* before they take effect. Try finding the *Federal Register* at your local newsstand someday.

There's nothing sinister about this. It's a necessary compromise needed to make democracy work in a complicated society with thousands of government programs, a $1,000,000,000,000 (one trillion dollar) budget, and only 535 congresspersons and senators to look over the whole thing. But it does mean that Medicare beneficiaries have to enter the fray along with the doctors, the hospitals, the insurers, and all the other interest groups if they want their wishes to be heard, let alone heeded.

So here's who runs the parts of the show:

*The Social Security Administration*

The **Social Security Administration** is charged with administering determinations of eligibility for Medicare. If you are applying on the basis of reaching age 65 and not on the basis of disability or end stage renal disease, this almost always amounts to proving that you are who you say you are and that you were born when you say you were. If you are applying on the basis of disability, things usually get sticky (see chapters 2 and 8). The moment you are found eligible, your concerns with the Social Security Administration end. It passes on information to beneficiaries, and local offices act as a contact point for Medicare, but once the Social Security Administration has determined that you're eligible, you immediately become the responsibility of the Health Care Financing Administration.

*The Health Care Financing Administration (HCFA)*

The **Health Care Financing Administration (HCFA)** was set up in the early days of the Carter administration to bring control of all federally funded health programs under one roof. (When we say "Medicare" in this book, we mean HCFA and the Medicare program as run by it.) The idea was that health financing issues should be dealt with as such, not as issues peculiar to the funding program, such as Medicare, Medicaid, the Indian Health Service, and so on. What happened in practice is that a lot of public servants who had been under different roofs were lodged under one roof. Medicare and Medicaid have shared good ideas and come to resemble each other a lot more than they once did, but nothing miraculous has happened, except for the **diagnosis-related groups (DRG) system.** This represents a major loss of power by the medical profession and hospitals, and a major gain for the government. It is a model for moving the health care system away from professional interests and toward public interests. It may or may not be repeated while HCFA is around. (Incoming presidents and cabinet secretaries love to reorganize things. It gives the appearance of action while they try to figure out what is going on and tears the reins of power out of the hands of the civil service, which gives the political appointees a chance to grab them, but only a chance. The civil service usually catches them again in the end.)

Medicare controls every aspect of what happens to you as a Medicare recipient from the moment you are determined eligible. You are not handed back to the Social Security Administration until you die, when the Social Security Administration makes the determination on survivors' benefits.

In the last fifteen years, HCFA has been charged with controlling the cost of medical care. In the course of trying to do that, it realized that Medicare and Medicaid laws only looked like they left a lot of decisions in the hands of the **carriers** and the medical profession. Medicare has begun to assert control in almost every area, including many that doctors and hospitals, or even the **Food and Drug Administration (FDA)**, another part of the federal government, consider their own. Medicare has decided to release figures on the death rates and readmission rates for patients in hospitals around the nation. It is safe to say that as pressure to reduce the federal deficit mounts, Medicare will discover more things in the law that it has the power to do. Again, there's nothing sinister about this. Medicare always had the power to do much of what has been done by regulation. It has always had the power to find the prices charged by some doctors "inherently unreasonable" and refuse to pay them. Only recently has it found the will to do so.

HCFA can usually be counted on to try to do the right thing. But the medical profession and health care providers still retain enormous power in political circles, even if that power has diminished in recent years. The mood in Congress, the pressure to control health care costs, and the activism of groups such as the People's Medical Society and the American Association of Retired Persons created a climate in which HCFA can be used as a lever to expand the power of consumers in the health care system. This situation is not guaranteed to last, and Medicare has to be watched. You can deal with it in two ways: first, as a member of an association that asserts the rights of Medicare beneficiaries, and second, as an individual beneficiary.

What HCFA cannot do on its own, Congress has often been willing to do. Congressional committee staffers and the civil servants in HCFA talk to each other, and ideas are passed around. The regulations that Medicare lawyers discovered that Medicare did not have the power to issue have shown a tendency to become laws in the very next Congress.

It is not editorializing, but just pointing to a fact, to say that this situation has come about because the hospitals and organized medicine have deeply offended some powerful congresspersons and senators in the last few years. Health care is so complicated that congresspersons who take the time to educate themselves about it are routinely deferred to by their colleagues. The current discord between Congress and organized medicine creates a great opportunity for ordinary people to have a very loud voice in the way Medicare operates.

*The Carriers and Intermediaries*

When the Medicare law was passed, health insurers demanded a role. Basically, they argued that Medicare was socialized medicine, and therefore unacceptable, if the federal government ran it itself, but was a boon to the public if the federal government gave them contracts to run it. They won, sort of.

Medicare contracts with health insurance organizations, called **carriers** and **intermediaries**, to process Medicare claims (intermediaries process Part A claims and carriers process Part B claims). A list of carriers and intermediaries for the various parts of the United States can be found in appendix A.

Medicare periodically holds competitions for the contract to be a Medicare carrier for a particular area. Those who want the contract write large, detailed proposals and submit them to Medicare. Medicare selects the one that looks like it can do the job at the lowest overall cost. Medicare then monitors the carrier's performance. A look at the list of carriers and intermediaries shows that the Blue Cross and Blue Shield plans were certainly not locked out, as they feared.

The carriers and intermediaries try to implement the results of changes in the law and regulations according to manuals issued by Medicare. Sometimes they fail. The key to dealing with them is accurate paperwork and meticulous record-keeping. We've provided a Medicare Claims Log in appendix B to simplify the job.

*The Peer Review Organizations*

The peer review organizations are groups of doctors who make decisions on the medical necessity of health care under contract with Medicare. We explain how to deal with them in chapter 6, which deals with hospitals, and in chapter 8. They are becoming an increasingly greater force within Medicare as the Health Care Financing Administration relies on them for cost control.

## How to Deal with All of the Above

In this section we discuss some points to remember in dealing with all of the above. We hope that things will go smoothly for you and that you will never have occasion to use them.

The most fundamental point is that *Medicare is not a gift. You paid for it while you were working.* Medicare owes you services in just the same way that a health insurer to whom you have paid premiums owes them to you. You still pay a premium for Part B (doctor insurance). There is a contractual obligation to provide you with the services you've paid for, even if the federal government is the one with whom you have the contract.

Second, *being a Medicare beneficiary does not deprive you of any right you would have as a holder of private health insurance.* In fact, as you'll see in chapter 8, you have *more* rights than holders of private health insurance in all but a few states. Third, the price of health care has reached a level that very few individuals can afford. Everyone is dependent on someone else — an employer, a parent, or the government — for health care. It has priced itself out of the private market. As far as health care is concerned, everyone is poor. Everyone needs help.

## The Rest of the Book

This book has seven more chapters. Chapter 2 gives you an essential overview. Chapter 3 tells you exactly what Medicare does and doesn't cover. Chapter 4 describes supplemental insurance. Chapter 5 tells you how to negotiate with your doctor about fees and treatment. Chapter 6 explains how to deal with hospitals and the peer review organizations. Chapter 7 covers Medicare and nursing homes. Chapter 8 covers the problems that can arise and what you can do to solve them yourself or how to get help when you need it. We've also provided fourteen appendices that contain other sources of help.

A final note: We believe that health care in one's later years should be a source of security and not one of endless worry. We hope that this book helps make it so.

In this chapter you will learn: How Social Security and Medicare are linked ▪ When you're eligible and how to apply ▪ How to overcome barriers and claim benefits you earned ▪ The correct forms to use to speed your application on its way ▪ What Medicare covers and what it doesn't ▪ How to file a claim for Social Security disability insurance

---

# 2. The Basics

Many are unaware of how relatively little of a person's necessary medical care Medicare covers. It's around 50 percent now, and that number is falling, for many reasons. Medical care has become more expensive than Congress anticipated, and legislation would be required to close the gap. At a time when federal deficits and the stability of the Medicare Trust Fund are major concerns, Congress is reluctant to increase benefits as long as beneficiaries will tolerate the situation. Doctors' fees have risen dramatically. Some of the nation's doctors still do not accept Medicare **assignment** for all patients, and Medicare has only recently begun to use its power to limit what it pays doctors. The combination of these factors drives up the doctor bill for both beneficiaries and the Medicare program. The situation is unlikely to get much better. One potential bright spot is a new physician payment system called the **Resources-Based Relative Value Scale (RBRVS)**. It's another attempt by Congress to get a handle on the ever-increasing cost of physician services; however, its effectiveness won't be known for several years.

This chapter deals, of necessity, with Social Security. Social Security and the Medicare program are entangled in the area of Medicare eligibility. Since we'll be talking about Social Security, it's worth noting that many people are unaware of how little of preretirement income Social Security is intended to replace — about 42 percent, on average.

(The proportion falls as preretirement earnings rise. Lower-paid workers have a much higher replacement ratio than more highly paid ones.)

For both these reasons, it is important to know your Medicare and Social Security status *before* you retire. It is equally important to know what Medicare covers before retiring — possibly losing any coverage you might have through your employer — or dropping any personal medical insurance coverage you might have.

## Who May Apply for Medicare and Who Is Eligible

Anyone who thinks he or she is in one of the groups that Medicare covers can apply for it. In fact, if there is any doubt at all — in your mind or in the mind of the representative of Social Security at the Social Security office where you apply for Medicare — about whether you are eligible, you should apply.

## The Basic Coverage Groups

Medicare was originally intended for "the elderly" — people 65 or older. It now covers the following:

- *The elderly* — those who are 65 or older
- Those who are **permanently and totally disabled**
- Those who have **end stage renal disease,** the medical term for kidney disease that is severe enough to require dialysis or a transplant

Of course, things are not really this simple. Most, but not all, of the elderly are covered. The permanently and totally disabled are covered, but only if they meet the Social Security Administration's current definition of "permanently and totally disabled" and have received Social Security disability payments for at least two years. Those with end stage renal (kidney) disease are covered, but only if they meet the current definition of end stage renal disease. For most people, becoming eligible is just a matter of turning 65 and applying. For a few, it can be a frustrating process involving lawyers, appeals, and a lot of expense and anguish. What we will try to do in this chapter is make the process as easy as possible for everyone involved.

The Medicare program consists of two distinct parts: Hospital Insurance or Part A, which provides payment for covered inpatient hospital care, post-hospital extended care, and home health care following hospitalization; and Supplementary Medical Insurance or Part B, which helps pay for physician's services, home health care services, hospital outpatient services, and other medical services and items not covered under Part A. There is a pronounced difference between these two parts with respect to entitlement, coverage, and payment.

The Part A program is financed primarily through payroll taxes under the Federal Insurance Contributions Act (FICA). You've probably seen these letters on the stubs from your payroll checks. The Part B program is financed through a combination of general revenues and monthly premiums paid by each Medicare beneficiary. This premium is deducted from your Social Security check, unless you specifically don't apply for Medicare Part B.

To be eligible for Medicare Part A, you must first be entitled to Social Security (insured) based on your own earnings or those of a spouse, parent, or child. To be insured, you must have a specified number of work credits, the exact number of which is dependent on whether you are filing for Medicare Part A based on age, disability, or end stage renal disease.

## Eligibility Requirements for Medicare Coverage

As mentioned earlier, Medicare is available to three basic groups of insured individuals — the aged, the disabled, and those with end stage renal disease. There are various eligibility requirements for each group.

To be eligible for Medicare, *you or your spouse must be entitled to payments under the Social Security Act or the Railroad Retirement Act.* This means, in general, that you must have worked for at least 10 years in a job that was covered under the Social Security Act, or be covered *based on the earnings record of someone who is covered. It is also possible to be eligible for Medicare if you are an alien lawfully admitted for permanent residence. (An alien lawfully admitted for permanent residency must have resided in the United States continuously for five years at the time of the application.)*

You must also be age 65 or older. If you are not yet 65, you may be eligible if you are permanently and totally disabled, or have end stage renal disease (ESRD). A common misconception is that you will be covered if you are receiving Social Security. *This is not true unless you meet the requirements above.* The age requirements for Social Security and Medicare are different. For example, it is possible to start receiving Social Security payments at age 62, but you will not be covered by Medicare until you reach 65.

You are "eligible" for Medicare as soon as, and whenever, you meet the eligibility requirements that apply to you. You are "entitled" to Medicare only after you have *filed an application and are officially determined to be eligible. (If you are turned down, you have the right to appeal.)*

## The Work Requirement

In order to be eligible for Social Security, and subsequently Medicare, you must earn a certain number of Social Security work credits called quarters of coverage, and pay your Social Security taxes. While it may seem obvious, you only earn quarters of coverage when you are employed by a business that is covered under the Social Security Act. Fortunately, just about everyone, including the self-employed, are covered under Social Security (certain federal, state and local government employees pay only the Medicare portion of the FICA tax. In addition there are some religious organizations that are exempt from paying Social Security taxes; if you have any doubt as to your status, contact the Social Security Administration.) Most people pay the full FICA tax, so the credits they earn are usable to insure them for both Social Security and Medicare benefits.

In order for a quarter in which you work to count for Social Security (and Medicare) purposes, you must have a certain amount of income during that quarter. At present, for every $640 in annual income you earn one quarter of coverage. Therefore, if you make at least $2,560 during the year, you earn the maximum of four quarters of coverage. *No more than four quarters of Social Security credit can be earned in any one year, regardless of your total income.*

This is very important because your eligibility for Social Security and Medicare is based on the number of quarters of coverage you've earned. Most people born after 1929 must earn 40 quarters of coverage (10 years of work) to be eligible for Social Security. This does not mean that you must work for 10 continuous years, rather it means that you must accumulate 40 quarters of coverage during your working years. Even if you have gaps in your work record, you don't lose the credits you've earned. Let's look at the following example:

*You work steadily for eight years and earn the maximum of 32 quarters of coverage; you then do not work again for three years. Since you were not working, you were not earning quarters of coverage during this three-year period. You then return to work and once again begin to earn quarters of coverage. Your count resumes at 32 as you eventually earn the 40 quarters of coverage needed for Social Security and Medicare eligibility.*

If you're like most people, you will earn more quarters of coverage than are required for Social Security eligibility. Earning additional credits doesn't increase the monthly benefit you receive (benefits are tied to your dollar earnings). A full discussion of your monthly benefit is beyond the scope of this book; however, we encourage you to use the form shown on page 24 to request a statement of your Social Security earnings and estimated future monthly benefit.

If you're not sure that you can qualify for Medicare on your work record and quarters of coverage, you may be eligible on the earnings record of someone who is insured. For example:

- *Wives* are eligible if they are age 65 or older and if their husbands are insured.

- *Husbands* are eligible under the same conditions as wives.

- *Divorced women* are eligible if they were married to the insured person for at least 10 years, are age 65 or older, and have not remarried.

- *Divorced men* are eligible under the same conditions as divorced women.

- *Widows and widowers* are eligible if they are 65 or older and were married to their insured spouse for at least one year before the death of the spouse.

- *Other family members* may be eligible if they meet certain conditions. (Contact the Social Security Administration to discuss your particular situation.)

These are the conditions under which most of us qualify for Social Security and Medicare. Medicare Part A begins the month in which you turn 65, provided you filed an application within six months of the month in which you became 65.

However, as mentioned earlier, there are two other ways to qualify: (1) if you are permanently and totally disabled (not able to work for 24 months), or (2) you have end stage renal disease and require dialysis (the mechanical filtering of blood) or a kidney transplant.

Qualifying for Social Security based on disability is not an easy task, because what you might consider a disability isn't always a disability to the Social Security Administration. Under existing law, Social Security considers disability *your inability to work, based on a medical condition. You will be considered disabled if you are unable to engage in any substantial gainful activity and only if your inability to work is also expected to last for at least a year or result in your death.* Only the Social Security Administration can determine if you are disabled based upon the information provided in your application for disability benefits. (See application, pages 28 through 33.)

The law requires that you have earned a certain number of quarters of coverage prior to your disability. The exact number of work credits you need for disability benefits depends on your age at the time you became disabled. Here's the formula for determining the quarters of coverage you need.

*Disabled before age 24: You need six quarters in the three-year period ending when your disability began.*

*Age 24–31: You need credit for having worked half the time between age 21 and the time you became disabled. If you became disabled at age 29 you would need four years of quarters.*

*Age 31 or older: You generally need the same number of quarters as needed for retirement, and you must have earned at least 20 of the credits in the 10 years prior to your becoming disabled.*

Contact the Social Security Administration for information on the years of work credit and quarters of coverage needed for your specific age.

If you are disabled and entitled to Social Security or Railroad Retirement benefits, you are automatically entitled to Medicare Part A after 24 months. After approval, there is also an additional five-month disability waiting period before you are covered by Medicare Part A, so you actually become covered after 29 months of disability.

To qualify for the ESRD program, you must require regular dialysis or have had a kidney transplant.

*In addition to having chronic renal failure, you must either be entitled to a monthly insurance benefit under Title II of the Social Security Act (or an annuity under the Railroad Retirement Act); be fully or currently insured (credited with 40 quarters of coverage, but not yet of retirement age) under Social Security (railroad work may count); or be the spouse or dependent child of a person who meets one of the previous requirements.*

Your first month of eligibility for Medicare Part A is the third month after the month in which a regular course of dialysis begins. However, this three-month waiting period can be waived if you participate in a course of self-dialysis training during those three months. If you receive a kidney transplant, your eligibility begins with the month of the transplant or it may begin up to two months earlier if you were hospitalized during this time in preparation for the transplant. For more information on the ESRD program contact the Social Security Administration and request HCFA publication number 10128, "Medicare: Coverage of Kidney Dialysis and Transplant Services."

Up to this point, our discussion has focused on the Social Security Administration and the role it has in determining your eligibility for benefits. Now we need to introduce you to another government agency and explain the role it plays in Medicare.

Until it is determined that you are eligible for Medicare, you are the responsibility of the Social Security Administration. Once you are eligible for Medicare, you deal with the **Health Care Financing Administration (HCFA)**, which runs Medicare and Medicaid. (For the sake of brevity and avoidance of alphabet soup, we'll use "Medicare" to refer to HCFA from now on, unless there's a clear need to distinguish the program from those who run it.) We'll discuss the application process later in this chapter. For the moment, please believe that we are not trying to confuse Social Security issues with Medicare issues. Until you are found eligible for Medicare, the two are tied together. Most of the advice we give on Medicare will also help you preserve or increase your benefits under Social Security.

## Enrollment Periods

There are three types of enrollment periods that apply to both Medicare Part A and Part B: the initial enrollment period, the general enrollment period, and the special enrollment period for aged and disabled individuals covered under group health plans.

The initial enrollment period begins with the first day of the third month before the month in which you meet the Part B or Part A eligibility requirements. This period runs for a total of seven months. What this means is that you may apply three months before you meet the eligibility requirement, usually age 65, to three months past your 65th birthday. The chart on page 38 will help you calculate when you should apply.

The general enrollment period is much less complicated. It always occurs during the first three months of a calendar year: January, February, and March. If you miss your initial enrollment period for any reason, you may always apply during this general enrollment period.

The special enrollment period applies if you are 65 or older or are disabled and you meet the following conditions:

- You are covered by your current employer's group health plan when you become eligible for Medicare.

- You are covered by your current employer's group health plan, or you are covered by your spouse's group health plan or, if you are disabled, you are covered under a group health plan of another family member. (Contact the Social Security Administration to discuss your particular situation.)

## What to Do If You Are Not Eligible Now

Remember, you cannot get Medicare unless you are eligible for Social Security. (There is an option to purchase Medicare as insurance if you're not eligible. We'll discuss this later.) In order to make sure you are eligible for Medicare, qualify for Social Security.

Two of the most common reasons why you would not qualify for Social Security are that you aren't old enough or you don't meet the work requirement. Only time will remedy these situations. (Remember you can qualify for Social Security at 62, but you can't get Medicare until you are 65.)

If you are found ineligible because you do not have enough covered work, there's only one answer: more work, earning the necessary quarters of coverage.

# SOCIAL SECURITY ADMINISTRATION

Form Approved
OMB No. 0960-0466

[ ] **SP**

## Request for Earnings and Benefit Estimate Statement

To receive a free statement of your earnings covered by Social Security and your estimated future benefits, all you need to do is fill out this form. Please print or type your answers. When you have completed the form, fold it and mail it to us.

1.  Name shown on your Social Security card:

    _____ _____
    First Name                              Middle
                                              Initial

    _____
    Last Name Only

2.  Your Social Security number as shown on your card:

    [ ][ ][ ] - [ ][ ] - [ ][ ][ ][ ]

3.  Your date of birth

    [ ][ ] [ ][ ] [ ][ ][ ][ ]
    Month  Day   Year

4.  Other Social Security numbers you have used:

    [ ][ ][ ] - [ ][ ] - [ ][ ][ ][ ]
    [ ][ ][ ] - [ ][ ] - [ ][ ][ ][ ]

5.  Your sex:   [ ] Male   [ ] Female

6.  Other names you have used
    (including a maiden name):

    _____

7.  Show your actual earnings for last year and your estimated earnings for this year. Include only wages and/or net self-employment income covered by Social Security.

    A.  Last year's actual earnings: (Dollars Only)

        $ [ ][ ][ ] , [ ][ ][ ] . [0][0]

    B.  This year's estimated earnings: (Dollars Only)

        $ [ ][ ][ ] , [ ][ ][ ] . [0][0]

8.  Show the age at which you plan to retire:

    [ ][ ]
    (Show only one age)

9.  Below, show the average yearly amount you think you will earn between now and when you plan to retire. We will add your estimate of future earnings to those earnings already on our records to give you the best possible estimate.

    Enter a yearly average, not your total future lifetime earnings. Only show earnings covered by Social Security. Do not add cost-of-living, performance or scheduled pay increases or bonuses. The reason for this is that we estimate retirement benefits in today's dollars, but adjust them to account for average wage growth in the national economy.

    However, if you expect to earn significantly more or less in the future due to promotions, job changes, part-time work, or an absence from the work force, enter the amount in today's dollars that most closely reflects your future average yearly earnings.

    **Most people should enter the same amount they are earning now (the amount in 7B).**
    Future average yearly earnings: (Dollars Only)

    $ [ ][ ][ ] , [ ][ ][ ] . [0][0]

10. Address where you want us to send the statement.

    _____
    Name

    _____
    Street Address (Include Apt. No., P.O. Box, or Rural Route)

    _____
    City                   State        Zip Code

11. [ ]  Please check this box if you want to get your statement in Spanish instead of English.

    I am asking for information about my own Social Security record or the record of a person I am authorized to represent. I understand that if I deliberately request information under false pretenses I may be guilty of a federal crime and could be fined and/or imprisoned. I authorize you to use a contractor to send the statement of earnings and benefit estimates to the person named in item 10.

    **Please sign your name (Do not print)**

    ▲ _____
      Signature

    _____
    Date              (Area Code) Daytime Telephone No.

Form SSA-7004-SM (2-93) Destroy Prior Editions

*Make Sure Your Earnings Record Is Accurate*

You can obtain a statement of your earnings record every three years by obtaining a Form 7004-SM (see form and instructions, page 24) from your local Social Security office and sending it to the Social Security Administration. You can also send a letter. The letter below is a suggested format for this.

> Your name
> Your street address
> Your city, state, and zip code
>
> Date

> Social Security Administration
> Wilkes Barre Data Operations Center
> P.O. Box 7004
> Wilkes Barre, PA 18767-7004

> Dear Madam or Sir:

> Please send me a copy of my earnings record. My Social Security number is [*fill in your number*]. My date of birth is [*fill in date*]. [*If you have used any other names:*] I am also known as [*fill in the other names*]. Thank you for your attention to this request.

> Sincerely yours,
> Your signature

If your earnings record does not show that you have enough covered quarters to be covered now, the first thing to do is make sure that the record is accurate. It can be in error regarding *whether or not* there were any earnings in a quarter. This can affect your eligibility for Social Security and Medicare. It can also be in error about the *amount* you earned. This can affect your eligibility for both programs and the amount of your Social Security benefits.

Errors in earnings records happen for a number of reasons. Failure of employers to report earnings to the **Social Security Administration (SSA)** is probably the most common reason now. In the past, there were many problems with making sure that each person working under Social Security had a unique number. In one case, a wallet manufacturer included a dummy Social Security card in its wallets. The number used was not obviously a fake one, such as 000-00-000, and the card looked just like the real thing. Many people who bought the wallets used the card and the number it carried as their **Social Security** number (SSN). In other cases, all members of a family used the same Social Security number.

To straighten out an earnings record that has errors in it, Social Security has to check it against other records that are correct. This is where the hard part begins. Ideally, you will have all the paycheck stubs or pay envelopes that were ever issued to you, and you will have all of your federal, state, and local tax returns for your entire working life. You will have the names and addresses of all your former employers. None of them will have shut down, moved, or changed its name. If all this is true, straightening out your earnings record will be snap.

The foregoing is almost never true. Fortunately, all you usually have to provide is information on the last five years of earnings, which are typically the highest-earning years (your SSA payment is based on the "high five"). Those five years contain twenty of the forty quarters you need to show that you worked, so all that is necessary is proving that you worked some in twenty other quarters.

Personnel at your local SSA district office can help you straighten out your earnings record. The SSA has specialists in this at regional offices if the local office can't help you, and your case can be sent to them as a last resort. The problem is that all of this will take time. For this reason, it is important to start early — before you need Medicare.

You may think you can see that your earnings record is right, but it's still a good idea to check it against your tax returns for the last five years. The figure recorded should equal the total of the Social Security Wages boxes on your W-2 forms. If you earned more than the maximum amount taxed for the year, only the maximum earnings for the year will be shown. If more is shown, you can apply to the IRS, via an amended tax return for the years in which too much was collected, to get a refund of the excess. See the example on page 27.

*Work,
More Work*

This is yet another reason to check your earnings record. Don't retire from your job, assuming that the SSA will provide more than enough to live on and Medicare will cover your medical bills, until you know you are eligible and what your benefits will be. Social Security has a form that you may request (by calling 1-800-772-1213) that allows you to estimate your benefit. Find out if you need more quarters of work to be covered.

This advice is obviously of no benefit if you have already quit and can't get your job back (or any job) or if you are permanently and totally disabled. We advise you to seek almost any sort of work you can do in order to obtain coverage. The benefits, although not as great as perhaps they should be, are well worth it.

---

**Excess Social Security Taxes: Getting a Refund**

In 1996, wages up to $62,700 were subject to a Social Security tax of 6.2 percent and a Medicare hospital tax of 1.45 percent for a combined tax rate of 7.65 percent. Earnings above $62,700 are subject only to the Medicare hospital tax.

By working two jobs, you earned $65,000. One paid $35,000 and the other $30,000. You did not reach $62,700 with either employer, so both continued to collect Social Security taxes.

You paid:                       $35,000 × 7.65% = $2,677.50

                                         $30,000 × 7.65% = $2,295.00

                                                Total = $4,972.50

You should have paid:     $62,700 × 7.65% = $4,796.55

                                        $ 2,300 × 1.45% = $    33.35

                                                Total = $4,829.90

Refund due:                $4,972.50 − 4,829.90 = $   142.60

Applying for a refund of this amount will not reduce your future Social Security benefits, because no more than $62,700 of income can be counted toward them in 1996.

---

If you feel you are disabled, you should apply for disability benefits. The necessary quarters of coverage are reduced, based on the year you became disabled.

*Proving That You Really Are Disabled*

You may be denied coverage if you do not qualify for Social Security benefits as a permanently and totally disabled person. Congress, in adding disabled person coverage, was acutely aware of the problems that had arisen in state Worker's Compensation programs, and structured the law so that only unquestionably disabled persons would qualify. The definition used to accomplish this seems absurdly strict:

*The term " disability" means (A) inability to engage in any substantial gainful activity by reason of any medically determined physical or mental impairment which can be expected to result in death or has lasted or can be expected to last for a continuous period of not less than 12 months, or (B) blindness; and the term "blindness" means central visual acuity of 20/200 or less in the better eye with the use of a correcting lens. (**Social Security Act, Sec. 216(i)(1)**)*

The application for disability insurance benefits is shown on pages 28–33.

## APPLICATION FOR DISABILITY INSURANCE BENEFITS

I apply for a period of disability and/or all insurance benefits for which I am eligible under title II and title XVIII of the Social Security Act, as presently amended.

### PART I—INFORMATION ABOUT THE DISABLED WORKER

1. (a) PRINT your name ⟶ FIRST NAME, MIDDLE INITIAL, LAST NAME

   (b) Enter your name at birth if different from item (a) ⟶

   (c) Check (√) whether you are ⟶ ☐ Male   ☐ Female

2. Enter your Social Security Number ⟶ _ _ _ / _ _ / _ _ _ _

3. (a) Enter your date of birth ⟶ MONTH, DAY, YEAR

   (b) Enter name of State or foreign country where you were born. ⟶

   If you have already presented, or if you are now presenting, a public or religious record of your birth established before you were age 5, go on to item 4.

   (c) Was a public record of your birth made before you were age 5?   ☐ Yes   ☐ No   ☐ Unknown

   (d) Was a religious record of your birth made before you were age 5?   ☐ Yes   ☐ No   ☐ Unknown

4. (a) What is your disabling condition? (Briefly describe the injury or illness that prevents, or has prevented, you from working.)

   (b) Is your injury or illness related to your work in any way? ⟶   ☐ Yes   ☐ No

5. (a) When did you become unable to work because of your disabling condition? ⟶ MONTH, DAY, YEAR

   (b) Are you still disabled? (If "Yes," go on to item 6.) (If "No," answer (c).) ⟶   ☐ Yes   ☐ No

   (c) If you are no longer disabled, enter the date your disability ended. ⟶ MONTH, DAY, YEAR

6. (a) Have you (or has someone on your behalf) ever filed an application for Social Security benefits, a period of disability under Social Security, supplemental security income, or hospital or medical insurance under Medicare? ⟶   ☐ Yes (If "Yes," answer (b) and (c).)   ☐ No (If "No," or "Unknown" go on to item 7.)   ☐ Unknown

   (b) Enter name of person on whose Social Security record you filed other application. ⟶

   (c) Enter Social Security Number of person named in (b). (If unknown, so indicate) ⟶ _ _ _ / _ _ / _ _ _ _

7. (a) Were you in the active military or naval service (including Reserve or National Guard active duty or active duty for training) after September 7, 1939 and before 1968? ⟶   ☐ Yes (If "Yes," answer (b) and (c).)   ☐ No (If "No," go on to item 8)

   (b) Enter dates of service ⟶ FROM: (month, year)   TO: (month, year)

   (c) Have you ever been (or will you be) eligible for a monthly benefit from a military or civilian Federal agency? (include Veterans Administration benefits only if you waived military retirement pay) ⟶   ☐ Yes   ☐ No

| 8. | Have you or your spouse worked in the railroad industry for 7 years or more? ⟶ | ☐ Yes | ☐ No |
|---|---|---|---|

| 9. | (a) Have you filed (or do you intend to file) for any other public disability benefits? (Include workers' compensation and Black Lung benefits) ⟶ | ☐ Yes (If "Yes," answer (b).) | ☐ No If "No," go on to item 10.) |
|---|---|---|---|

(b) The other public disability benefit(s) you have filed (or intend to file) for is (Check as many as apply):

☐ Veterans Administration Benefits     ☐ Welfare

☐ Supplemental Security Income     ☐ Other (If "Other," complete a Workers' Compensation/Public Disability Benefit Questionnaire)

| 10. | (a) Have you ever engaged in work that was covered under the social security system of a country other than the United States? (If "Yes," answer (b).) (If "No," go on to item 11.) ⟶ | ☐ Yes | ☐ No |
|---|---|---|---|

(b) List the country(ies): ⟶

**11.** Enter below the names and addresses of all the persons, companies, or Government agencies for whom you have worked this year, last year, and the year before last.
If the above does not apply, write "NONE" below and go on to item 13.

| NAME AND ADDRESS OF EMPLOYER (If you had more than one employer, please list them in order beginning with your last (most recent) employer) | Work Began | | Work Ended (If still working show "Not ended") | |
|---|---|---|---|---|
| | MONTH | YEAR | MONTH | YEAR |
| | | | | |
| | | | | |
| | | | | |

(If you need more space, use "Remarks" space on page 3.)

| 12. | May the Social Security Administration or the State agency reviewing your case ask your employers for information needed to process your claim? ⟶ | ☐ Yes | ☐ No |
|---|---|---|---|

**13.** THIS ITEM MUST BE COMPLETED, EVEN IF YOU WERE AN EMPLOYEE.

| (a) Were you self-employed this year, last year, or the year before? (If "Yes," answer (b).) (If "No," go on to item 14.) ⟶ | ☐ Yes | ☐ No |
|---|---|---|

| (b) Check the year or years in which you were self-employed | In what kind of trade or business were you self-employed? (For example, storekeeper, farmer, physician) | Were your net earnings from your trade or business $400 or more? (Check "Yes" or "No") |
|---|---|---|
| ☐ This Year | | |
| ☐ Last Year | | ☐ Yes   ☐ No |
| ☐ Year before last | | ☐ Yes   ☐ No |

| 14. | (a) How much were your total earnings last year? (Count both wages and self-employment income. If none, write "None.") ⟶ | Amount $ _____ |
|---|---|---|
| | (b) How much have you earned so far this year? (If none, write "None.") ⟶ | Amount $ _____ |
| | (c) Did you receive any money from an employer(s) on or after the date in item 5(a) when you became unable to work because of your disability? (If "Yes," give amounts and explain in "Remarks" on page 3.) ⟶ | ☐ Yes   ☐ No Amount $ _____ |
| | (d) Do you expect to receive any additional money from an employer such as sick pay, vacation pay, other special pay? (If "Yes," please give amounts and explain in "Remarks" on page 3.) ⟶ | ☐ Yes   ☐ No Amount $ _____ |

FORM SSA-16-F6 (1-85)  Page 2

## PART II — INFORMATION ABOUT THE DEPENDENTS OF THE DISABLED WORKER

| 15. | Have you ever been married? (If "Yes," answer item 16) (If "No," go on to item 17.) | ☐ Yes ☐ No |
|---|---|---|

**16.** (a) Give the following information about your current marriage. If not currently married, show your last marriage below.

| To whom married | When (Month, day, year) | Where (Name of City and State) |
|---|---|---|

| Your current or last marriage | How marriage ended (If still in effect, write "Not ended.") | When (Month, day, year) | Where (Name of City and State) |
|---|---|---|---|
| | Marriage performed by:<br>☐ Clergyman or public official<br>☐ Other (Explain in Remarks) | Spouse's date of birth (or age) | If spouse deceased, give date of death |
| | Spouse's Social Security Number (If none or unknown, so indicate) — — — / — — / — — — — | | |

(b) Give the following information about each of your previous marriages. **(If none, write "None.")**

| To whom married | When (Month, day, year) | Where (Name of City and State) |
|---|---|---|

| Your previous marriage | How marriage ended | When (Month, day, year) | Where (Name of City and State) |
|---|---|---|---|
| | Marriage performed by:<br>☐ Clergyman or public official<br>☐ Other (Explain in Remarks) | Spouse's date of birth (or age) | If spouse deceased, give date of death |
| | Spouse's Social Security Number (If none or unknown, so indicate) — — — / — — / — — — — | | |

*(Use a separate statement for information about any other marriages.)*

**17.** If your claim for disability benefits is approved, your children (Including natural children, adopted children, and stepchildren) or dependent grandchildren (including stepgrandchildren) may be eligible for benefits based on your earnings record.

List below FULL NAME OF ALL such children who are now or were in the past 12 months UNMARRIED and:
- UNDER AGE 18 ● AGE 18 TO 19 AND ATTENDING SECONDARY SCHOOL
- DISABLED OR HANDICAPPED (age 18 or over and disability began before age 22)

**(IF THERE ARE NO SUCH CHILDREN, WRITE "NONE" BELOW AND GO ON TO ITEM 18.)**

| 18. | Do you have a dependent parent who was receiving at least one-half support from you when you became unable to work because of your disability? (If "Yes," enter name and address in "Remarks.") | ☐ Yes ☐ No |
|---|---|---|

REMARKS (You may use this space for any explanation. If you need more space, attach a separate sheet.)

# IMPORTANT INFORMATION ABOUT DISABILITY INSURANCE BENEFITS —
## PLEASE READ CAREFULLY

**I. SUBMITTING MEDICAL EVIDENCE:** I understand that as a claimant for disability benefits, I am responsible for providing medical evidence showing the nature and extent of my disability. I may be asked either to submit the evidence myself or to assist the Social Security Administration in obtaining the evidence. If such evidence is not sufficient to arrive at a determination, I may be requested by the State Disability Determination Service to have an independent examination at the expense of the Social Security Administration.

**II. RELEASE OF INFORMATION:** I authorize any physician, hospital, agency or other organization to disclose to the Social Security Administration, or to the State Agency that may review my claim or continuing disability, any medical record or other information about my disability.

I also authorize the Social Security Administration to release medical information from my records, only as necessary to process my claim, as follows:

- Copies of medical information may be provided to a physician or medical institution prior to my appearance for an independent medical examination if an examination is necessary.
- Results of any such independent examination may be provided to my personal physician.
- Information may be furnished to any contractor for transcription, typing, record copying, or other related clerical or administrative service performed for the State Disability Determination Service.
- The State Vocational Rehabilitation Agency may review any evidence necessary for determining my eligibility for rehabilitative services.

**THIS MUST BE ANSWERED** ➤ 19. DO YOU UNDERSTAND AND AGREE WITH THE AUTHORIZATIONS GIVEN ABOVE? ☐ Yes ☐ No     (If "No,", explain why)

_____
_____
_____
_____
_____
_____
_____

**III. REPORTING RESPONSIBILITIES:** I agree to promptly notify Social Security if:

- My MEDICAL CONDITION IMPROVES so that I would be able to work, even though I have not yet returned to work.
- I GO TO WORK whether as an employee or a self-employed person.
- I apply for or receive a decision on benefits under any WORKERS' COMPENSATION law or plan (including Black Lung benefits from the Department of Labor.) or other public benefit based on disability.
- I am imprisoned for conviction of a felony.

The above events may affect my eligibility to disability benefits as provided in the Social Security Act, as amended.

**I know that anyone who makes or causes to be made a false statement or representation of material fact in an application or for use in determining a right to payment under the Social Security Act commits a crime punishable under Federal law by fine, imprisonment or both. I affirm that all information I have given in this document is true.**

| SIGNATURE OF APPLICANT | Date (Month, day, year) |
|---|---|
| Signature (First name, middle initial, last name) (Write in ink)<br><br>SIGN HERE ➤ | Telephone Number(s) at which you may be contacted during the day. (Include the area code) |

Mailing Address (Number and street, Apt. No., P.O. Box, or Rural Route) (Enter resident address in "Remarks" if different)

| City and State | ZIP Code | Enter Name of County (if any) in which you now live |
|---|---|---|
| | | |

Witnesses are required ONLY if this application has been signed by mark (X) above. If signed by mark (X), two witnesses to the signing who know the applicant must sign below, giving their full addresses. Also, print the applicant's name in the Signature block.

| 1. Signature of Witness | 2. Signature of Witness |
|---|---|
| Address (Number and street, City, State, and ZIP Code) | Address (Number and street, City, State, and ZIP Code) |

Form SSA-16-F6 (1-85) Page 4

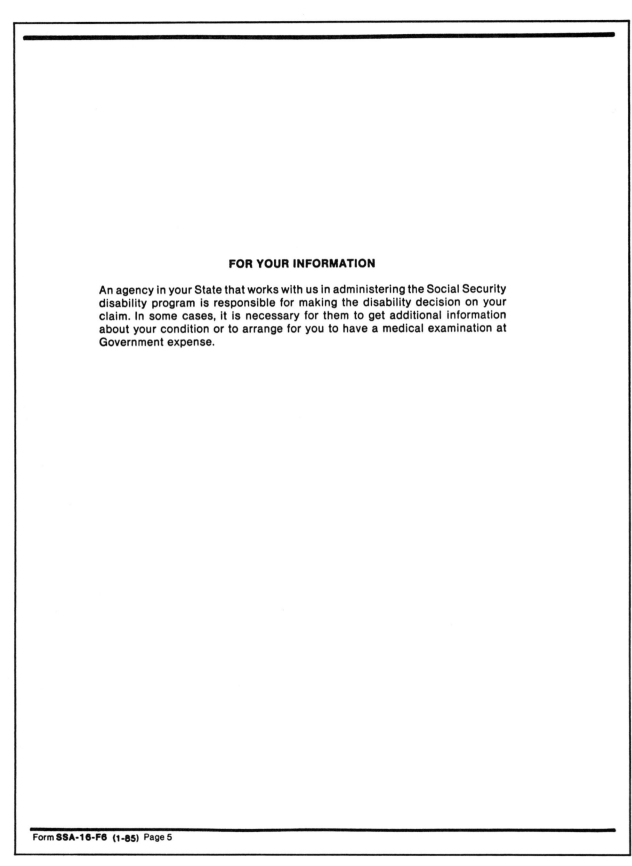

**FOR YOUR INFORMATION**

An agency in your State that works with us in administering the Social Security disability program is responsible for making the disability decision on your claim. In some cases, it is necessary for them to get additional information about your condition or to arrange for you to have a medical examination at Government expense.

## RECEIPT FOR YOUR CLAIM FOR SOCIAL SECURITY DISABILITY INSURANCE BENEFITS

| PERSON TO CONTACT ABOUT YOUR CLAIM | SSA OFFICE | DATE CLAIM RECEIVED |
|---|---|---|
| TELEPHONE NUMBER (INCLUDE AREA CODE) | | |

Your application for Social Security disability benefits has been received and will be processed as quickly as possible.

You should hear from us within _____ days after you have given us all the information we requested. Some claims may take longer if additional information is needed.

In the meantime, if you change your address, or if there is some other change that may affect your claim, you - or someone for you - should report the change. The changes to be reported are listed below.

Always give us your claim number when writing or telephoning about your claim.

If you have any questions about your claim, we will be glad to help you.

| CLAIMANT | SOCIAL SECURITY CLAIM NUMBER |
|---|---|
| | |

### CHANGES TO BE REPORTED AND HOW TO REPORT
### FAILURE TO REPORT MAY RESULT IN OVERPAYMENTS THAT MUST BE REPAID

▶ You change your mailing address for checks or residence. To avoid delay in receipt of checks you should ALSO file a regular change of address notice with your post office.

▶ You go outside the U.S.A.

▶ Any beneficiary dies or becomes unable to handle benefits.

▶ Custody Change — Report if a person for whom you are filing or who is in your care dies, leaves your care or custody, or changes address.

▶ You are confined to jail, prison, penal institution, or correctional facility for conviction of a felony.

▶ Change of Marital Status — Marriage, divorce, annulment of marriage.

▶ You return to work (as an employee or self-employed) regardless of amount of earnings.

▶ Your condition improves.

▶ If under age 65, you begin to receive workers' compensation or another public disability benefit (including Black Lung benefits) or the amount of your present Workers' compensation or public disability benefit changes.

**HOW TO REPORT**

You can make your reports by telephone, mail, or in person, whichever you prefer.

If you are awarded benefits, and one or more of the above changes occur, the change(s) should be reported by calling

_____
(Telephone Number—Include Area Code)

### Collection and Use of Information From Your Application — Privacy Act Notice/Paperwork Act Notice

The Social Security Administration is authorized to collect the information on this form under sections 202(b), 202(c), 205(a), and 1872 of the Social Security Act, as amended (42 U.S.C. 402(b), 402(c), 405(a), and 1395ii). While it is VOLUNTARY, except in the circumstances explained below, for you to furnish the information on this form to Social Security, no benefits may be paid unless an application has been received by a Social Security office. Your response is mandatory where the refusal to disclose certain information affecting your right to payment would reflect a fraudulent intent to secure benefits not authorized by the Social Security Act. The information on this form is needed to enable Social Security to determine if you and your dependents are entitled to insurance coverage and/or monthly benefits. Failure to provide all or part of this information could prevent an accurate and timely decision on your claim or your dependent's claim, and could result in the loss of some benefits or insurance coverage. Although the information you furnish on this form is almost never used for any other purpose than stated in the foregoing, there is a possibility that for the administration of the Social Security programs or for the administration of programs requiring coordination with the Social Security Administration, information may be disclosed to another person or to another governmental agency as follows: 1. to enable a third party or an agency to assist Social Security in establishing rights to Social Security benefits and/or coverage; 2. to comply with Federal laws requiring the release of information from Social Security records (e.g., to the General Accounting Office and the Veterans Administration); and 3. to facilitate statistical research and audit activities necessary to assure the integrity and improvement of the Social Security programs (e.g., to the Bureau of the Census and private concerns under contract to Social Security).

Form **SSA-16-F6** (1-85) Page 6      ☆ U.S. GOVERNMENT PRINTING OFFICE 1984 461-398/10024

The regulations implementing the Social Security Act specifically prescribe that if you are able to perform any gainful work at all, you are not disabled for Social Security purposes. If the disability examiners judge that you could do some work, you are not disabled. You may protest that you do not know how to do the work the examiners believe you can do, that you have no chance of getting any training for it, and that the only shop that does that kind of work is in Shanghai. No matter. Practical difficulties like this aren't considered — only your state of body and mind. The definition leads to paradoxes: persons likely to live a long time, but not "able-bodied" in any sense, are denied benefits.

There is obviously a large subjective component to an examiner's determination as to whether or not a person is disabled in the sense the SSA law requires. There is no exact medical standard that determines, for example, that a person who has only partial use of one hand is capable or incapable of running a telephone answering service from home. The task is made harder because some disabled persons have achieved more than the vast majority of the nondisabled: Some who have only the use of their eyes and mouth have written novels and painted; a quadriplegic who has lost the ability to speak, but can still make sounds, is one of the world's leading astrophysicists. Usually such individuals have a good deal of support (for buying special equipment and hiring assistants). Disabled persons who have this level of support and the drive to make use of it are rare. But the fact that they exist makes it all the easier for examiners to deny benefits to disabled applicants.

Examiners in the same office, to say nothing of examiners in different parts of the country, arrive at completely opposite judgments about whether or not specific persons meet the requirements for disability benefits. And politics seems to enter the picture as well. Different presidential administrations have placed great emphasis on strict applications of the rules; others have not. Courts in different **federal judicial districts** have made different decisions about disability cases, and the **Department of Health and Human Services**, which includes the Social Security Administration and Medicare, is picking and choosing among them in an effort to keep costs down. Your chance of being found eligible for benefits on the basis of disability depends, unfortunately, on the luck of the draw: what your doctor says, which examiner you get, which federal judicial district you live in, and which **Administrative Law Judge (ALJ)** hears your appeal.

If you are denied benefits because you are found not disabled, we strongly urge you to appeal. At the same, you should realize that time and costs will be involved and that you will probably need the help of a lawyer. We cover how to appeal decisions in chapter 8.

## If All Else Fails, You Don't Have to Be Eligible to Buy It: What You Can Buy From Medicare

Persons 65 years old who do not otherwise qualify for Medicare can purchase Medicare coverage just like private insurance. The 1997 premium for the combined Part A Hospital Insurance ($311) and Part B Medical Insurance ($43.80) is $354.80 per month. If, for some reason, you do not have 40 quarters of Social Security coverage, you may still be able to purchase Medicare Part A. New regulations permit those persons with at least 30 quarters of coverage to buy into Medicare Part A for $187 per month. Their Part B premium would be the same at $43.80 per month. Contact a Social Security office for more information about this program.

You are permitted to purchase Part B of Medicare (insurance for doctor bills) if you are a resident of the United States, are 65 or over, and are either a citizen or an alien lawfully admitted for permanent residence who has resided in the United States for the last five years. (It is under this rule that everyone enrolls in Part B.) If you are not eligible for Part A of Medicare, enrolling for Part B entitles you to purchase it, so you have to buy Part B to get Part A.

Examples:

*Victoria Smith-Jones's brother Cedric is entranced by Victoria's letters about life in the United States and decides to move here in late 1992. He is lawfully admitted for permanent residence. Being independently wealthy, he decides not to work. He loses most of his fortune in the 1997 stock market crash and can no longer afford his extremely expensive medical insurance. He is 65 in early 1998 and discovers that he is not automatically eligible for Medicare because he has never worked (anywhere, anytime). He decides to purchase Medicare. He calls his local Social Security office, establishes that he is not eligible but will meet the requirements for purchase, requests that an application to purchase Part B and Part A be sent to him, and signs up.*

*Marge's sister, Amber Smith Citron, aged 66, was married to her former husband, Harold Citron, for nine years and 361 days. She would have been eligible for Medicare on his earnings record had she been married to him for ten years. She has been working and has earned 34 quarters of coverage, but still needs 40 for full eligibility. She meets the requirements of age (65 or over), and current U.S. residence, and, like Cedric, signs up to purchase Medicare. Unlike Cedric, she will be eligible in early 1998. When she is eligible, she will no longer pay the Part A premium and will pay a reduced Part B premium.*

## How and When to Apply

Once more, being between ages 62 and 65 does not *entitle* you to Medicare. Being 65 or over does not *enroll* you for Medicare. It may take action on your part when you turn 65. Some people are automatically enrolled; others are given notices that they need to enroll. Automatic enrollment and notification are administrative actions of the Social Security Administration, not requirements of the law. The categories of those who are enrolled automatically have changed, and they could change again. *If you want Medicare, apply for it.* The worst that can happen is that you'll find out your enrollment is already taken care of.

- If you are 65 or over and have been receiving Social Security benefits, you will automatically be enrolled for participation in Parts A and B (the hospital and doctor insurance portions of Medicare). You will receive a notice and your card (shown on page 37) about three to four months before your sixty-fifth birthday. Your card will not be valid until you turn 65. You are covered for Medicare even if you do not have your card; the hospital can bill under your Social Security number even if you do not have the card. You can obtain a Temporary Notice of Medicare Eligibility from your Social Security office.

- If you are 65 or over when you apply for Social Security benefits, you will automatically be enrolled as part of the application process for Social Security. Your card will be sent to you in the mail automatically. You are covered for Medicare even if you do not have your card if you are over 65 and have been found eligible for Social Security.

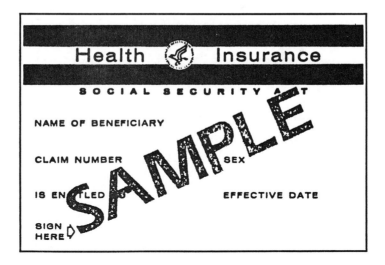

- End-stage-renal-disease patients are automatically enrolled if they are receiving Social Security disability benefits; otherwise, they must apply.

Your card also shows your health insurance claim number. Sometimes this claim number is referred to as your Medicare number. The claim number has nine digits and a letter. On some cards, there may also be another number after the letter. Your full claim number must always be included on all Medicare claims and correspondence. When a husband and wife both have Medicare, each will receive a separate card and claim number. Each spouse must use the exact name and claim number shown on his or her card.

It is important that you remember to

1. Always show your Medicare card when you receive services that Medicare can help you pay for.
2. Always write your health insurance claim number (including the letter) on any bills you send in and on any correspondence about Medicare. Also, you should have your Medicare card available when you make a telephone inquiry.
3. Carry your card with you whenever you are away from home. If you ever lose it, immediately ask your Social Security office to get you a new one.
4. Use your Medicare card only after the effective date shown on it.
5. Never permit someone else to use your Medicare card.

If you enrolled for Social Security and began receiving benefits before you were 65, *you must take action to enroll in Medicare.* Formerly, people were notified by mail when they were eligible to enroll.

This service has been dropped as a cost-cutting measure. You will have to keep track of the time yourself.

You can apply for Part B Medicare coverage *to begin on your 65th birthday* anytime between three months before your 65th birthday and three months after. If you apply later than this, your Part A (hospital insurance) coverage will begin on the date you apply, not on your birthday. Your "personal enrollment period," as the SSA calls it, is these seven months. The chart below may help.

## Get It, Because You Can't Always Get What You Want

If you do not apply for Part B (doctor insurance) when you apply for Part A, you will not be eligible to apply until the next **general enrollment period**, which runs from January 1 to March 31 of each year.

| MONTH IN WHICH 65TH BIRTHDAY OCCURS | EARLIEST MONTH TO APPLY | LATEST MONTH TO APPLY |
| --- | --- | --- |
| April 1997 | January 1997 | July 1997 |
| May 1997 | February 1997 | August 1997 |
| June 1997 | March 1997 | September 1997 |
| July 1997 | April 1997 | October 1997 |
| August 1997 | May 1997 | November 1997 |
| September 1997 | June 1997 | December 1997 |
| October 1997 | July 1997 | January 1998 |
| November 1997 | August 1997 | February 1998 |
| December 1997 | September 1997 | March 1998 |
| January 1998 | October 1997 | April 1998 |
| February 1998 | November 1997 | May 1998 |
| March 1998 | December 1997 | June 1998 |
| April 1998 | January 1998 | July 1998 |
| May 1998 | February 1998 | August 1998 |
| June 1998 | March 1998 | September 1998 |
| July 1998 | April 1998 | October 1998 |
| August 1998 | May 1998 | November 1998 |
| September 1998 | June 1998 | December 1998 |
| October 1998 | July 1998 | January 1999 |
| November 1998 | August 1998 | February 1999 |
| December 1998 | September 1998 | March 1999 |

Your premium will be raised 10 percent for each year you wait to apply. In addition, your coverage will not begin until July 1 of the year you enroll.

We recommend that you apply for Part B coverage at the same time you apply for Part A, if you can afford it. Failure to take Part B will make any supplemental insurance you buy harder to obtain and will make your premium higher. The Part B premium is tax-deductible, just like any other medical insurance premium.

## Application Forms and Process

Whether or not you are receiving Social Security, you should apply for Medicare three months before your sixty-fifth birthday. This will allow ample time for all the paperwork to be processed, any questions about your eligibility to be cleared up, and the like so that you obtain coverage as soon as you are eligible.

The first step is to telephone your local **Social Security office**. These offices are commonly listed under the federal government section in the blue pages of your local phone directory, and under "United States Government" in the white pages. If you can't find a listing, call the information operator and ask for any Social Security office. Calling any Social Security office will enable you to find out which one you should go to.

Call that office. Tell them you want to apply for Medicare (and Social Security, if you are not already receiving it). The SSA is making a determined effort to carry out as much business as possible over the phone. This is generally more efficient, and it saves you a visit to the Social Security office. At the same time, if you have trouble dealing with matters like this over the phone (if, for example, you have trouble hearing and don't have an amplified phone), you can insist on a face-to-face visit.

Whichever way you apply, the Social Security office representative will fill out most of the forms for you. This is done to ensure that the type of answers the SSA needs to make a decision are obtained on the forms involved. After the representative has filled out the forms, you should read them — and insist on the correction of any errors — before you sign them. If you need special assistance (if, for example, you are deaf), special help will be made available to you. You may have to go to another Social Security office to find the right person to help you. The representative at the first Social Security office you go to will give you instructions. If you think you will need special help, you should mention this when you first call.

The representative will ask you to bring certain documents when you come to the Social Security office, usually, the following:

- Proof of age
- Records of earnings, such as W-2 forms (or tax returns for the self-employed) for the past two years
- Your Social Security card

If you are applying because you think you are disabled, you will be asked to bring some documents relating to your medical problems. The Social Security office representative will tell you what they are.

*Keep your originals. Keep your originals. Keep your originals.* Need we say more?

The form of proof of age that the Social Security office wants is a birth certificate or a hospital birth record. If you can't obtain either of these, don't worry:

- The census records of 1910, 1920, or 1930 are accepted.
- Any school record that gives your age and was recorded before you were 21 is acceptable.
- Newspaper birth announcements are accepted.
- **Immigration and naturalization records** are acceptable.
- If all else fails, **notarized affidavits** from people who are in a position to know your age are acceptable.

The SSA will accept a number of other varieties of proof.

There are three reasons for asking you to bring in proof of earnings. First, it lets the representative at the Social Security office determine quickly, between the earnings on your Social Security earnings record and the proofs of earnings that you bring in, whether or not you have the required quarters of coverage. If you're close, having this information when you apply can eliminate a lot of worry and another phone call or trip. Second, your Social Security benefit is supposed to be based on the highest five years of your earnings, and having current information avoids having to give you a smaller benefit now, and a catch-up check and bigger benefits later, when the SSA computers get fed the information. Third, you may be receiving reduced Social Security. Suppose you chose to retire at age 62, applied for reduced benefits, and then took a job, or continued to work after 65 and earned enough to have your benefits reduced. In these cases, you are supposed to have your benefits recomputed periodically to take into account your additional earnings.

You also need not worry if you have lost your Social Security card. If you can remember the number, you can apply for a duplicate. If you can't remember the number, it is likely to be on a number of other documents around your house, such as payroll stubs, credit card bills, and insurance policies. If all else fails, the Social Security office has access to a computer system that will retrieve your name or any that sound like it from the Social Security computer system. This considerably narrows the search for your real number.

The forms you will face when you get to the Social Security office, and instructions for filling them out, are shown on pages 42–54. We also provide copies of some forms that are used for requesting reconsideration of denials of coverage and payment. The use of these forms is explained in chapters 6 and 8.

## What Medicare Covers and What It Doesn't

A common misconception about Medicare is that it has a wide scope of coverage, comparable with the best private insurance plans. While it does cover hospital and physician services, there are limitations on days of care and rather large copayments if you encounter a lengthy hospital stay. In addition, there is no limit on your out-of-pocket expenses for services provided under Medicare Part B. Other items, such as hearing aids, eyeglasses, prescription drugs, dental care, and custodial care, are not covered.

Many health maintenance organizations offer much better coverage — in fact, unlimited coverage on most services — to individuals and families for less than the cost of the Medicare Part A and Part B buy-in monthly premium combined (see page 35).

DEPARTMENT OF HEALTH AND HUMAN SERVICES
Social Security Administration

TOE 120/145/155

Form Approved.
OMB No. 0960-0007

**(Do not write in this space)**

## APPLICATION FOR RETIREMENT INSURANCE BENEFITS

I apply for all insurance benefits for which I am eligible under Title II (Federal Old-Age, Survivors, and Disability Insurance) and Title XVIII (Health Insurance for the Aged and Disabled) of the Social Security Act, as presently amended.

☐ Supplement. If you have already completed an application entitled "APPLICATION FOR WIFE'S OR HUSBAND'S INSURANCE BENEFITS", you need complete only the circled items. All other claimants must complete the entire form.

| | | |
|---|---|---|
| ① (a) | PRINT your name | FIRST NAME, MIDDLE INITIAL, LAST NAME |
| (b) | Enter your name at birth if different from item (a)➡ | FIRST NAME, MIDDLE INITIAL, LAST NAME |
| (c) | Check (✓) whether you are ➡ | ☐ Male ☐ Female |

② Enter your Social Security Number ➡ ___ - ___ / ___ - ___ / ___ - ___

3. (a) Enter your date of birth ➡ MONTH, DAY, YEAR

   (b) Enter name of State or foreign country where you were born. ➡

If you have already presented, or if you are now presenting, a public or religious record of your birth established before you were age 5, go on to item 4.

   (c) Was a public record of your birth made before you were age 5? ☐ Yes ☐ No ☐ Unknown

   (d) Was a religious record of your birth made before you were age 5? ☐ Yes ☐ No ☐ Unknown

4. (a) Have you (or has someone on your behalf) ever filed an application for Social Security benefits, a period of disability under Social Security, supplemental security income, or hospital or medical insurance under Medicare?
   ☐ Yes (If "Yes," answer (b) and (c).)   ☐ No (If "No," go on to item 5.)

   (b) Enter name of person on whose Social Security record you filed other application. ➡ (First name, middle initial, last name)

   (c) Enter Social Security Number of person named in (b). (If unknown, so indicate) ➡ ___ - ___ / ___ - ___ / ___ - ___

Do not answer 5 if you are age 66 and 5 months, or older. Go on to question 6.

5. (a) Are you so disabled that you cannot work or was there some period during the last 14 months when you were so disabled that you could not work? ➡ ☐ Yes ☐ No

   (b) If "Yes," enter the date you became disabled. ➡ MONTH, DAY, YEAR

6. (a) Were you in the active military or naval service (including Reserve or National Guard *active* duty or active duty for training) after September 7, 1939 and before 1968? ➡
   ☐ Yes (If "Yes," answer (b) and (c).)   ☐ No (If "No," go on to item 7.)

   (b) Enter dates of service. ➡ From (Month, year) | To (Month, year)

   (c) Have you *ever* been (or will you be) eligible for a monthly benefit from a military or civilian Federal agency? (include Veterans Administration benefits *only* if you waived military retirement pay) ➡ ☐ Yes ☐ No

7. Have you or your spouse worked in the railroad industry for 7 years or more? ➡ ☐ Yes ☐ No

Form SSA-1-F6 (1-86) Destroy prior editions          Page 1          (Over)

42

| 8. | (a) | Have you ever engaged in work that was covered under the social security system of a country other than the United States? ➤ | ☐ Yes ☐ No *(If "Yes," answer (b).) (If "No," go on to item 9.)* |
|---|---|---|---|
| | (b) | If "Yes," list the country(ies). ➤ | |

| 9. | Have you ever been married? ➤ | ☐ Yes ☐ No *(If "Yes," answer item 10.) (If "No," go to item 12.)* |
|---|---|---|

**10.** (a) Give the following information about your current marriage. If not currently married, show your last marriage below.

| To whom married | | When *(Month, day, year)* | Where *(Name of City and State)* |
|---|---|---|---|
| Your current or last marriage | How marriage ended *(If still in effect, write "Not ended.")* | When *(Month, day, year)* | Where *(Name of City and State)* |
| | Marriage performed by: ☐ Clergyman or public official ☐ Other *(Explain in Remarks)* | Spouse's date of birth (or age) | If spouse deceased, give date of death |
| | Spouse's Social Security Number (If none or unknown so indicate) __ __ __ / __ __ / __ __ __ __ | | |

(b) Give the following information about each of your previous marriages. **(IF NONE, WRITE "NONE")**

| To whom married | | When *(Month, day, year)* | Where *(Name of City and State)* |
|---|---|---|---|
| Your previous marriage (Use a separate statement for information about any other marriages) | How marriage ended | When *(Month, day, year)* | Where *(Name of City and State)* |
| | Marriage performed by: ☐ Clergyman or public official ☐ Other *(Explain in Remarks)* | Spouse's date of birth (or age) | If spouse deceased, give date of death |
| | Spouse's Social Security Number (If none or unknown so indicate) __ __ __ / __ __ / __ __ __ __ | | |

**11.** If you are currently married, answer this question only if your spouse is within 3 months of age 62 or older, or has a child-in-care who is eligible on your earnings record.
Do you wish this application to protect your spouse's right to Social Security benefits? ☐ Yes ☐ No

**12.** List below FULL NAME OF ALL your children (including natural children, adopted children, and stepchildren) or dependent grandchildren (including stepgrandchildren) who are now or were in the past 6 months UNMARRIED and:
- UNDER AGE 18 • AGE 18 TO 19 AND ATTENDING SECONDARY SCHOOL
- DISABLED OR HANDICAPPED (age 18 or over and disability began before age 22)

Also list any student who is between the ages of 18 to 23 if such student was both: 1. Previously entitled to Social Security benefits on any Social Security record for August 1981, and 2. Was also in full-time attendance at a post-secondary school prior to May 1982.
**(IF THERE ARE NO SUCH CHILDREN, WRITE "NONE" BELOW AND GO ON TO ITEM 13.)**

| | |
|---|---|
| | |

**13.** Enter below the names and addresses of all the persons, companies, or government agencies for whom you have worked this year, last year, and the year before last.
**IF NONE, WRITE "NONE" BELOW AND GO ON TO ITEM 15.**

| (a) NAME AND ADDRESS OF EMPLOYER *(If you had more than one employer, please list them in order beginning with your last (most recent) employer)* | Work Began | | Work Ended *(If still working, Show "Not ended")* | |
|---|---|---|---|---|
| | Month | Year | Month | Year |
| | | | | |
| | | | | |
| | | | | |

| (b) Are you an officer of a corporation, or are you related to an officer of a corporation? ➤ | ☐ Yes ☐ No |
|---|---|

| **14.** May we ask your employers for wage information needed to process your claim? ➤ | ☐ Yes ☐ No |
|---|---|

Form SSA-1-F6 (1-86) Page 2

| (15) | THIS ITEM MUST BE COMPLETED, EVEN IF YOU ARE AN EMPLOYEE | | ☐ Yes *(If "Yes," answer (b).)*  ☐ No *(If "No," skip to item 16.)* |
| --- | --- | --- | --- |
| | (a)  Were you self-employed this year, last year, or the year before? ➡ | | |

| (b)  Check the year or years in which you were self-employed | In what kind of trade or business were you self-employed? *(For example, storekeeper, farmer, physician)* | Were your net earnings from your trade or business $400 or more? *(Check "Yes" or "No")* | |
| --- | --- | --- | --- |
| ☐ This year | | ░░░░░░░░░░░░ | |
| ☐ Last year | | ☐ Yes | ☐ No |
| ☐ Year before last | | ☐ Yes | ☐ No |

**16.** (a) How much were your total earnings last year? ➡ $

(b) Place an "X" in each block for EACH MONTH of last year in which you did not earn more than * $_____ in wages, and did not perform substantial services in self-employment. These months are exempt months. If no months were exempt months, place an "X" in "NONE". If all months were exempt months, place an "X" in "ALL".

\* Enter the appropriate monthly limit after reading the instructions, "How Your Earnings Affect Your Benefits".

| NONE | | ALL | |
| --- | --- | --- | --- |
| Jan. | Feb. | Mar. | Apr. |
| May | Jun. | Jul. | Aug. |
| Sept. | Oct. | Nov. | Dec. |

**17.** (a) How much do you expect your total earnings to be this year? ➡ $

(b) Place an "X" in each block for EACH MONTH of this year in which you did not or will not earn more than * $_____ in wages, and did not or will not perform substantial services in self-employment. These months are exempt months. If no months are or will be exempt months, place an "X" in "NONE". If all months are or will be exempt months, place an "X" in "ALL".

\* Enter the appropriate monthly limit after reading the instructions, "How Your Earnings Affect Your Benefits".

| NONE | | ALL | |
| --- | --- | --- | --- |
| Jan. | Feb. | Mar. | Apr. |
| May | Jun. | Jul. | Aug. |
| Sept. | Oct. | Nov. | Dec. |

**18.** Answer this item ONLY if you are now in the last 4 months of your taxable year (Sept., Oct., Nov., and Dec., if your taxable year is a calendar year).

(a) How much do you expect to earn next year? ➡ $

(b) Place an "X" in each block for EACH MONTH of next year in which you do not expect to earn more than * $_____ in wages, and do not expect to perform substantial services in self-employment. These months will be exempt months. If no months are expected to be exempt months, place an "X" in "NONE". If all months are expected to be exempt months, place an "X" in "ALL".

\* Enter the appropriate monthly limit after reading the instructions, "How Your Earnings Affect Your Benefits".

| NONE | | ALL | |
| --- | --- | --- | --- |
| Jan. | Feb. | Mar. | Apr. |
| May | Jun. | Jul. | Aug. |
| Sept. | Oct. | Nov. | Dec. |

An ANNUAL REPORT of earnings must be filed with the Social Security Administration within 3 months and 15 days after the end of any taxable year in which you earn more than the yearly limit, if you are under age 70 for at least 1 full month of that year and receive some benefits during the taxable year. I AGREE TO FILE AN ANNUAL REPORT OF EARNINGS. THE ANNUAL REPORT IS REQUIRED BY LAW AND FAILURE TO REPORT MAY RESULT IN A MONETARY PENALTY.

**19.** If you use a fiscal year, that is, a taxable year that does not end December 31 (with income tax return due April 15), enter here the month your fiscal year ends. ➡ (Month) _____

IF YOU ARE AGE 65 AND 6 MONTHS, OR OLDER, DO NOT ANSWER ITEM 20. GO ON TO ITEM 21.

**PLEASE READ CAREFULLY THE INFORMATION ON THE OPPOSITE PAGE AND ANSWER ONE OF THE FOLLOWING ITEMS.** ➡

**20.** (a) I want benefits beginning with the earliest possible month that will be the most advantageous. ➡ ☐

(b) I am age 65 (or will be age 65 within 4 months) and I want benefits beginning with the earliest possible month that will be the most advantageous providing there is no permanent reduction in my ongoing monthly benefit. ➡ ☐

(c) I want benefits beginning with _____ . I understand that either a higher initial payment or a higher continuing monthly benefit amount may be possible, but I choose not to take it. ➡ ☐

Form SSA-1-F6 (1-86) Page 3          (Turn to Page 4)

If this claim is approved and you are still entitled to benefits at age 65, you will automatically have hospital insurance protection under Medicare at age 65. If you are not also eligible for automatic enrollment in the Supplementary Medical Insurance Plan, this application may be used for voluntary enrollment.

**COMPLETE THIS ITEM ONLY IF YOU ARE WITHIN 3 MONTHS OF AGE 65 OR OLDER**

ENROLLMENT IN MEDICARE'S SUPPLEMENTARY MEDICAL INSURANCE PLAN: The medical insurance benefits plan pays for most of the costs of physicians' and surgeons' services, and related medical services which are not covered by the hospital insurance plan. Coverage under this SUPPLEMENTARY MEDICAL INSURANCE PLAN does not apply to most medical expenses incurred outside the United States. Your Social Security district office will be glad to explain the details of the plan and give you a leaflet which explains what services are covered and how payment is made under the plan.

Once you are enrolled in this plan, you will have to pay a monthly premium to cover part of the cost of your medical insurance protection. The Federal Government contributes an equal amount or more toward the cost of your insurance. Premiums will be deducted from any monthly Social Security, railroad retirement, or civil service benefit checks you receive. If you do not receive such benefits, you will be notified about when, where, and how to pay your premiums. If you are eligible for automatic enrollment, you will be automatically enrolled unless you indicate, by checking the "NO" block below, that you do not want to be enrolled.

| **21.** DO YOU WISH TO ENROLL IN THE MEDICARE SUPPLEMENTARY MEDICAL INSURANCE PLAN? ⟶ | ☐ Yes | ☐ No |
|---|---|---|

Answer question 22 ONLY if you were born January 2, 1924, or later. Otherwise, go on to question 23.

| **22.** | (a) Are you entitled to, or do you expect to become entitled to, a pension or annuity based on work after 1956 not covered by Social Security? | ☐ Yes (If "Yes," answer (b) and (c).) | ☐ No (If "No," go on to item 23.) |
|---|---|---|---|
| | (b) ☐ I became entitled, or expect to become entitled, beginning ⟶ | MONTH | YEAR |
| | (c) ☐ I became eligible, or expect to become eligible, beginning ⟶ | MONTH | YEAR |

I agree to notify the Social Security Administration if I become entitled to a pension or annuity based on employment after 1956 not covered by Social Security, or if such pension or annuity stops.

It is possible for your Social Security monthly payments to be forwarded directly to your bank, savings and loan, credit union, or other financial organization for deposit to your account. This method of payment is known as direct deposit. If you wish direct deposit you will have to contact your financial organization to complete the necessary form. We will advise you when your direct deposit request is processed. If you do not wish direct deposit your benefits will be paid by check to your mailing address.

| **23.** Do you plan to file a form through your financial organization to begin direct deposit payments? ⟶ | ☐ Yes | ☐ No |
|---|---|---|

It is possible that your claim will be ready to be paid before the direct deposit form is returned by your financial organization. Your claim will be processed and any payments due will be sent to you until your direct deposit request is received.

REMARKS *(You may use this space for any explanations. If you need more space, attach a separate sheet.)*

_____

_____

_____

_____

_____

_____

**I know that anyone who makes or causes to be made a false statement or representation of material fact in an application or for use in determining a right to payment under the Social Security Act commits a crime punishable under Federal law by fine, imprisonment or both. I affirm that all information I have given in this document is true.**

| SIGNATURE OF APPLICANT | Date *(Month, day, year)* |
|---|---|
| Signature *(First name, middle initial, last name) (Write in ink)* | Telephone number (s) at which you may be contacted during the day |
| (SIGN HERE ▶) | _____ _____ _____ Area Code |

Mailing Address *(Number and street, Apt. No., P.O. Box, or Rural Route) (Enter Resident Address in "Remarks", if Different.)*

| City and State | ZIP Code | Enter Name of County (if any) in which you now live |
|---|---|---|

Witnesses are required ONLY if this application has been signed by mark (X) above. If signed by mark (X), two witnesses who know the applicant must sign below, giving their full addresses. Also, print the applicant's name in the Signature block.

| 1. Signature of Witness | 2 Signature of Witness |
|---|---|
| Address *(Number and street, City, State and ZIP Code)* | Address *(Number and street, City, State and ZIP Code)* |

Form SSA-1-F6 (1-86) Page 4

## CHANGES TO BE REPORTED AND HOW TO REPORT
Failure to report may result in overpayments that must be repaid, and in possible monetary penalties

▶ You change your mailing address for checks or residence. To avoid delay in receipt of checks you should ALSO file a regular change of address notice with your post office.

▶ You go outside the U.S.A.

▶ Any beneficiary dies or becomes unable to handle benefits.

▶ Work Changes-On your application you told us you expect total earnings for 19___ to be $_____.

You (are) (are not) earning wages of more than $_____a month.

You (are) (are not) self-employed rendering substantial services in your trade or business.

(Report AT ONCE if above work pattern changes)

▶ You are confined to jail, prison, penal institution, or correctional facility for conviction of a felony.

▶ You become entitled to a pension or annuity based on employment after 1956 not covered by Social Security, or if such pension or annuity stops.

▶ Custody Change—Report if a person for whom you are filing or who is in your care dies, leaves your care or custody, or changes address.

▶ Change of Marital Status—Marriage, divorce, annulment of marriage.

**HOW TO REPORT**

You can make your reports by telephone, mail, or in person, whichever you prefer.

WHEN A CHANGE OCCURS AFTER YOU RECEIVE A NOTICE OF AWARD, YOU SHOULD REPORT BY CALLING THE APPROPRIATE TELEPHONE NUMBER SHOWN NEAR THE TOP OF PAGE 6.

In addition, an annual report of earnings must be filed with the Social Security Administration within 3 months and 15 days after the end of any taxable year in which you earned more than the annual exempt amount.

THE ANNUAL REPORT OF EARNINGS IS REQUIRED BY LAW AND FAILURE TO REPORT MAY RESULT IN A MONETARY PENALTY.

---

## PLEASE READ THE FOLLOWING INFORMATION CAREFULLY
## BEFORE YOU ANSWER QUESTION 20.

Benefits may be payable for some months prior to the month in which you file this claim (but not for any month before the first month you will be age 62 for the entire month) if:

(1) you have a child or spouse entitled to unreduced benefits based on your earnings during any of the past 6 months;

—OR—

(2) you will earn over the exempt amount this year. (For appropriate exempt amount, see the instructions, "How Your Earnings Affect Your Benefits".

If your first month of entitlement is prior to age 65, your benefit rate will be reduced. However if you do not actually receive your full benefit amount for one or more months before age 65 because benefits are withheld due to your earnings, your benefit will be increased at age 65 to give credit for this withholding. Thus, your benefit amount at age 65 will be reduced only if you receive one or more full benefit payments prior to the month you are 65.

## RECEIPT FOR YOUR CLAIM FOR SOCIAL SECURITY RETIREMENT INSURANCE BENEFITS

| TELEPHONE NUMBER(S) TO CALL IF YOU HAVE A QUESTION OR SOMETHING TO REPORT | BEFORE YOU RECEIVE A NOTICE OF AWARD | SSA OFFICE | DATE CLAIM RECEIVED |
|---|---|---|---|
| | AFTER YOU RECEIVE A NOTICE OF AWARD | | |

Your application for Social Security benefits has been received and will be processed as quickly as possible.

You should hear from us within____ days after you have given us all the information we requested. Some claims may take longer if additional information is needed.

In the meantime, if you change your address, or if there is some other change that may affect your claim, you—or someone for you—should report the change. The changes to be reported are listed on page 5.

Always give us your claim number when writing or telephoning about your claim.

If you have any questions about your claim, we will be glad to help you.

| CLAIMANT | SOCIAL SECURITY CLAIM NUMBER |
|---|---|
| | |

### Collection and Use of Information From Your Application — Privacy Act/Paperwork Act Notice

The Social Security Administration is authorized to collect the information on this form under sections 202(a), 205(a) and 1872 of the Social Security Act, as amended (42 U.S.C. 402(a), 405(a), and 1395ii). While it is voluntary, except in the circumstances explained below, for you to furnish the information on this form to Social Security, no benefits may be paid unless an application has been received by a Social Security office. Your response is mandatory where the refusal to disclose certain information affecting your right to payment would reflect a fraudulent intent to secure benefits not authorized by the Social Security Act. The information on this form is needed to enable Social Security to determine if you and your dependents are entitled to insurance coverage and/or monthly benefits. Failure to provide all or part of this information could prevent an accurate and timely decision on your claim or your dependent's claim, and could result in the loss of some benefits or insurance coverage. Although the information you furnish on this form is almost never used for any other purpose than stated in the foregoing, there is a possibility that for the administration of the Social Security programs or for the administration of programs requiring coordination with the Social Security Administration, information may be disclosed to another person or to another governmental agency as follows: 1. to enable a third party or an agency to assist Social Security in establishing rights to Social Security benefits and/or coverage; 2. to comply with Federal laws requiring the release of information from Social Security records (e.g., to the General Accounting Office and the Veterans Administration); and 3. to facilitate statistical research and audit activities necessary to assure the integrity and improvement of the Social Security programs (e.g., to the Bureau of the Census and private concerns under contract to Social Security).

## APPLICATION FOR ENROLLMENT IN MEDICARE
### THE MEDICAL INSURANCE PROGRAM

(TID)  **SMI**

1. SOCIAL SECURITY CLAIM NUMBER

(CAN) ☐ ☐ ☐ — ☐ ☐ — ☐ ☐ ☐ ☐

2. FOR AGENCY USE ONLY

(BIC) ☐ ☐ ☐

3. DO YOU WISH TO ENROLL FOR MEDICAL INSURANCE UNDER MEDICARE?

(DEC)  YES ☐

4. CLAIMANT'S NAME

(CLN)

| Last name | First name | Middle initial |

5. PRINT SOCIAL SECURITY NUMBER HOLDER'S NAME IF DIFFERENT FROM YOURS

6. MAILING ADDRESS (NUMBER AND STREET, P.O. BOX, OR ROUTE)

IF THIS IS A CHANGE OF ADDRESS, CHECK HERE ☐

7. CITY, STATE, AND ZIP CODE

8. TELEPHONE NUMBER

9. WRITTEN SIGNATURE (DO NOT PRINT)

SIGN HERE ➡ _____

10. DATE SIGNED

(DOF) __ __ / __ __ / __ __
MONTH   DAY   YEAR

## IF THIS APPLICATION HAS BEEN SIGNED BY MARK (X), A WITNESS WHO KNOWS THE APPLICANT MUST SUPPLY THE INFORMATION REQUESTED BELOW

11. SIGNATURE OF WITNESS

12. DATE SIGNED

13. ADDRESS OF WITNESS

14. REMARKS

(TOA)  1

TO: (Circle one)

| (1)<br>NEPSC | (2)<br>MATPSC | (3)<br>SEPSC | (4)<br>GLPSC | (5)<br>WNPSC | (6)<br>MAMPSC | (7)<br>ODO | (8)<br>DIO |

FORM HCFA-40B (3/86)

48

## PRIVACY ACT NOTICE

The following information is given pursuant to the Privacy Act of 1974. The Social Security Administration is authorized to collect information about your medical insurance enrollment. While completing this form is voluntary, failure to provide all or part of this information will result in your not being enrolled for medical insurance under Medicare. The routine uses for information obtained are fully explained and published annually in the Federal Register. The Social Security Administration will further explain these uses upon request.

## SPECIAL MESSAGE FOR INDIVIDUAL APPLYING
## FOR MEDICAL INSURANCE UNDER MEDICARE

This form is your application for the medical insurance part of Medicare. It can be used either during your personal enrollment period or during any general enrollment period.

Your personal enrollment period lasts for 7 months. It begins 3 months before the month you reach age 65 (or 3 months before the 25th month you have received social security disability benefits) and it ends 3 months after you reach age 65 (or 3 months after the 25th month you have received social security disability benefits). To have medical insurance start in the month you are 65 (or the 25th month of disability insurance benefits), you must sign up in the first 3 months of your personal enrollment period. If you sign up in any of the remaining 4 months, your medical insurance starting date will be later.

If you do not file during your personal enrollment period, you can file any time after that during a general enrollment period which is the first 3 months of every year. If you sign up in a general enrollment period, your medical insurance begins July 1 of that year. However, when you file in a general enrollment period, your premium may be subject to a penalty increase. For each 12 month period elapsing between the end of your personal enrollment period and the general enrollment period in which you file, your premium will be increased 10 percent.

★ U.S.G.P.O.: 1988 –491–258/53764

Form Approved
OMB No. 72-R0705

(Do not write in this space)

## APPLICATION FOR HOSPITAL INSURANCE

(This application form may also be used to
enroll in Supplementary Medical Insurance)

I apply for entitlement to Medicare's hospital insurance under Part A of title XVIII of the Social Security Act, as presently amended, and for any cash benefits to which I may be entitled under title II of that Act.

**1.**
(a) Print your name ➤ | (First name, middle initial, last name)

(b) Enter your sex (check one) ➤ | ☐ Male ☐ Female

(c) Enter your Social Security Number ➤ | __ __ __ / __ __ / __ __ __ __

**2.** Enter your name at birth if different from item 1 ➤

**3.**
(a) Enter your date of birth (Month, day, year) ➤

(b) Enter name of State or foreign country where you were born ➤
If you have already submitted a public or religious record of your birth made before you were age 5, go on to item 4)

(c) Was a public record of your birth made before you were age 5? | ☐ Yes ☐ No ☐ Unknown

(d) Was a religious record of your birth made before you were age 5? | ☐ Yes ☐ No ☐ Unknown

**4.**
(a) Have you (or has someone on your behalf) ever filed an application for social security benefits, a period of disability under social security, supplemental security income, or hospital or medical insurance under Medicare? ➤ | ☐ Yes  ☐ No
If "Yes," answer (b) and (c).)  (If "No," go on to item 5.)

(b) Enter name of person on whose social security record you filed other application. ➤

(c) Enter Social Security Number of person named in (b). (If unknown, so indicate) ➤ | __ __ __ / __ __ / __ __ __ __

**5.**
(a) Were you in the active military or naval service (including Reserve or National Guard *active* duty or active duty for training) after September 7, 1939? ➤ | ☐ Yes  ☐ No
If "Yes," answer (b) and (c).)  (If "No," go on to item 7.)

(b) Enter dates of service ➤ | From: (Month, year) | To: (Month, year)

(c) Have you *ever* been (or will you be) eligible for a monthly benefit from a military or civilian Federal agency? (Include Veterans Administration benefits *only* if you waived military retirement pay) ➤ | ☐ Yes  ☐ No

**6.** Did you work in the railroad industry any time on or after January 1, 1937? ➤ | ☐ Yes  ☐ No

Form SSA-18 F5 (3-80) Previous editions of this form are obsolete   Page 1                    (Over)

50

| 7. | (a) Have you ever engaged in work that was covered under the social security system of a country other than the United States? ⟶ | ☐ Yes ☐ No |
|---|---|---|
| | (b) If "Yes," list the country(ies). ⟶ | |

| 8. | (a) How much were your total earnings last year? ⟶ (If none, write "None") | Earnings $ |
|---|---|---|
| | (b) How much do you expect your total earnings to be this year? ⟶ (If none, write "None") | Earnings $ |

| 9. | Are you a resident of the United States? ⟶ (To reside in a place means to make a home there.) | ☐ Yes ☐ No |
|---|---|---|

| 10. | (a) Are you a citizen of the United States? ⟶ (If "Yes," go on to item 11.) (If "No," answer (b) and (c) below.) | ☐ Yes ☐ No |
|---|---|---|
| | (b) Are you lawfully admitted for permanent residence in the United States? ⟶ | ☐ Yes ☐ No |

(c) Enter below the information requested about your place of residence in the last 5 years:

| ADDRESS AT WHICH YOU RESIDED IN THE LAST 5 YEARS (Begin with the most recent address. Show actual date residence began even if that is prior to the last 5 years.) | DATE RESIDENCE BEGAN | | | DATE RESIDENCE ENDED | | |
|---|---|---|---|---|---|---|
| | Month | Day | Year | Month | Day | Year |
| | | | | | | |
| | | | | | | |
| | | | | | | |
| | | | | | | |

*(If you need more space, use the "Remarks" space on the third page or another sheet of paper)*

| 11. | Are you currently married? ⟶ | ☐ Yes ☐ No |
|---|---|---|
| | *(If "Yes," give the following information about your current marriage.) (If "No," go on to item 12.)* | |

**YOUR CURRENT MARRIAGE**

| To whom married *(Enter your wife's maiden name or your husband's name)* | When *(Month, day, year)* |
|---|---|
| Spouse's date of birth (or age) | Spouse's Social Security Number *(If none or unknown, so indicate)* __ __ __ / __ __ / __ __ __ __ |

| 12. | If you had a previous marriage and your spouse died, OR if you had a previous marriage which lasted 10 or more years, give the following information. *(If you had no previous marriage (s), enter "NONE.")* |
|---|---|

**YOUR PREVIOUS MARRIAGE**

| To whom married *(Enter your wife's maiden name or your husband's name).* | When *(Month, day, year)* |
|---|---|
| Spouse's date of birth (or age) | Spouse's Social Security Number *(If none or unknown, so indicate)* __ __ __ / __ __ / __ __ __ __ |
| If spouse deceased, give date of death ⟶ | |

*(Use "Remarks" space on page 3 for information about any other marriages.)*

Form SSA-18 F5 (3-80) Page 2

| 13. | Is or was your spouse a railroad worker, railroad retirement pensioner, or a railroad retirement annuitant? ⟶ | ☐ Yes | ☐ No |
|---|---|---|---|
| 14. | (a) Were you or your spouse a civilian employee of the Federal Government after June 1960? ⟶ (If "Yes," answer (b).) (If "No," omit (b), (c), and (d).) | ☐ Yes | ☐ No |
| | (b) Are you or your spouse now covered under a medical insurance plan provided by the Federal Employees Health Benefits Act of 1959? ⟶ (If "Yes," omit (c) and (d).) (If "No," answer (c).) | ☐ Yes | ☐ No |
| | (c) Are you **and** your spouse barred from coverage under the above Act because your Federal employment, or your spouse's was not long enough? ⟶ (If "Yes," omit (d) and explain in "Remarks" below.) (If "No," answer (d).) | ☐ Yes | ☐ No |
| | (d) Were either you or your spouse an employee of the Federal Government after February 15, 1965? ⟶ | ☐ Yes | ☐ No |

Remarks:

_____

_____

_____

_____

_____

_____

_____

| 15. | If you are found to be otherwise ineligible for hospital insurance under Medicare, do you wish to enroll for hospital insurance on a monthly premium basis (in addition to the monthly premium for supplementary medical insurance)? ⟶ (If "Yes," you MUST also sign up for medical insurance.) | ☐ Yes | ☐ No |
|---|---|---|---|

### INFORMATION ON MEDICAL INSURANCE UNDER MEDICARE

Medical insurance under Medicare helps pay your doctor bills. It also helps pay for a number of other medical items and services not covered under the hospital insurance part of Medicare.

If you sign up for medical insurance, you must pay a premium for each month you have this protection. If you get monthly social security, railroad retirement, or civil service benefits, your premium will be deducted from your benefit check. If you get none of these benefits, you will be notified how to pay your premium.

The Federal Government contributes to the cost of your insurance. The amount of your premium and the Government's payment are based on the cost of services covered by medical insurance. The Government also makes additional payments when necessary to meet the full cost of the program. (Currently, the Government pays about two-thirds of the cost of this program.) You will get advance notice if there is any change in your premium amount.

If you have questions or would like a leaflet on medical insurance, call any Social Security office.

_____

| SEE OTHER SIDE TO SIGN UP FOR MEDICAL INSURANCE |

If you become entitled to hospital insurance as a result of this application, you will be enrolled for medical insurance automatically unless you indicate below that you do not want this protection. If you decline to enroll now, you can get medical insurance protection later only if you sign up for it during specified enrollment periods. Your protection may then be delayed and you may have to pay a higher premium when you decide to sign up.

The date your medical insurance begins and the amount of the premium you must pay depend on the month you file this application with the Social Security Administration. Any social security office will be glad to explain the rules regarding enrollment to you.

| 16. | **DO YOU WISH TO ENROLL FOR SUPPLEMENTARY MEDICAL INSURANCE?** ⟶<br><br>*(If "Yes," answer question 17.)* | ☐ Yes    ☐ No<br><br>☐ Currently Enrolled |
|---|---|---|
| 17. | Are you or your spouse receiving an annuity under the Federal Civil Service Retirement Act, or other law administered by the Office of Personnel Management? ⟶ | ☐ Yes    ☐ No |
|  | *(If "Yes," enter Civil Service annuity number here. Include the prefix "CSA" for annuitant, "CSF" for survivor.)* | Your No.<br><br>Spouse's No. |
|  | If you entered your spouse's number, is he (she) enrolled for supplementary medical insurance under social security? ⟶ | ☐ Yes    ☐ No |

**I know that anyone who makes or causes to be made a false statement or representation of material fact in an application or for use in determining a right to payment under the Social Security Act commits a crime punishable under Federal law by fine, imprisonment or both. I affirm that all information I have given in this document is true.**

| SIGNATURE OF APPLICANT | Date *(Month, day, year)* |
|---|---|
| Signature *(First name, middle initial, last name) (Write in ink)*<br><br>**SIGN HERE** ▶ | Telephone Number(s) at which you may be contacted during the day |

Mailing Address *(Number and street, Apt. No., P.O. Box, or Rural Route)*

| City and State | ZIP Code | Enter Name of County (if any) in which you now live |
|---|---|---|

Witnesses are required ONLY if this application has been signed by mark (X) above. If signed by mark (X), two witnesses to the signing who know the applicant must sign below, giving their full addresses.

| 1. Signature of Witness | 2. Signature of Witness |
|---|---|
| Address *(Number and street, City, State, and ZIP Code)* | Address *(Number and street, City, State, and ZIP Code)* |

## A REMINDER TO APPLICANTS FOR THE SOCIAL SECURITY HOSPITAL INSURANCE

| NAME OF PERSON TO CONTACT ABOUT YOUR CLAIM | SSA OFFICE | DATE |
|---|---|---|
| TELEPHONE NO. | | |

### RECEIPT FOR YOUR CLAIM

Your application for the hospital insurance has been received and will be processed as quickly as possible.

You should hear from us within      days after you have given us all the information we requested. Some claims may take longer if additional information is needed.

In the meantime, if you change your mailing address, you should report the change.

Always give us your claim number when writing or telephoning about your claim.

If you have any questions about your claim, we will be glad to help you.

| CLAIMANT | SOCIAL SECURITY CLAIM NUMBER |
|---|---|
| | |

### COLLECTION AND USE OF INFORMATION FROM YOUR APPLICATION — PRIVACY ACT NOTICE

PRIVACY ACT NOTICE: The Social Security Administration (SSA) is authorized to collect the information on this form under sections 226 and 1818 of the Social Security Act, as amended (42 U.S.C. 426 and 1395-17) and section 103 of Public Law 89-97. The information on this form is needed to enable social security and the Health Care Financing Administration (HCFA) to determine if you and your dependents may be entitled to hospital and/or medical insurance coverage and/or monthly benefits. While you do not have to furnish the information requested on this form to social security, no benefits or hospital or medical insurance can be provided until an application has been received by a social security office. Failure to provide all or part of the information requested could prevent an accurate and timely decision on your claim or your dependent's claim, and could result in the loss of some benefits or hospital or medical insurance. Although the infor-

mation you furnish on this form is almost never used for any other purpose than stated above, there is a possibility that for the administration of the social security or HCFA programs or for the administration of programs requiring coordination with SSA or HCFA, information may be disclosed to another person or to another governmental agency as follows: 1) to enable a third party or an agency to assist social security or HCFA in establishing rights to social security benefits and/or hospital or medical insurance coverage; 2) to comply with Federal laws requiring the release of information from social security and HCFA records (e.g., to the General Accounting Office and the Veterans Administration); and 3) to facilitate statistical research and audit activities necessary to assure the integrity and improvement of the social security and HCFA programs (e.g., to the Bureau of the Census and private concerns under contract to social security and HCFA).

Form **SSA-18 F5** (3-80) Page 5

54

FORM APPROVED
OMB NO 66–R0123

## APPLICATION FOR HEALTH INSURANCE BENEFITS
## UNDER MEDICARE FOR INDIVIDUAL
## WITH CHRONIC RENAL DISEASE

I hereby request that my right to health insurance benefits be determined under Section 226 (A) of the Social Security Act.

| | | |
|---|---|---|
| 1. | Print Your Full Name *(First name, middle initial, last name)* | Enter your Social Security Number |
| 2. | Check ( ✓ ) whether you are:  ☐ Male  ☐ Female | Enter your maiden name *(if applicable)* |
| 3. | Enter your date of birth (Month, day, year) ⟶ | |
| 4. | (a) Have you received regularly scheduled dialysis? ⟶ *(If "Yes," answer (b).)* *(If "No," go to 6.)* | ☐ Yes  ☐ No |
| | (b) Enter beginning date(s) and ending date(s) (if applicable) of all periods of regularly scheduled dialysis *(month, year)* ⟶ | Dialysis Began:  |  Ended: |
| 5. | (a) Have you participated (or do you expect to participate) in a self-dialysis training program? ⟶ *(If "Yes," answer (b).)* *(If "No," go to 6.)* | ☐ Yes  ☐ No |
| | (b) Enter date self-dialysis training began (or is expected to begin) *(month, year)* ⟶ | |
| 6. | (a) Have you received a kidney transplant? ⟶ *(If "Yes," answer (b).)* *(If "No," go to (e).)* | ☐ Yes  ☐ No |
| | (b) Enter date(s) of transplant(s) *(month, year)* ⟶ | |
| | (c) Were you in a hospital for transplant surgery or for necessary procedures preliminary to transplant before the month you actually received the transplant? ⟶ *(If "Yes," answer(d).)* *(If "No," go to 7.)* | ☐ Yes  ☐ No |
| | (d) Enter dates of hospitalization for 6(c) *(month, day, year)* ⟶ | From:  |  To: |
| | (e) If you are scheduled to receive a transplant, enter date *(month, year)* ⟶ | |

55

7. ENROLLMENT IN THE SUPPLEMENTARY MEDICAL INSURANCE PLAN: The medical insurance benefits plan pays for most of the costs of physicians' and surgeons' services, and other covered medical services such as OUTPATIENT MAINTENANCE DIALYSIS TREATMENTS, which are not covered by the hospital insurance plan. This plan covers outpatient treatment provided in a hospital or a facility which meets prescribed conditions. It also COVERS HOME DIALYSIS, including the rental or purchase of home dialysis machine, and the purchase of disposable equipment and supplies needed for the dialysis.

Coverage under this SUPPLEMENTARY MEDICAL INSURANCE PLAN does not apply to most medical expenses incurred outside the United States. Your social security district office will be glad to explain the details of the plan and give you a leaflet which explains what services are covered and how payment is made under the plan.

Once you are enrolled in this plan, you will have to pay a monthly premium to cover part of the cost of your medical insurance protection. The Federal Government contributes an equal amount or more toward the cost of your insurance. Premiums will be deducted from any monthly social security, railroad retirement, or civil service benefit checks you receive. If you do not receive such benefits, you will be notified about when, where, and how to pay your premiums.

YOU WILL BE AUTOMATICALLY ENROLLED IN THIS PLAN UNLESS YOU INDICATE, BY CHECKING THE "NO" BLOCK BELOW, THAT YOU DO NOT WANT TO BE ENROLLED.

(a) DO YOU WISH TO ENROLL IN THE SUPPLEMENTARY MEDICAL INSURANCE PLAN? *(If"No", go to 8.)*————▶  ☐ Yes   ☐ No

(b) If your application is processed within 5 months after the first month in which you meet all the requirements for your Medicare entitlement, your coverage will begin with that first month.
If your application is processed more than 5 months after your first possible month of entitlement, you may choose one of the following for your first month of coverage. (Please check one):

•The earliest possible month of entitlement, if you are willing and able to pay all premiums for past months of coverage   ☐
OR
•The month in which this application is filed, if it is the same as, or later than, your first possible month of entitlement   ☐
OR
•The month in which this enrollment will be processed————▶   ☐

ITEMS 8 THROUGH 16 REQUEST INFORMATION NEEDED TO DETERMINE INSURED STATUS FOR MEDICARE ENTITLEMENT.

8. (a) Have you (or has someone on your behalf) ever filed an application for social security benefits, a period of disability under social security, or hospital or medical insurance under Medicare?————————————▶
*(If"Yes," answer(b) and (c).)*
*(If"No," go to 9.)*   ☐ Yes   ☐ No

(b) Enter name of person(s) on whose social security record(s) you filed other application(s)————————▶   *(First, middle initial, last)*

(c) Enter social security number(s) of person(s) named in (b). *(If unknown, so indicate.)*————————▶

9. (a) Have you (or has someone on your behalf) ever filed an application for monthly benefits or hospital or medical insurance under Medicare with the Railroad Retirement Board?————————▶
*(If "Yes," answer (b) and (c).)*
*(If "No," go to 10.)*   ☐ Yes   ☐ No

(b) Enter the name of person(s) on whose railroad record you filed other application(s)————————▶   *(First, middle initial, last)*

(c) Enter Railroad Number of person named in (b). *(If unknown, so indicate.)*————————▶

Form **HCFA-43** (11-78)  (Page 2)

IF YOU ARE ALREADY ENTITLED TO A MONTHLY SOCIAL SECURITY BENEFIT OR A MONTHLY RAILROAD ANNUITY, DO NOT COMPLETE ITEMS 10 THROUGH 16.

| 10. | (a) Were you in the active military or naval service (including Reserve or National Guard active duty or active duty for training) after September 7, 1939? ➔ *(If "Yes," answer (b).) (If "No," go to 11.)* | ☐ Yes ☐ No |
|---|---|---|
| | (b) Enter dates of service ➔ | FROM: _(Month, year)_  TO: _(Month, year)_ |
| 11. | Have you worked in the railroad industry any time on or after January 1, 1937? ➔ | ☐ Yes ☐ No |

12. 
- Enter below the names and addresses of all the persons, companies, or Government agencies for whom you worked during the last 12 months.
- If you worked in agricultural employment, give this information for this year and last year.
- If neither of the above applies, write "None" below and go to 14.

| Name and address of employer *(If you had more than one employer, please list them in order beginning with your last (most recent) employer.)* | Work began | | Work ended *(If still working, show "Not Ended")* | |
|---|---|---|---|---|
| | Month | Year | Month | Year |
| | | | | |
| | | | | |
| | | | | |
| | | | | |
| *(If you need more space, use "Remarks" space on back page.)* | | | | |

| 13. | May we ask your employers for wage information needed to process your claim? ➔ | ☐ Yes ☐ No |
|---|---|---|
| 14. | (a) Were you self-employed this year, last year, or the year before? *(If "Yes," answer (b).) (If "No," go to 15.)* ➔ | ☐ Yes ☐ No |

| (b) Check the year or years in which you were self-employed. | In what kind of trade or business were you self-employed? *(For example, storekeeper, farmer, physician)* | Were your net earnings from your trade or business $400 or more? *(Check "Yes" or "No")* |
|---|---|---|
| ☐ This year | | |
| ☐ Last year | | ☐ Yes ☐ No |
| ☐ Year before last | | ☐ Yes ☐ No |

Form **HCFA-43** (11-78) (Page 3)

IF YOU HAVE BEEN CONTINUALLY EMPLOYED FOR 2 OR MORE YEARS IN THE LAST 3 YEARS, DO NOT COMPLETE ITEMS 15 AND 16.

**15.** (a) Check your Marital Status. *(If single, go to 16.)*

☐ MARRIED ☐ WIDOWED ☐ DIVORCED ☐ SINGLE

| (b) Enter your wife's maiden name or your husband's name | Date of marriage | Date of divorce *(if divorced)* | Date of death *(if deceased)* | Your wife's or your husband's Social Security or Railroad Number *(If none or unknown, so indicate.)* |
|---|---|---|---|---|
|  |  |  |  |  |

(c) Check ( ✓ ) whether your marriage was performed by:
☐ Clergyman or authorized public official, or ☐ Other *(Explain in Remarks)*

(d) Were you married before your present marriage?
*(If "Yes," give the following information about each of your previous marriages. If you need more space, use "Remarks" section below or attach a separate sheet.)* ☐ Yes ☐ No

| YOUR PREVIOUS MARRIAGE | To Whom Married | When *(Month, day, and year)* | Where *(Enter name of city & State)* |
|---|---|---|---|
|  | How Marriage Ended | When *(Month, day, and year)* | Where *(Enter name of city & State)* |

**16.** Complete the following if you are single.

| MOTHER'S NAME | MOTHER'S SOCIAL SECURITY OR RAILROAD NUMBER |
|---|---|
| FATHER'S NAME | FATHER'S SOCIAL SECURITY OR RAILROAD NUMBER |

REMARKS: _____
_____
_____
_____

IMPORTANT: Medicare coverage based on kidney failure will end with either:

a. The last day of the 36th month after the month in which a kidney transplant is received, or

b. The last day of the 12th month after the month in which a regular course of dialysis is discontinued, unless another course of dialysis is initiated or another transplant is received before the last day of

I AGREE TO NOTIFY THE SOCIAL SECURITY ADMINISTRATION IF THE COURSE OF DIALYSIS ENDS OR A KIDNEY TRANSPLANT IS RECEIVED.

**I know that anyone who makes or causes to be made a false statement or representation of material fact in an application or for use in determining a right to payment under the Social Security Act commits a crime punishable under Federal law by fine, imprisonment or both. I affirm that all information I have given in this document is true.**

| SIGNATURE OF APPLICANT | Date *(Month, day, year)* |
|---|---|
| Signature *(First name, middle initial, last name) (Write in ink)*  SIGN HERE ► | Telephone Number(s) at which you may be contacted during the day |

Mailing Address *(Number and street, Apt. No., P.O. Box, or Rural Route)*

| City and State | ZIP Code | Enter Name of County (if any) in which you now live |
|---|---|---|

Witnesses are required ONLY if this application has been signed by mark (X) above. If signed by mark (X), two witnesses to the signing who know the applicant must sign below, giving their full addresses.

| 1. Signature of Witness | 2. Signature of Witness |
|---|---|
| Address *(Number, Street, City, State, and ZIP Code)* | Address *(Number, Street, City, State, Zip Code)* |

Form HCFA-43 (11-78)  (Page 4)                                    ☆U.S. G.P.O. 1980-311-171/3015

**PLEASE DETACH THIS PAGE AND KEEP FOR YOUR RECORDS**

### APPLICATION FOR HEALTH INSURANCE BENEFITS
### UNDER MEDICARE FOR INDIVIDUAL
### WITH CHRONIC RENAL DISEASE
#### Collection and Use of Information from Your Application

The Privacy Act of 1974 requires the Social Security Administration to give the following facts to individuals from whom information about themselves is requested:
- the statutory authority for the request,
- whether it is mandatory or voluntary to give the information,
- the principal purpose(s) for which the information is needed,
- the effects of not providing the information, and
- the routine uses which may be made of the information.

These items are explained in the following sections. If you have any questions about your rights under the Privacy Act, you may contact any social security office.

I. The Social Security Administration is authorized to collect the information on this form under 205(a), 226(A), and 1872 of the Social Security Act, as amended (42 U.S.C. 405(a), 426, and 1395ii).

II. While it is not mandatory, except in the circumstances explained below, for you to furnish the information on this form to social security, health insurance entitlement cannot be established unless an application has been received by a social security office. Your response is mandatory where the refusal to disclose certain information affecting your entitlement would reflect a fraudulent intent to secure benefits not authorized by the Social Security Act.

III. The information on this form is needed to enable social security to determine if you are entitled to health insurance coverage.

IV. Failure to provide all or part of this information could prevent an accurate and timely decision on your claim, and could result in the loss of some insurance coverage.

V. Although the information you furnish on this form is almost never used for any other purpose than stated in Part III, above, there is a possibility that for the administration of the social security programs or for the administration of programs requiring coordination with the Social Security Administration, information may be disclosed to another person or to another governmental agency as follows:

1. To enable a third party or an agency to assist social security in establishing rights to health insurance coverage.

2. To comply with Federal laws requiring the release of information from social security records (e.g., to the General Accounting Office and the Veterans' Administration).

3. To facilitate statistical research and audit activities necessary to assure the integrity and improvement of the social security programs (e.g., to the Bureau of the Census and private concerns under contract to social security.)

Form **HCFA-43** (11-78)

**PLEASE DETACH THIS PAGE AND KEEP FOR YOUR RECORDS**

DEPARTMENT OF HEALTH, EDUCATION, AND WELFARE
HEALTH CARE FINANCING ADMINISTRATION

Form Approved.
OMB No. 066-R-0067

## REQUEST FOR RECONSIDERATION OF PART A HEALTH INSURANCE BENEFITS

INSTRUCTIONS: *Please type or print firmly.* Leave the block empty if you cannot answer it. Take or mail the WHOLE form to your Social Security office which will be glad to help you. Please read the statement on the reverse side of page 2.

| 1. BENEFICIARY'S NAME | 2. HEALTH INSURANCE CLAIM NUMBER |
|---|---|

3. REPRESENTATIVE'S NAME, IF APPLICABLE

☐ RELATIVE  ☐ ATTORNEY  ☐ OTHER PERSON)  ☐ PROVIDER FILING

### 4. PLEASE ATTACH A COPY OF THE NOTICE(S) YOU RECEIVED ABOUT YOUR CLAIM TO THIS FORM.

5. THIS CLAIM IS FOR

☐ INPATIENT HOSPITAL   ☐ SKILLED NURSING FACILITY (SNF)   ☐ HEALTH MAINTENANCE ORGANIZATION (HMO)
☐ EMERGENCY HOSPITAL   ☐ HOME HEALTH AGENCY (HHA)

| 6. NAME AND ADDRESS OF PROVIDER (Hospital, SNF, HHA, HMO) | CITY AND STATE | PROVIDER NUMBER |
|---|---|---|

| 7. NAME OF INTERMEDIARY | CITY AND STATE | INTERMEDIARY NUMBER |
|---|---|---|

| 8. DATE OF ADMISSION OR START OF SERVICES | 9. DATE(S) OF THE NOTICE(S) YOU RECEIVED |
|---|---|

10. I DO NOT AGREE WITH THE DETERMINATION ON MY CLAIM. PLEASE RECONSIDER MY CLAIM BECAUSE

11. YOU MUST OBTAIN ANY EVIDENCE (For example, a letter from a doctor) YOU WISH TO SUBMIT.

☐ I HAVE ATTACHED THE FOLLOWING EVIDENCE:

☐ I WILL SEND THIS EVIDENCE WITHIN 10 DAYS:

☐ I HAVE NO ADDITIONAL EVIDENCE OR OTHER INFORMATION TO SUBMIT WITH MY CLAIM.

13. ONLY ONE SIGNATURE IS NEEDED. THIS FORM IS SIGNED BY:

☐ BENEFICIARY  ☐ REPRESENTATIVE  ☐ PROVIDER REP.

SIGN HERE ▶

14. STREET ADDRESS

12. IS THIS REQUEST FILED WITHIN 60 DAYS OF THE DATE OF YOUR NOTICE?

☐ YES  ☐ NO

IF YOU CHECKED "NO" ATTACH AN EXPLANATION OF THE REASON FOR THE DELAY TO THIS FORM.

CITY, STATE, ZIP CODE

| TELEPHONE | DATE |
|---|---|

15. If this request is signed by mark (X), TWO WITNESSES who know the person requesting reconsideration must sign in the space provided on the reverse side of this page of the form.

### DO NOT FILL IN BELOW THIS LINE — FOR SOCIAL SECURITY USE — THANK YOU

16. ROUTING

☐ INTERMEDIARY

☐ HCFA, RO-MEDICARE

☐ BSS, ODR

18. SSA OR INTERMEDIARY DATE STAMP

17. ADDITIONAL INFORMATION

FORM **HCFA-2649** (8-79  FORMERLY SSA-2649)
DESTROY PRIOR EDITIONS

INTERMEDIARY

Page 1 of 4

60

DEPARTMENT OF HEALTH,
EDUCATION, AND WELFARE
SOCIAL SECURITY ADMINISTRATION
BUREAU OF HEARINGS AND APPEALS

## REQUEST FOR HEARING
## <u>PART A</u> HEALTH INSURANCE BENEFITS
### Take or mail original and all copies to your local Social Security office.

| CLAIMANT'S NAME | CLAIM FOR |
|---|---|
| | ☐ Hospital Services |
| WAGE EARNER'S NAME (Leave blank if same as above) | ☐ Extended Care Facility Services |
| | ☐ Home Health Agency Services |
| HI CLAIM NUMBER | ☐ Emergency Services |
| | PERIOD IN QUESTION |
| | FROM:            TO: |
| NAME AND ADDRESS OF INTERMEDIARY | NAME AND ADDRESS OF PROVIDER |

I disagree with the determination made on the above claim and request a hearing before a hearing examiner of the Bureau of Hearings and Appeals. My reasons for disagreement are: (additional pages may be added if necessary.)

Check one of the following:

☐ I have additional evidence to submit.
(Attach such evidence to this form or forward to the Social Security Office within 10 days.)

☐ I have <u>no</u> additional evidence to submit.

Check <u>ONLY ONE</u> of the statements below.

☐ I wish to appear in person before the hearing examiner.

☐ I waive my right to appear and give evidence, and hereby request a decision on the evidence before the hearing examiner.

Signed by:    (Either the claimant or representative should sign-Enter addresses for both. If claimant's representative is not an attorney, complete Form SSA-1696)

| SIGNATURE OR NAME OF CLAIMANT'S REPRESENTATIVE<br>☐ ATTORNEY ☐ NON-ATTORNEY | CLAIMANT'S SIGNATURE |
|---|---|
| ADDRESS | ADDRESS |
| CITY, STATE, AND ZIP CODE | CITY, STATE, AND ZIP CODE |
| TELEPHONE NUMBER | DATE: | TELEPHONE NUMBER |

Claimant should not fill in below this line

Is this request filed within 6 months of the reconsideration determination?    ☐ Yes    ☐ No
If "No" is checked: (1) attach claimant's explanation for delay, (2) attach any pertinent letter, material, or information in the Social Security Office.

### ACKNOWLEDGMENT OF REQUEST FOR HEARING

Your request for a hearing was filed on_____at _____
The hearing examiner will notify you of the time and place of the hearing at least 10 days prior to the date which will be set for the hearing.

| Hearing Examiner Copy | TO:<br>☐ Hearing Examiner _____ (Location) | For the Social Security Administration |
|---|---|---|
| Claim File Copy | TO:<br>☐ BHI, Reconsideration Branch<br><br>☐ BHI, Regional Office _____<br>(Only emergency services in other than Federal Hospitals) | By: _____<br>(Signature)        (Title)<br><br>_____<br>(Street Address)<br><br>(City)    (State)    (ZIP Code) |

Interpreter Needed_____     Servicing District Office Code_____
(Language)

Form HA 501.1
(2-72)

HEARING  EXAMINER

Form Approved
OMB No. 0938-0033

# REQUEST FOR REVIEW OF PART B MEDICARE CLAIM
## Medical Insurance Benefits - Social Security Act

NOTICE—Anyone who misrepresents or falsifies essential information requested by this form may upon conviction be subject to fine and imprisonment under Federal Law.

| Carrier's Name and Address | **1** Name of Patient |
|---|---|
| The name and address of the Carrier for your state will be listed in this space. | **2** Health Insurance Claim Number |

**3** I do not agree with the determination you made on my claim as described on my Explanation of Medicare

Benefits dated:

**4** MY REASONS ARE: *(Attach a copy of the Explanation of Medicare Benefits, or describe the service, date of service, and physician's name—NOTE.—If the date on the Notice of Benefits mentioned in item 3 is more than six months ago, include your reason for not making this request earlier.)*

_____

_____

_____

_____

_____

_____

_____

**5** ☐ I have additional evidence to submit. *(Attach such evidence to this form)*

☐ I do not have additional evidence.

COMPLETE ALL OF THE INFORMATION REQUESTED. SIGN AND RETURN THE FIRST COPY AND ANY ATTACHMENTS TO THE CARRIER NAMED ABOVE. IF YOU NEED HELP, TAKE THIS AND YOUR NOTICE FROM THE CARRIER TO A SOCIAL SECURITY OFFICE, OR TO THE CARRIER. KEEP THE DUPLICATE COPY OF THIS FORM FOR YOUR RECORDS.

**6** SIGNATURE OF **EITHER** THE CLAIMANT **OR** HIS REPRESENTATIVE

| Representative ➡ | Claimant ➡ |
|---|---|
| Address | Address |
| City, State, and ZIP Code | City, State, and ZIP Code |
| Telephone Number | Date | Telephone Number | Date |

Form HCFA-1964 (1-78) (Formerly SSA-1964)      **CARRIER'S COPY**      (over)

DEPARTMENT OF HEALTH AND HUMAN SERVICES
HEALTH CARE FINANCING ADMINISTRATION

Form Approved
OMB No. 0938-0034

# REQUEST FOR HEARING - PART B MEDICARE CLAIM
## Medical Insurance Benefits - Social Security Act

NOTICE—Anyone who misrepresents or falsifies essential information requested by this form may upon conviction be subject to fine and imprisonment under Federal Law.

| Carrier's Name and Address | **1** Name of Patient |
|---|---|
| The name and address of the Carrier for your state will be listed in this space. | **2** Health Insurance Claim Number |

**3** I disagree with the review determination on my claim, and request a hearing before a hearing officer of the insurance carrier named above.

MY REASONS ARE: *(Attach a copy of the Review Notice. NOTE.—If the review decision was made more than 6 months ago include your reason for not making this request earlier)*

_____

_____

_____

_____

**4** Check one of the Following:

☐ I have additional evidence to submit. *(Attach such evidence to this form or forward it to the carrier within 10 days.)*

☐ I do not have additional evidence.

Check <u>Only One</u> of the Statements Below:

☐ I wish to appear in person before the Hearing Officer.

☐ I do not wish to appear and hereby request a decision on the evidence before the Hearing Officer.

**5** EITHER THE CLAIMANT OR REPRESENTATIVE SHOULD SIGN IN THE APPROPRIATE SPACE BELOW:

| Signature or Name of Claimant's Representative ➡ | Claimant's Signature ➡ |
|---|---|
| Address | Address |
| City, State, and ZIP Code | City, State, and ZIP Code |
| Telephone Number     Date | Telephone Number     Date |

*(Claimant should not write below this line)*

## ACKNOWLEDGMENT OF REQUEST FOR HEARING

Your request for a hearing was received on _____. You will be notified of the time and place of the hearing at least 10 days before the date of the hearing.

| Signed | Date |
|---|---|

Form **HCFA-1965** (8-79) (Formerly SSA-1965)

CARRIERS COPY

63

*The Meaning of "Coverage"*

Coverage under Medicare is limited three ways, first by the services that are covered at all. By "covered" we mean that Medicare is willing to pay something for the service — not necessarily the full amount the **provider** wants, not necessarily enough to relieve you of all the burden of payment, not necessarily enough to attract enough providers to make the service routinely available, but something. (A provider is a person or institution of a sort for whose services Medicare makes payments. Some providers are people; some are institutions, such as hospitals.) Services for which Medicare will pay nothing are "not covered." The chart on pages 65 and 66 provides a brief summary of what is covered and what is not.

## THE MEDICARE PROGRAM....
## WHAT IT PAYS....WHAT YOU PAY

Program services, as well as deductibles and copayments, are subject to change on a yearly basis. For the most current information, consult the latest edition of *Your Medicare Handbook,* available at most Social Security Administration offices.

| Medicare Services | Benefit Period | Medicare Pays | You Pay |
|---|---|---|---|
| **Part A: Hospital Insurance** | | | |
| **Hospital Services*** | First 60 days | All but deductible | Deductible of $760 |
| Semiprivate room rate Miscellaneous hospital | 61 to 90 days | All but $190/day | $190/day |
| services & supplies | 91 to 150 days | All but $380/day | $380/day |
| Dietary & meal services Special care units Diagnostic procedures, X rays, etc. Laboratory services Operating & recovery rooms Anesthesia & supplies Rehabilitation services | Beyond 150 days | Nothing | All costs |
| **Skilled Nursing Facility Care** | First 20 days | All costs | Nothing |
| In approved facility after a 3-day hospital stay and | 21 to 100 days | All but $95/day | $95/day |
| admitted to the facility within 30 days of discharge | Beyond 100 days | Nothing | All costs |
| **Home Health Care** | Unlimited as medically necessary | All costs | Nothing |
| **Hospice Care** | Two 90-day periods One 30-day period | All costs but outpatient drugs and respite care | Limited drug costs and respite care |
| **Blood Service** | As needed | All but first 3 pints | First 3 pints |

\* Includes inpatient psychiatric care of 190 lifetime days.

| Medicare Services | Benefit Period | Medicare Pays | You Pay |
|---|---|---|---|
| **Part B: Medical Insurance** | | | |
| Physician & surgeon fees<br>Therapists (physical/speech/ occupational)<br>Diagnostic tests<br>Medical supplies<br>Ambulatory services<br>Ambulance service | As medically necessary | 80% of approved amount after $100 deductible | $100 deductible and 20% of the Medicare-approved charge (plus any cost above approved charge) |
| **Outpatient Hospital Services** | As medically necessary | 80% of approved amount after $100 deductible | 20% of approved charge after deductible |
| **Home Health Care** | As medically necessary | All costs | Nothing |
| **Immunosuppressive Drugs** | As medically necessary | One year of drugs used in immunosuppressive therapy after transplant | 20% of the cost |
| **Blood Service** | As needed | 80% of the cost after first 3 pints | First 3 pints and 20% of cost |

*Nursing Homes Are Partially Covered*

Medicare does not cover what we usually think of as "nursing home care." There are three levels of nursing home care:

- **Skilled nursing facilities (SNFs)** offer care delivered by registered and licensed practical nurses on the orders of an attending physician. They offer services such as oxygen therapy, intravenous and tube feedings, care of catheters and wound drains, and physical, occupational, and speech therapy.

- **Intermediate care facilities (ICFs)** provide less intensive care than skilled nursing facilities. Patients are generally more mobile, and rehabilitation therapies are stressed.

- **Sheltered, or custodial, care** is nonmedical. Residents do not require constant attention from nurses and aides but need assistance with one or more daily activities or no longer want to be bothered with keeping up a house. The social needs of residents are met in a secure environment free of as many anxieties as possible.

Medicare covers nursing home care at the skilled nursing facility (SNF, pronounced *sniff*) level only. Further, Medicare will pay for skilled nursing facility services *only* if the following conditions are met:

- The nursing home must be a skilled nursing facility, and it must be certified to participate in the Medicare program.
- A three-day prior hospitalization is required, and a physician must certify that the person requires skilled care.
- There must be ongoing utilization review to determine if the person is receiving skilled nursing services.
- If a determination is made that skilled care is no longer required, Medicare coverage ceases.

You should be aware that Medicare is not a long-term solution to paying for nursing home care, because it does not cover intermediate or sheltered care (the two most common levels of care required). Medicare coverage for skilled care is as follows:

| TIME IN DAYS | MEDICARE PAYS | YOU PAY |
| --- | --- | --- |
| 1–20 | All costs | Nothing |
| 21–100 | All but $95/day | $95/day |
| 101+ | Nothing | All costs |

Let's consider an example:

*The Smith family's aged grandmother, Iphigenia, has had a stroke and broken her hip when falling down. She had to have the hip replaced with an artificial one and has been in and out of the hospital with infections and failure of the bone to solidify around the hip. The last stay in the hospital seems to have finally fixed her hip, but she is currently unable to walk and has trouble with bowel and bladder control, and tends to get dehydrated very easily. She needs a long stay in a nursing home for recuperation, with almost constant nursing attention to make sure that her wound does not get reinfected and her fluid intake is adequate, and occupational and speech therapy. As things turn out, she has to stay in the nursing home for an entire year after her last discharge from the hospital.*

Let's see what Medicare paid: The nursing home charged $100 per day for skilled nursing facility services. (This figure included the room charge plus estimated ancillary charges, for items such as medicine, equipment, and the like.) Medicare paid for the first 20 days and all costs above $95 for days 21 through 100. That leaves 265 days to pay for.

| | |
|---|---|
| What's the portion paid by Medicare, and what's the portion paid by the Smiths? | |
| Total cost: $100 × 365 = | $36,500 |
| Medicare payment for first 20 days: | |
| 20 × $100 = | $ 2,000 |
| Smiths' copayment for days 21–100: | |
| 80 × $95 = | $ 7,600 |
| Medicare payment for days 21–100: | |
| 80 × $5 ($100 − $95) = | $    400 |
| Smiths' payment for days 101–365: | |
| 265 × $100 = | $26,500 |
| Medicare paid | $ 2,400 (7%) |
| The Smiths paid | $34,100 (93%) |

As we can see from this example, Medicare is *not* the answer to financing long-term nursing home care. Let's see what happens when the copayment remains at $95 per day and the daily rate increases to $125.

| | |
|---|---|
| Total cost: $125 × 365 = | $45,625 |
| Medicare payment for first 20 days: | |
| 20 × $125 = | $ 2,500 |
| Smiths' copayment for first 20 days: | $     0 |
| Medicare payment for days 21–100: | |
| 80 × $30 ($125 − $95) = | $ 2,400 |
| Smiths' copayment for days 21–100: | |
| 80 × $95 = | $ 7,600 |
| Medicare payment for days 101–365: | $     0 |
| Smiths' payment for days 101–365: | |
| 265 × $125 = | $33,125 |
| Medicare paid: | $ 4,900 (11%) |
| The Smiths paid: $45,625 − $4,900 = | $40,725 (89%) |

Note that even though Medicare paid a slightly larger percentage of the total cost, the Smiths continued to bear the majority of the nursing home cost. Medicare is not the answer to funding long-term care.

Another common misconception is that "Medicare will take care of you until you're well." This is not true. Most Medicare recipients recover sufficiently to leave the hospital, but they are discharged when they no longer need hospital services — not when they are completely well. Some never get completely well. Some never recover sufficiently to leave a skilled nursing facility. In recognition of this, Medicare imposes a cutoff point for skilled nursing facility services. Longer-term needs are taken care of by federal/state programs such as **Medicaid** and **Supplemental Security Income (SSI)**. There is a growing recognition on the part of the policymakers that some of the needs of the elderly, such as the need for help in eating and dressing, are not medical needs. They're not medical because medicine can't do anything for them. They are social problems that ought to be handled outside the medical model. The federal government has sponsored a few experiments with **social health maintenance organizations (SHMOs)** to test ways to provide care outside the medical model, but this sort of work is still in its infancy. For the moment, don't assume that Medicare will take care of any need you have for long-term care. It won't.

What options are available when Medicare runs out? The chief one is Medicaid, a program that is jointly funded by the states and the federal government. States have a wide range of latitude in whom they cover, what services they cover, and the income and resource limits they use. For these reasons, it is hard to be too specific with numerical examples. It is possible to state the general principles.

The Medicaid program does cover nursing home care, but Medicaid is intended for the *very* poor who have nowhere else to turn. Not all of the very poor are covered. Medicaid is a state-run program that receives federal funds. States make most of the rules, and the trend in recent years has been to make requirements more stringent. The old law virtually guaranteed that the spouse who stayed at home would have to impoverish himself or herself to pay for the care of the spouse in the nursing home.

Legislation passed in 1988 greatly reduces the burden but can still lead to a substantial loss of assets.

- In any month in which a married person is in a nursing home, no income of the at-home spouse is to be considered available to the spouse in the nursing home.

- Income is considered the property of the person to whom it is paid. Income paid to both spouses is attributed 50 percent to each.

- The home, household goods, and personal effects of both spouses are not counted in considering Medicaid eligibility.

- All assets other than these will be counted and divided in two. If the at-home spouse has less than $15,000, the spouse in the nursing home may transfer assets to him or her to make up to $15,000 available to the at-home spouse. (States may, at their option, raise this figure to any amount less than $76,000. The $15,000 amount will be indexed to inflation.)

- The assets that remain in the name of the spouse in the nursing home are considered available to pay for his or her nursing home care. All assets in excess of $76,000 are attributed to the spouse in the nursing home and are considered available to pay for nursing home care.

- States must allow nursing home residents to retain certain sums for medical expenses not covered by Medicare or Medicaid before contributing to the expense of their nursing home care. The states may place "reasonable limits" on the amounts spent.

- States must allow the at-home spouse sufficient income from the other spouse to bring total household income of the at-home spouse to at least 150 percent of the federal poverty level for a two-person household. States will not be required to allow more than $1,918 per month, except by court order or change in regulations.

One very important point: Your spouse and parents do not *actually* have to give anything toward the cost of your care, but your *eligibility* is determined as though they do. Even though the legislation makes things much more uniform across the nation than they were, the exact requirements, as well as the exact amount of liquid assets and income you may retain and still be eligible, will vary from state to state because of the range ($15,000–$76,000) in which Congress allows states to set the level. Check the list of Medicaid state offices in appendix N to find out where to call to determine the exact eligibility requirements for your state.

You are *automatically* eligible for Medicaid if you are eligible for, or receiving, **Supplemental Security Income (SSI)** payments for the aged, blind, and disabled, but you must apply at a state welfare office. If you meet the requirements for SSI, there is little chance that you would have to give up additional income or assets to qualify for Medicaid.

If your income, less certain deductions and medical bills, is within certain (low) limits, you may be eligible for Medicaid as **medically needy.** You must "spend down" (deduct medical bills from income) to the point at which you are eligible. If you have low enough income, high enough medical bills, and meet certain other tests, Medicaid pays for all medical bills. You can contact your state Medicaid agency, listed in appendix N, to find out about application procedures and eligibility requirements in your state.

Certain low-income Medicare beneficiaries may be eligible to have their state's Medicaid program pay for their Part B coverage. **Qualified Medicare Beneficiaries,** or QMBs, are eligible to have the state pay their Part B premium and, in most cases, the deductibles and copayments. Contact your nearest welfare or Social Security office for more information.

In general, you must meet these eligibility requirements:

- You must be entitled to Medicare Hospital Insurance (Part A).

- Your monthly income must be at or below the federal poverty level for an individual or couple, and your resources may not exceed $6,000 (amounts are slightly higher in Alaska and Hawaii).

If you don't qualify for the QMB program based on income, you may be eligible for assistance under the **Specified Low-Income Medicare Beneficiary** program. Individuals and couples are eligible for assistance if their incomes are up to 120 percent of the poverty level (amounts are slightly higher in Alaska and Hawaii). If you qualify, your state will pay your Medicare Part B premium, but not the deductibles and copayments.

*What Medicare Means by "Services"*

Medicare covers "hospital services," but not all of them. **Private rooms, private duty nursing**, radios, televisions, and telephones are among the services offered by hospitals, but Medicare does not automatically pay for them the way it does, say, for operating room charges. Medicare doesn't pay for private rooms unless they are prescribed by doctors or no other room is available. The same is true for private duty nursing. Radios, televisions, and telephones are never covered. Medicare will not pay for the first three pints of blood used in blood transfusions in a year, but it will pay for all blood used after those first three. Any blood deductible paid under Part A or Part B applies, so you will have to pay for no more than three pints of blood in any year. The deductible is waived if you or someone else replaces the blood. Check with the local blood bank or the hospital blood bank on how to have a pint credited to your deductible.

Drugs administered in the hospital are normally covered, but those that have not been judged "safe and effective" by the Food and Drug Administration are not covered.

All insurance plans have reserved the right, from their inception, to pay for what the carrier defines as covered, not anything a doctor may choose to prescribe or a patient may want. So, too, with Medicare. As the cost of medical care rises, limitations on payment by insurance companies and Medicare will increase, not decrease. Medicare and private insurers are likely to insist on more, rather than less, proof of safety and effectiveness before paying for a new service.

In the following sections, we discuss what is covered and what is not for each type of service. Chapter 3 explains the **copayments** and **deductibles** that are involved. These are charges that you or your insurance company have to cover. Depending on the details of your supplemental insurance for Medicare (if you own such a policy), only part of the copayment or deductible may be paid. You pay the remainder. (See chapter 4 for a discussion of insurance to supplement Medicare.)

*Services Covered: Hospitals*

Medicare covers the following services for **inpatient hospital care:**

- Semiprivate room (no more than two beds to a room)
- All meals, including any special diets that are needed, plus **hyperalimentation**
- Nursing services regularly provided by the unit you are in (Medicare pays for nursing services in the **intensive care unit,** even though they are more expensive than those on the **general medical/surgical floors.**)
- Intensive care, intensive care units, and care in other **special care units** (for example, a brain surgery unit)
- Drugs furnished in the hospital, unless they are excluded because the Food and Drug Administration has not found them "safe and effective"
- Blood transfusions, except for the cost of the first three pints of blood (As we noted before, the cost of the blood can be met under the Part A or Part B deductible, and will be waived if the blood is replaced.)
- Hospital charges for lab tests
- Hospital charges for **X rays** and **radiotherapy**
- Medical supplies, such as dressing, casts, splints, **catheters,** and **intravenous (IV) lines**
- Use of **durable medical equipment,** such as wheelchairs and crutches, while in the hospital
- All hospital **operating room** and **recovery room** charges
- Rehabilitation services, such as physical therapy, speech pathology, and the like, provided during the inpatient stay

The charges of **hospital-based physicians,** such as **pathologists, radiologists, physiatrists, nuclear medicine** and **pulmonary specialists,** to name a few, are not covered under the hospital insurance portion of Medicare but are paid by Part B, doctor insurance. This splitting of charges between the hospital and the physician for what looks like a hospital-provided service can often be confusing. The Claims Log we provide for you (see appendix B) will help you keep all of this straight and make sure that you pay no more than you absolutely have to.

Medicare once again pays for a limited number of hospital days per benefit period (see page 65), and has reinstated the spell of illness deductible. Each time you experience a spell of illness and are admitted to a hospital, you are responsible for the Part A hospital deductible. Remember, Medicare will only pay for services that are deemed to be **medically necessary.**

Before the enactment of the **Diagnosis-Related Group (DRG)** prospective payment system, limitations on days paid for by Medicare could have affected your hospital stay. The diagnosis-related groups system provides a set payment for each condition. In addition, there is a process that allows the hospital to apply for more money if your case is unusually expensive. Now you can be discharged only when hospital care is no longer medically necessary. The deal between the hospital and Medicare under the DRG system requires that the hospital provide as much service as Medicare patients' doctors deem necessary for their care.

You may think that Medicare pays for care anywhere in the world. It doesn't. Only care in hospitals in the fifty states and the District of Columbia, Puerto Rico, and the last two U.S. territories — Guam and the Virgin Islands — is paid for. Care you receive in Europe, Canada, Mexico, and the rest of the world is *not* covered. The only exception is if you are close to the Canadian or Mexican border and in need of emergency care, and the nearest hospital is a Canadian or Mexican one. In this situation, Medicare will pay for services in a Canadian or Mexican hospital.

Another limitation on hospital services, mentioned briefly earlier, is **medical necessity.** We'll discuss this more in chapter 8. For the moment, the general idea is this: Medicare will not pay for anything it does not consider dictated by the needs of good, professional medicine as applied to your case. Sometimes, for example in certain types of surgery that are often abused, the **medical necessity determination** is made before you go into the hospital or have the operation. In other instances, it is made after Medicare-mandated reviewers of coverage, such as the **peer review organizations (PROs)**, review your chart and decide that your case has not been handled as it should have been.

Medicare has been experimenting with ways to hold down costs ever since the program began to cost much more than anticipated, in the late 1960s. The peer review organizations are the latest example. Peer review organizations are groups of doctors who contract with Medicare to make sure that the care given to Medicare beneficiaries is of acceptable quality and is really needed. The requirement that care be "reasonable and necessary" has always been in the law. The peer review organizations are just the latest means of enforcing it. They review some cases before care is given, if local or national evidence indicates a high level of inappropriate use. In these situations, approval is required before Medicare pays. In other cases, they look at charts after the patient has been discharged and make decisions about the appropriateness of what was done. Finally, they review requests from hospitals for extra payment (over and above the amount the diagnosis-related groups system pays) and extra days of care.

*Unless you have received an official notice that a service is not considered medically necessary before you have it done, or that additional hospital days are not necessary before you decide to stay,* you never have to pay for medically unnecessary care. We discuss in chapter 8 what to do when you receive such notices.

## *Physicians and Related Services*

Medicare pays for most services of physicians — holders of the degrees of **Doctor of Medicine (M.D.)** or **Doctor of Osteopathy (D.O.)** — and some of the services of **podiatrists** (foot doctors), some of the services of **chiropractors**, and dental surgery performed by **dentists** in a hospital. Some services of **optometrists** (those licensed to prescribe eyeglasses and contact lenses) are covered as well.

Most **outpatient treatments** and tests, such as **electrocardiograms (EKGs)**, X rays, and physical therapy, are covered. When the Medicare law was passed, most such services were performed in the outpatient departments of hospitals. Now most of them are available in physicians' offices and are covered by Medicare.

For coverage of nonhospital services (or Medicare services in general), the usual rule is that routine services, such as annual physicals, that are not aimed at treating a specific illness are not covered, and that services designed to improve appearance or bodily function, such as cosmetic surgery, are not covered unless they are needed to restore a state of health that existed before illness or injury.

Outpatient psychiatric services are covered, but require a 50 percent copayment. The limit on total lifetime inpatient psychiatric hospital days has been raised to 190.

At present, drugs and **biologicals** (**hormones, serums, vaccines,** and such) are covered only if administered by the treating professional. They are not covered if they are prescribed for self-administration. Prescription drugs that the doctor prescribes for you to administer to yourself are generally not covered. The only exceptions are immunosuppressive drugs, such as cyclosporine, an antirejection drug prescribed for kidney transplant patients under the end stage renal disease portion of Medicare.

*Services Covered:*
*Nursing Homes*

As we discussed earlier, Medicare coverage for a skilled nursing facility is limited to 100 days per benefit period, with full payment for the first 20 days and a copayment for days 21 through 100 (the copayment for 1997 is $95). *Medicare does not pay for nursing home care that is needed simply because you can no longer care for yourself.* The limited payment for skilled nursing facility services actually functions as a money-saver: If you need skilled nursing services to recover, but can safely have them outside a hospital, it makes sense for the government to cover them in a lower-cost setting like a nursing home.

The enormous expense of nursing home services — more than $60 billion annually — indicates that they have certainly helped many people who could not care for themselves. But the care given in many nursing homes is, frankly, of uncertain quality. Quality of nursing home care is not well monitored. Medicare has only recently decided to require that some sort of nurse (a **registered nurse** or a **licensed practical nurse** or **licensed vocational nurse**) be available on all shifts in all nursing homes. We have much more to say about nursing homes in chapter 7.

*Other Covered*
*Services*

*Home health care:* Home health care is covered for up to 21 consecutive days; there is no limit on the total number of visits. The major restriction is that the visits must be for medical care only. Homemaker-type services are not included. After 21 consecutive days, there must be a break of at least one day before another series will be paid for.

*Flu shots:* Medicare covers the cost of flu shots.

*Durable medical equipment:* A number of pieces of **durable medical equipment**, such as wheelchairs and hospital beds for home use, are covered. If a doctor prescribes it, Medicare will usually approve the equipment and pay 80 percent of the cost.

*Therapeutic shoes for diabetics:* If prescribed by a doctor, 80 percent is covered.

*Eyeglasses, contact lenses, and hearing aids:* Eyeglasses, contact lenses, and hearing aids are covered only if needed following eye or ear surgery, or as a result of eye or ear disease other than normal visual or hearing defects such as astigmatism, myopia, or age-related hearing loss.

## How to Maximize Your Medicare Benefits

In this section, we talk about some of the ways that are emerging to get more out of Medicare. Most are the results of experiments by the federal government to make market forces play a bigger role in health care, and experiments in health care cost containment or in approaches to paying for health care that have worked well for people under 65.

*Medicare Supplemental Insurance*

One of the most effective ways to maximize the value of your Medicare dollar is to purchase Medicare supplemental insurance. A good supplemental policy will cover all of the Medicare deductibles and copayments, and protect you from large out-of-pocket expenses. However, selecting the right policy has been far from an easy chore because there was very little, if any, standardization among policies — a situation that has finally been addressed by Congress.

The National Association of Insurance Commissioners was directed by Congress to design standard supplemental policies in an effort to make it easier for beneficiaries to comparison shop. To achieve this goal, the commissioners designed one basic supplemental package and also provided for the development of up to nine other plans. Each plan contains a core of basic coverage that includes: Part A hospital copayment days, Part B copayment, blood deductible, and hospital coverage beyond Medicare. The additional nine plans offer expanded coverage. (See Appendix D.) In addition, regulations require that:

- You be given a 30-day free-look period, during which you may cancel a policy and receive a full refund.
- Benefits paid out must equal 65 percent of premiums on individual policies and 75 percent for group policies.
- Certified insurers must submit their advertising to state insurance commissioners for review.

We suggest that, at a minimum, you purchase a policy that covers *all* the deductibles and copayments for hospital and doctor bills. This means that you will have to pay only what Medicare does not reimburse, and it limits your expense to relatively minor items (with the exception of nursing home care). To protect yourself from this expense, the policy should also cover the skilled nursing facility copayment for days 21 through 100. You should also look for policies that cover physician charges in excess of the Medicare-approved charge. Policies that cover these expenses should pay at least 80 percent of the excess fee up to the full balance billing limits for nonparticipating doctors. This offers you further protection from large out-of-pocket expenses, which already cost Medicare beneficiaries billions of dollars each year.

The only way to protect yourself against excess fees is by always using a participating physician; however, we recognize that this is not always possible. Contact your nearest Social Security Administration office and ask for the directory of doctors who accept assignment. Another way to avoid excess fees is to negotiate with the nonparticipating physician and ask him/her to accept the Medicare-approved payment (See chapter 5, Negotiating With Your Doctor).

Here are some insurance policy features to look for:

- Guaranteed renewability
- No more than a six-month exclusion for preexisting conditions
- No limitations to single diseases, such as cancer, etc.
- Payment for services in full, rather than a fixed amount
- No waiting periods for coverage

In chapter 4, we explain more about supplemental insurance and give you a means of comparing policies.

*Negotiating with Your Doctor*

Another way to make the most of Medicare is to talk with your doctor about your care. We go into great depth in this area in chapter 5. Among the reasons you should negotiate your care (and his or her fees) with your doctor(s) are these:

- Most American experience their first serious illness only when they are over 50 or thereabouts.
- Because of this, the most expensive illnesses will come when people have reduced incomes, and when they are dependent on Medicare for health coverage.

- Medicare pays, on average, only about half of the health care expenses of elderly and disabled people, and that percentage is falling each year.
- Almost no form of supplementary insurance covers everything that people will need.
- The cost of treatment, the physical and psychological burdens of treatment, and the effect on relatives are *all* determined mostly by the doctor.
- The doctor, in large measure, determines how and when people die.

You should fight the tendency — which is forced on Americans by their culture — to think of Medicare as some sort of charity. Medicare beneficiaries paid premiums for Part A through their work in the past and are paying premiums for Part B now. In dealing with your doctor, think of Medicare as just like any other insurance. Medicare may not pay everything that the doctor might like, but the doctor's prices, which are largely unaffected by market forces, are a sort of wish list to begin with. It's probable that *no* insurance company is paying the doctor everything he or she wants.

Even better, don't think of the insurance issue at all. Doctors make their living by selling their services, and the satisfaction of their customers should be a big concern to them. When it comes right down to it, if a doctor loses you as a patient, any and all fees he or she might have gotten from you are lost. If the doctor keeps you as a patient and accepts Medicare **assignment** to help you pay only a bearable portion of your income for medical expenses, all that is lost is the difference between the doctor's wishes and the Medicare payment. If you have to point this out, do so. Your doctor may learn something.

## *Health Maintenance Organizations (HMOs)*

**Health Maintenance Organizations (HMOs)** are a proven approach to medical care delivery. When they were first started, they were bitterly opposed by doctors and medical organizations, because they either required the doctors to become employees and accept a salary, or because they limited what doctors could charge. In the 1930s, a group of consumers in Washington, D.C., set up an HMO, which they owned and controlled (and still do). The doctors were hired by a board elected from the membership, and were actually (and still are) employees of their patients. The **American Medical Association (AMA)** sued them, and the case reached the Supreme Court. The Court said that if a group of people wanted to hire a group of doctors to take care of them, they could not be prevented from doing so.

Even though HMOs are growing rapidly, only about half of the Medicare beneficiaries in the nation live in the service areas of those with Medicare contracts. Because such organizations are new to many, we'll explain in some detail how they work with Medicare.

Most HMOs are not consumer-owned. Whether or not they are for-profit or nonprofit, they are "owned" by a self-perpetuating board of trustees, the same way **nonprofit voluntary hospitals** are. Regardless of who owns them, they usually make at least a pretense of seeking member involvement in the way the HMO is run.

The basic idea behind health maintenance organizations is that health care will, overall, be cheaper if preventive services are covered and if there is no need for people to worry about the cost before seeking care. This makes sense. HMOs have clearly demonstrated that they can save at least 25 percent over the cost of care provided in a **fee-for-service system**, like Medicare, in which doctors are paid something for each service they provide. It is thought that this provides a **perverse incentive** for the doctor to give care that is not really needed. Much research evidence suggests that this is true.

The opposite side of the coin, of course, is the risk that HMO doctors may be tempted to undertreat people to save money. This has happened, but rarely. Studies of HMO patients in general have found that their health is just as good as, and perhaps a little bit better than, the health of patients treated by doctors in private practice. Studies have also shown that the quality of care given in HMOs is, in the main, just as good as or just a little bit better than the care given by doctors in private practice.

As a Medicare patient in an HMO, you will most likely get more services, at a lower cost, than you will as a patient of doctors in private practice. HMOs usually offer what those in the health insurance industry call a "Cadillac" package of services, with few or no copayments or deductibles, depending on the organization. Prescription drugs are often provided at no or low cost. This alone can make an HMO worth considering for someone who must take several expensive drugs. They do this both because they believe in the original ideal of supplying services to maintain health, rather than just cure illness, and because they need to attract patients.

Some people do not like certain features of health maintenance organizations, so HMOs compete in other ways, often by offering more benefits than do traditional insurance plans. The same features that deter some people often attract other people. For one thing, your choice of doctors is limited to doctors who are employees of the HMO (if it is a **staff model health maintenance organization**), to those who are in the **group practices** that the HMO has contracted with (if it is a **group model health maintenance organization**), or to doctors in private practice who have signed on as members of an **individual practice association (IPA) model health maintenance organization**. Opponents of HMOs make a big issue of the supposed denial of freedom of choice. It is little understood that Blue Shield, still the major supplier of insurance for doctors' services in the country, works on essentially the same principle: it will pay in full only for the services of doctors on the Blue Shield panel. The difference in HMOs is that no payment is made for services of doctors not on the HMO panel, unless an HMO doctor calls them in as a consultant or refers you to them.

A group or staff model HMO is far more convenient for a person, especially a moderately sick one, than seeing a physician in private practice. Usually, **primary care physicians (general practitioners, family practitioners,** general **internists, pediatricians,** and **obstetrician-gynecologists)** are located in the same building with **specialists.** Often, but not always, it is possible to see a specialist immediately if the primary care physician thinks one is needed. **Outpatient surgery** suites, **chemotherapy** rooms, X-ray departments, laboratories, and pharmacies are often located in the same building as the doctors' offices. HMOs pioneered "one-stop shopping" in medicine primarily as a means of cost control and as a convenience to their doctors, but it is a great convenience for patients as well. Some large HMOs even have their own emergency rooms, located in their clinics.

An IPA model HMO uses the offices of private physicians who have agreed to see HMO patients in addition to their private patients. Office care in an IPA model HMO feels just like going to a doctor in private practice. Otherwise, all the following comments regarding hospital care and the like apply.

On the negative side (and not all agree that it is a negative), your choice of hospitals as an HMO member will be limited to those that the HMO has contracted with. Since HMOs are looking to control costs, these often will not be what are perceived to be the best hospitals in the city. The HMO management will learn which hospitals are the cheapest and have the best records for particular diseases and types of patients. You may find that you are admitted to one hospital, treated for one condition, and then transferred to another hospital for treatment of a second. If you need specialized surgery, you may have the surgery in a university medical school hospital and be transferred to a small community hospital to recuperate. Saving money in this way enables HMOs to offer the Cadillac plan at a rate that employers, patients — and Medicare — are willing to pay.

Health maintenance organizations usually offer high-option and low-option plans. A typical high-option plan can include all physician services for any purpose, all drugs for any purpose with no or a small copayment, unlimited hospital care, all emergency care, and all out-patient care, as well as podiatric services, eyeglasses, and hearing aids. Low-option plans vary widely. An increasingly common one is one small copayment — $5 to $10 — for everything. This greatly simplifies the HMO's bookkeeping and billing operations. It can mean, however, that one owes $200–$300 for a heavy day that included a visit with the primary care physician, a referral to a specialist, a welter of lab tests, a special X-ray series, a visit to the HMO nurse for shots and treatment, and five or six prescriptions. Even so, this is a very small amount compared to the out-of-pocket expenses for a Medicare beneficiary with no supplemental insurance or a plan that imposes heavy copayments and deductibles.

In some HMOs, the low option is limited to only the services covered by Medicare, but with the HMO covering all of Medicare copayments and deductibles and imposing none of its own. This is like a Medicare supplemental insurance plan that covers all the gaps in Medicare coverage but adds nothing else.

Premiums vary greatly, depending on the package of services chosen, the HMO's experience with Medicare patients, how many Medicare beneficiaries are enrolled versus younger (and usually healthier) people, who are cheaper to care for, the hospitals the HMO contracts with, going rates for doctors in the area, and so on. HMO enrollment is growing rapidly, and HMOs are experimenting with ways to enroll and retain people, so shopping around, especially in urban areas, is possible. It is safe to say that you will always be able to obtain *all* of the care you need in a HMO more cheaply than with a supplemental insurance plan, and certainly more cheaply than the cost of Medicare Part B premiums plus the copayments and deductibles.

Some people think that joining a health maintenance organization requires turning over their Social Security check to it. This is not true.

When you enroll in an HMO that accepts Medicare patients, Medicare makes a regular monthly payment to the HMO. You continue to pay the Part B premium and may also have to pay a premium to the HMO to pay for services which Medicare does not cover. This extra premium may be larger or smaller than the Part B premium. It is just like the premium you pay for supplemental medical insurance to an insurance company.

Some HMO patients on a low-option plan that imposes a copayment for each service who are very sick and use a large amount of outpatient services will find themselves spending thousands of dollars out of pocket. It may even be cheaper (for them, not the HMO) to be treated in the hospital. This, paradoxically, is something that HMOs were set up to avoid. Such situations are teaching HMOs something that providers of employee benefit plans have known for years — that it is important to provide a maximum **out-of-pocket limit,** or **stop-loss provision,** for persons who have **catastrophic illnesses.**

There are other aspects of being an HMO member that you may or may not find to your liking. Virtually all HMOs require that they approve **out-of-area care** before it is provided, except in life-threatening emergencies. This may leave you sitting in the emergency room in Dubuque while the emergency room doctor and your HMO doctor in Los Angeles argue about whether you really need to be admitted. This stressful situation, which HMOs pioneered, is becoming more common as private insurance plans and Medicare itself have started requiring the same sort of preapproval for many services.

Some, but not all, HMOs try to make maximum use of **physician extenders,** such as **nurse practitioners, medical technicians,** and **physicians' assistants.** They do this based on research that shows that persons with these sorts of training can do as well as, or better than, doctors for a limited range of situations and can be trusted to recognize situations they can't handle and call in the doctor. If you think of them as specialists in low-end routine care, you can be comforted by the evidence that they sometimes are better than M.D.'s. If your image of proper medical care is having one specialist to look at your eyes, another to listen to your heart, a third to talk about your arthritis, and a fourth to talk about your kidneys, a visit with the nurse practitioner will not make you happy. From the HMO's viewpoint, using physician extenders cuts costs, enables more people to be seen, gives them a sympathetic ear for problems that the doctor seems too busy to listen to, and makes the best use of expensive physicians' time.

Some HMOs have a lot of general internists on staff and have **pro-**

**tocols** that require the other primary physicians to refer patients to them as special situations develop. This may lead to having your horse switched in midstream for no apparent reason while you are assured that there is no need to refer you to a specialist. Others treat internists as specialists in the use of drugs to treat disease of the internal organs — their original self-definition as specialists, before they got turned into a species of generalists. Still others make no distinction at all between the types of primary care providers. Some are quite happy to let your gynecologist attend to all your medical needs. Others are very strict about limiting gynecologists to **gynecological problems** only.

It is safe to say three things about the kind of care you will receive in a health maintenance organization. First, no matter how friendly it is, it will appear a little more regimented and impersonal than care in a private physician's office. It will feel a bit like a clinic, no matter how hard the HMO works at atmosphere. Second, your choice of primary care doctor will be limited to those who have signed up with the HMO, either as employees of a staff model HMO, members of a group practice HMO, or individual practice association HMO doctors. Third, you will get more care for the dollar than in traditional insurance plans, and your out-of-pocket expenses will be less. Whether you like the trade-offs is up to you. The rate of withdrawal — dropping out after signing up — is quite low. Most of those who get as far as enrolling seem to think the trade-offs are worth it.

*Conditions for HMO Enrollment as a Medicare Beneficiary*

Health maintenance organization membership was not available for Medicare beneficiaries until recently. Now it is almost routine. To be an HMO member as a Medicare beneficiary,

- You must be enrolled in *both* Part A and Part B of Medicare.
- You can join only an HMO that has a contract with Medicare, not just any one.
- You must live in the **service area** of the HMO, that is, the geographical area from which the HMO is licensed to enroll members.
- You must enroll during the open enrollment period of the HMO you have chosen. This may be all year, or it may be limited to a few months.
- You can drop out at any time by notifying the HMO in writing, on a form it prescribes for this purpose. A letter will not do, unless the organization specifically allows withdrawal requests by letter. You must submit the withdrawal request by the tenth day of the month to be returned to the regular Medicare program on the first of the

next month. Requests received after the tenth will result in return to the regular program on the first of the month after next. In either case, the HMO will continue to provide you with services.

You have certain protections as an HMO member. Medicare requirements for HMO beneficiaries may go beyond what the state requires to license an HMO.

- You cannot be denied enrollment because of your state of health. The HMO *is* allowed to deny *high-option* coverage to persons with some medical conditions.
- All Medicare-covered services must be available with reasonable promptness when needed. Emergency facilities must be available around the clock.
- The HMO cannot terminate your membership because of poor health or because of the cost of treating you.
- If the HMO ends its contract with Medicare — thereby dropping all Medicare beneficiaries — you must be given at least sixty days' notice.
- The HMO must have written procedures for resolving complaints.
- You have the same rights to appeal decisions about your care in an HMO as you do for regular services (see chapter 8).
- You can withdraw from the HMO at any time by notifying it in writing. If the HMO requires that a special form be used to withdraw, you must use it.

Since the absence of freedom of choice is the one big negative associated with HMOs, many are experimenting with **freedom of choice options**. Usually, this means that you can see any doctor you want, provided that he or she has credentials satisfactory to the HMO, but must pay a copayment to see one who is not on the HMO panel.

The HMO is required to maintain a certain ratio between Medicare and non-Medicare patients. It is almost impossible to avoid a situation in which the younger, healthier members of an HMO are partially subsidizing the care of older, sicker ones. (This is true in HMOs that do not enroll Medicare members. The healthier patients who use few services subsidize those who are sicker. If this were not the case, a different premium would have to apply to every individual, and sick people could not afford care. There is nothing shady about this; it's part of the basic concept of insurance.) Medicare payment to the HMO, which is based on the average Medicare expenditure per person in the region, may not cover the cost of all HMO services. Because of this, the HMO may have closed enrollment and will allow no more Medicare recipients to join until the ratio is adjusted.

A chart you can use to compare different HMOs is provided in chapter 4, on supplemental health insurance for Medicare beneficiaries.

*Competitive Medical Plans*

**Competitive medical plans** (**CMPs**) are insurance plans that contract with Medicare to provide all Medicare-covered services for a flat fee paid to them by Medicare. They can charge a premium, over and above the cost of Medicare, for services not covered by Medicare. Some competitive medical plans are health maintenance organizations, but they are not required to follow the HMO model.

*Medicare Choices*

Medicare is launching a new managed-care project called **Medicare Choices** that will be available to residents of California, Florida, Georgia, Louisiana, Montana, New York, North Carolina, Ohio, Pennsylvania, Texas and Virginia. Medicare Choices is a demonstration project designed to bring managed care to those areas where Medicare beneficiaries currently have little, if any, access. Many of the participants are hospitals, although some of the plans selected are physician-sponsored. Plans selected for the Medicare Choices project must offer the same coverage as regular Medicare; however, they may also offer additional services.

*MIGs at Twelve O'Clock — Medicare Insured Groups*

Congress has appropriated funds for three **Medicare insured groups**, or **MIGs**. These are experiments in which a purchaser of health insurance for those under 65, such as an employer or a union health plan, undertakes to provide health insurance to Medicare beneficiaries on the same basis, in return for a payment from the federal government. If the experimental MIGs work well, they will probably be written into the Social Security act as one more option for receiving health care under Medicare, along with health maintenance organizations and competitive medical plans.

Medicare has a pamphlet on various prepaid health coverage plans, "Medicare and Managed Care Plans," which can be obtained at your local Social Security office. If they have none, ask them to order HCFA publication number 02195.

In this chapter you will learn: What is covered by Medicare Part A hospital insurance ▪ What is covered by Medicare Part B medical insurance ▪ What is meant by deductibles and copayments ▪ What is meant by benefit period ▪ When you are not responsible for the cost of services received ▪ When you are responsible for the cost of services received ▪ How to read an Explanation of Medicare Benefits ▪ How the Diagnosis-Related Groups system affects hospital payment and you ▪ What your rights are while a hospital patient

# 3. What Medicare Does (and Doesn't) Pay For

The purpose of this chapter is to explain, in terms that are as clear as the complexity of the program permits, exactly what Medicare pays for and what you (or your insurer, or both) have to pay for.

Medicare pays in full for only a few items. Even if you have insurance that supplements Medicare, the insurance plan may require you to pay part of the cost. The same is true if you belong to a **Health Maintenance Organization (HMO)** through which you obtain Medicare services. The phrase "what you pay for" in this chapter should be understood to include what has to be paid, regardless of who pays it. You may have other sources of payment for what Medicare doesn't cover — payments made by your insurer or HMO (plus what you pay out-of-pocket).

What gets paid for, how much, and when, under Medicare, is an odd combination of the following:

- The *services* that providers agree to provide in their contracts with Medicare
- The *amount* of the services that Medicare covers
- Medicare's commitment to *cost-sharing* through copayment and deductibles

- *How* the law establishing Medicare (Title XVIII of the Social Security act) dicates that each type of **provider** be paid
- The *medical necessity* of the services you actually received

The regulations that govern Medicare are *not* set up this way. As a result, it is very hard to discover exactly what is paid, or not paid, under what conditions, by reading them. But the ways we have cut them up, above, really do cover all the issues that are involved in determining what you wind up paying for. In each of the sections that begin on page 93, we discuss what Medicare pays and what you pay under related headings:

- Covered Services
- Limitations on Services
- Cost-sharing
- How Payment Is Made
- Medical Necessity Determinations

## When You Never Have to Pay

There are numerous situations in which Medicare decides not to pay a provider, or to pay less than the provider wanted. It's important to understand when you don't have to pay for something that Medicare has refused to pay a provider for: *You are never obligated to pay for a service unless you can reasonably have been expected to know that the service was not covered, or was not (medically) reasonable and necessary. You are never obligated to pay more than Medicare has decided to pay the provider if the provider has agreed to accept* **assignment.**

## "Reasonably Have Been Expected to Know"

"Reasonably have been expected to know" is a legal phrase. What it means, basically, is this: if you have not been informed *in writing* by an appropriate review authority, the provider, a Medicare intermediary or carrier, or Medicare itself that a service is not covered or is not (medically) reasonable and necessary, and you could not be expected to know it from official sources (such as pamphlets that you were given when you signed up for Medicare, or from prior notices that such services were not covered), then you are protected from having to pay for it, even if Medicare doesn't. The key word is *reasonably.* What you can reasonably be expected to know is that which a reasonable person would expect an individual like you, in your situation, having received the information you received, to know. The working definition, as Medicare's **administrative law judges** and the courts use it, resides in **case law** and is continuously evolving. As it stated in the regulations, there are two important parts: you have to receive *a written notice*, and you have to receive it from *an appropriate source*.

Some examples may help here:

Example 1: *You go into the hospital for surgery. The operation (or procedure; we'll call all procedures "operations" for the sake of simplicity) is one that Medicare normally requires be done in an* **outpatient** *facility, because it has been proven that this can be done safely and at lower cost than in the hospital. Your doctor believes that he can show that your case required* **inpatient** *surgery. The* **Peer Review Organization (PRO)** *that reviews such cases disagrees. The hospital gets paid nothing. You do not have to pay anything. Why? Because you cannot reasonably have been expected to know exactly which operations are required to be done as outpatient operations, or to know the steps your doctor should have followed to check.*

Example 2: *You go into the hospital for surgery. The operation is one that Medicare normally requires be done only after the peer review organization has approved it. (This may be because there is disagreement among doctors about when the operation is needed or whether it works, or because there is wide variation across the country in the number of operations done on similar groups of people. It may also be because the peer review organization has determined that many of the operations performed in your area turn out to be unnecessary.) The hospital does not obtain approval. The hospital is paid nothing, but you are not required to pay anything. You could not reasonably have been expected to know which operations were on the preapproval list.*

Example 3: *You have carefully searched for a doctor who accepts* **assignment**. *The doctor you chose is on the list of* **Medicare-participating physicians** *that your local Social Security office provided you. You specifically ask her if she takes assignment. She says that she does. The old year passes, and the new one begins. You suddenly begin getting bills from her for more than 20 percent of Medicare's charge for her services. It turns out that she has not renewed her* **participating-physician agreement** *with Med-*

*icare and has taken no steps to inform her patients. You call the office to complain, and find out that she no longer accepts assignment. You do not have to pay more than 20 percent of the Medicare-approved charge until you learn this. You are required to pay the extra costs for services received after you learn this.*

Example 4: *You are discharged from the hospital but need further therapy before you can go home. You are admitted to a nursing home for some physical therapy and daily changing of a dressing. The peer review organization determines that you could have been treated at home, or at the doctor's office, so your stay is not* **medically necessary.** *The nursing home is paid nothing, but you do not have to pay anything.*

Don't worry if you didn't understand everything in the examples. What you need to understand is the general principle: when Medicare makes a payment, all sorts of wheels turn which you cannot reasonably be expected to know about. You are protected from the consequences of behind-the-scenes decisions if you are not informed of them. *The fact that Medicare has refused payment doesn't mean that you have to pay.*

On the other hand, there *are* situations in which you *can* "reasonably be expected to know" something or other, and you must act to make sure that you do not have to pay more than is necessary. Some examples, parallel to the ones above, should help make this clear:

Example 1: *You go into the hospital for surgery. The operation is one that Medicare normally requires be done in an* **outpatient** *facility, because it has been proven that this can be done safely and at lower cost than in the hospital. Your doctor believes that he can show that your case requires* **inpatient** *surgery. He checks with the appropriate personnel at the hospital. They advise him that your condition does not require hospitalization and can safely be done in an outpatient facility (a clinic, an* **ambulatory surgery** *center, or the doctor's office). You are informed of this in* writing. *You do not appeal. You decide to go to the hospital. As expected, the* Peer Review Organization (PRO) *will recommend that nothing be paid for the hospital stay. You are so informed,* in writing. *You do not appeal. You have to pay the hospital bill and any doctors' bills associated with doing the operation in the hospital. Why? You could reasonably have been expected to* *know that this operation was required to be done as an outpatient operation; you were informed in writing.*

*Example 2: You go into the hospital for surgery. The operation is one that Medicare normally requires be done only after the peer review organization has approved it. The hospital does not obtain approval. Your doctor tells you this, in writing. You do not insist that a formal determination be made, or one is made and you do not appeal it. You decide to go ahead with the operation. You have to pay the hospital bill plus any additional doctors' fees. Why? You could reasonably have been expected to know that Medicare would not pay for the operation; you were informed in writing.*

*Example 3: You have carefully searched for a doctor who accepts* **assignment**. *The doctor you chose is on the list of* **Medicare-participating physicians** *that your local Social Security office provided you. You specifically ask her if she takes assignment. She says that she does. The old year passes, and the new one begins. The doctor informs all her patients,* in writing, *by letter, that she will no longer accept assignment for all Medicare patients. You suddenly begin getting bills from her for more than the 20 percent of the Medicare-approved charge. Are you responsible for the additional amount over and above the 20 percent copayment? Yes. Why? Because you could have reasonably been expected to know that the physician no longer accepts assignment since you were informed in writing. However, you are protected from excessive* **balance billing** *by a Medicare regulation that limits what the physician may charge you.*

Medicare regulations limit the maximum fee that a nonparticipating physician may charge you and also limit the amount of balance billing that he or she may do. Using the Medicare-approved amount as the base, a physician's maximum fee for a service will be limited to a markup of 115 percent. You do not have to pay any amount that exceeds the maximum charge.

*Example 4: You are discharged from the hospital but need further therapy before you can go home. You are admitted to a nursing home for some physical therapy and daily changing of a dressing.*

*The Peer Review Organization determines that you could have
been treated at home, or at the doctor's office, so your stay is not
medically necessary. You are informed of this in writing, and you
elect not to appeal the decision or you lose your appeal. You have
to pay for the nursing home stay. Why? You could reasonably have
been expected to know that Medicare would not pay; you were
informed in writing.*

Again, don't worry about the technicalities here. We'll inform you
about what you can appeal, and how to do it, below. Chapter 8 provides more detail about the appeal process. For the moment, remember
three things:

- First, an oral notice to you isn't worth the paper it's printed on. Only
  *written* notifications have effect.
- Second, the written notice must come from an appropriate source:
  the Peer Review Organization, the Medicare intermediary or carrier,
  or the provider (doctor, hospital, nursing home official).
- Third, once you have been informed that a service is not covered,
  you are expected to know that it is not covered in the future.

## Dealing with Claims, Bills, and Carriers

We aren't saying that hospitals and doctors are unethical, but — like
most of us — they prefer getting money to not getting money. They
do not see it as their job to determine exactly what has and hasn't been
approved and bill you only for your share of the approved charges.
However, a recent change in Medicare regulations does make doctors
responsible for filing *all* Medicare claims — even those who do not accept Medicare assignment. This means that you no longer need to fill
out and submit a HCFA form 1490S; however, we recommend that you
use the Medicare Claims Log found in appendix B to keep track of these
claims in the event of a problem.

The **Explanation of Medicare Benefits** sent to you by the Medicare
carrier, and the information you receive from your insurance company
should be used to complete the claims log.

The **intermediaries** and **carriers** who handle Medicare payments see
it as their primary duty to get the checks and the bills out. The peer
review organization is interested in making determinations of medical
necessity, and arguing with Medicare to get more money in its next
review contract. *So none of these parties has, as its main concern,
making sure that you get billed for only what you really have to pay*

*for. You have to look out for yourself.* Because the payment system under Medicare is so complicated, it is virtually certain that at least one of your encounters with a health care provider will result in a bill for something you don't really owe. Because of this same complexity, and because there can be a considerable time lag before your case is reviewed (if it needs to be) or the hospital is audited, a long time can pass before who gets what, and who has to pay for what, is finally decided.

Your Medicare carrier or intermediary is required, as part of its contract with Medicare, to maintain a mailing address you can write to about amounts that you think you don't owe. Most of them also provide a telephone number. Your Medicare Supplemental Insurance carrier should have such an address and a telephone number, and is usually required by state insurance laws to have both. (Addresses and telephone numbers of the various Medicare intermediaries and carriers are provided in appendix A. Where to write with insurance complaints for each of the states is provided in appendix C.) Your health maintenance organization, if you belong to one, is required by both state and federal laws to have a procedure for resolving disputes and usually will maintain an address and a telephone number. Don't hesitate to call them. We can guarantee you that more than one of the explanations they send you won't make sense. (A sample Explanation of Medicare Benefits is shown on page 95.)

## Hospitals

*Covered Services*

You may want to examine the Medicare coverage chart on page 98 before proceeding any further. We want to call your attention to the column labeled "benefit period." As a result of the recent changes to Medicare, benefit periods are once again a part of Medicare hospital services.

A benefit period is a way of measuring your use of services under Medicare hospital insurance. Your first benefit period starts when you enter a hospital and after your hospital coverage begins. A benefit period ends when you have been out of the hospital or other facility (SNF, rehabilitation center, or whatever) for 60 days.

It's very important that you understand the benefit period, because it will help you determine when you are liable for the Part A deductible. For example, if you are admitted to the hospital for the first time on January 15th and are discharged on the 25th, you would pay the Part A deductible and during this benefit period you use 10 days. If you are readmitted on February 5th, you would not pay the deductible because it has been less than 60 days since your previous hospitalization and your readmission date would be day 11 in your benefit period.

On the other hand, if you are not hospitalized again until October 1st and are discharged on the 23rd, you are liable for the one-day Part A deductible, because more than 60 days have elapsed since your previous hospitalization.

Medicare's discussion of covered services for hospitals is basically an attempt to describe, at length, the services that hospitals normally provide to all patients. Bed and board, nursing services, use of hospital facilities, medical social services, drugs, biologicals, use of supplies and equipment, diagnostic and therapeutic services, and the services of **house staff** (**interns** and **residents** in training) are covered.

*Limitations on Services*

Private rooms are not covered unless your medical condition requires you to be isolated or there are no semiprivate or ward rooms available. Medicare will pay until you no longer need the private room or until you can be transferred to a semiprivate room or ward. You do not have to pay for the private room unless it was requested by you or a member of your family who was told, at the time the request was made, that there would be an additional charge. (Please note that the notice here does not need to be a written one.)

Medicare will not pay for the services of a **private duty nurse** unless the hospital normally provides one for patients in your condition.

# Explanation of Your Medicare Part B Benefits

Name of Beneficiary

Iphigenia Smith
4321 Edgar Allen Poe Drive
San Diego, CA 99110

Your Medicare number:   120-99-6789

A summary about this notice dated December 30, 1996.

| | |
|---|---|
| Total charges: | $1,755.00 |
| Total Medicare approved: | $1,339.00 |
| Medicare paid your provider: | $1,071.20 |
| You are responsible for: | $  367.80 |

---

## Details about this claim (See the back of this notice for more information.)

You received these services from your provider;
Dr. Sherman T. Potter, claim-#9876-1234-2468

Midway Medical Clinic, 2552 Baskerville Rd.,
San Diego, CA 99110

This indicates amount billed and approved.

| Services and Service Codes | Dates | Charge | Medicare approved | Notes |
|---|---|---|---|---|
| 65850 surgery, incision of eye | Nov 15, 1996 | $975.00 | $780.00 | a |
| 90040 brief office visit | Nov 19, 1996 | $100.00 | $  0 | b |
| 90070 extended office visits | Nov 17–29, 1996 | $600.00 | $516.00 | a |
| 90040 brief office visit | Nov 30, 1996 | $ 40.00 | $ 21.50 | a |
| 90040 brief office visit | Dec 15, 1996 | $ 40.00 | $ 21.50 | a |
| | Total | $1,755.00 | $1,339.00 | |

This indicates the service and date provided.

Notes:

a   We based the approved amount on the fee schedule for this service.

b   Medicare did not pay for this test. Medicare pays for this only when the laboratory is certified for this type of test.

This tells you if assignment was taken and the dollar amount billed.

Here's an explanation of this claim:

| | | |
|---|---|---|
| Of the total charges, Medicare approved | $1,339.00 | The provider accepted this amount. See #4 on the back of this notice. |
| The deductible you still owe | $  0 | You have met the $100 deductible for 1996. |
| | $1,339.00 | Medicare pays 80 percent of this total. |
| | × .80 | |
| We are paying the provider | $1,071.20 | Your copayment is 20 percent or $267.80. |
| Of the amount approved | $1,339.00 | |
| Subtract what we pay the provider | $1,071.20 | |
| You are responsible for | $ 267.80 | |
| plus charges not covered by Medicare | $ 100.00 | |
| The total you are responsible for: | $ 367.80 | The provider may bill you for this amount. If you have other insurance, the other insurance may pay this amount. |

This indicates whether or not you have met the $100 deductible this year.

This explains what you pay.

---

If you have questions about this notice, call Blue Cross Blue Shield of Maryland at 410-861-2273 or toll free at 800-662-5170 or visit us at 1946 Greenspring Drive, Timonium, Maryland.
You'll need this notice when you call or visit us about this claim.
If you want to appeal this claim, see #5 on the other side. You must write us by June 30, 1997.

This gives you the time frame to file any appeal.

This is your Part B carrier. If you suspect a mistake, contact this office.

# Important Information You Should Know About Your Medicare Part B Benefits

**This part of the notice answers some common questions that people ask about collecting Medicare benefits. If you have other questions, see your copy of *The Medicare Handbook* or call us for more information.**

**1. What should I do if I have questions about this notice?**

If you have questions about this notice, call, write, or visit us and we will tell you the facts that we used to decide what and how much to pay. Turn to the front of this notice: our address and phone number are on the bottom of the page.

**2. Can I appeal how much Medicare paid for these services?**

If you do not agree with what Medicare approved for these services, you may appeal our decision. To make sure that we are fair to you, we will not allow the same people who originally processed these services to conduct this review.

However, in order to be eligible for a review, you **must** write to us within **6 months** of the date of this notice, unless you have a good reason for being late (for example, if you had an extended illness which kept you from being able to file on time).

Turn to the front of this notice: the deadline date and our address are on the bottom of the page. It may help your case if you include a note from your doctor or supplier (provider) that tells us what was done and why.

If you want help with your appeal, you can have a friend, lawyer, or someone else help you. Some lawyers do not charge unless you win your appeal. There are groups, such as lawyer referral services, that can help you find a lawyer. There are also groups, such as legal aid services, who will give you free legal services if you qualify.

**3. How much does Medicare pay?**

The details on the front of this notice explain how much Medicare paid for these services. See your copy of *The Medicare Handbook* for more information about the benefits you are entitled to as a beneficiary in the Medicare Part B program. If you need another copy of the handbook, call or visit your local Social Security office.

Medicare may make adjustments to your payment. We may reduce the amount we pay for services by a certain percentage (Balanced Budget Law). If your provider accepted assignment, you are not liable to pay the amount of this reduction. We pay interest on some claims not paid within the required time.

All Medicare payments are made on the condition that you will pay Medicare back if benefits are also paid under insurance that is primary to Medicare. Examples of other insurance are employer group health plans, automobile medical, liability, no fault, or workers' compensation. Notify us immediately if you have filed or could file a claim with insurance that is primary to Medicare.

**4. How can I reduce my medical costs?**

Many providers have agreed to be part of **Medicare's participation program.** That means that they will always accept the amount that Medicare approves as their full payment. Write or call us for the name of a participating provider or for a free list of participating providers.

A provider who accepts assignment can charge you only for the part of the annual deductible you have not met and the copayment which is the remaining 20 percent of the approved amount.

If you are treated by one of these doctors you can save money. See *The Medicare Handbook* for more information about how you can reduce your medical costs.

**5. How can I use this notice?**

You can use this notice to:
- Contact us immediately if you think Medicare paid for a service you did not receive

- Show your provider how much of your deductible you have met

- Claim benefits with another insurance company. If you send this notice to them, make a copy of it for your records.

---

**Keep this notice for your records.**
*Health Care Financing Administration*

Medicare will pay only for drugs used in the hospital. The hospital may give you a limited supply of drugs to take with you if this will facilitate your discharge and the drug is needed until you can obtain a continuing supply.

Medicare will pay for all supplies and equipment used in the hospital. It will pay for supplies taken out of the hospital for outpatient use only if use must continue after you leave (example: a heart pacemaker) or they are required to assist your departure (example: crutches).

The chart on pages 98–99 should make it obvious that there is a good reason to have some Medicare Supplemental Insurance. The trick is to get what you need while paying no more than you have to. We discuss how to find good insurance in chapter 4.

There is a separate blood deductible for Parts A and B. You are responsible for paying for the first three units of whole blood or **packed red cells** received in a hospital or skilled nursing facility. You must either pay for the blood or have it replaced. You are considered to have it replaced if an acceptable donor offers to replace it in your behalf, whether or not the provider or its blood supplier accepts the offer. If you have paid for or replaced blood under Medicare hospital insurance (Part A), you do not need to pay for or replace that blood again under Medicare medical insurance (Part B).

*How Payment Is Made*

Payment for hospitals under Medicare was always complicated. It has recently gotten more so, because of changes to the Medicare law passed by Congress that established the **prospective payment system** for hospitals. Prospective payments to hospitals are made through the **diagnosis-related groups (DRG) system.**

*Why Prospective Payment?* Consider an example. Suppose you go to an auto dealer and ask whether or not you need a car. If the answer is yes, you want the dealer to decide what kind of car a person like you should have, get it for you, and bill you, without regard to price. The chances are you will get a Mercedes, with all the options. Consider another. You go to the car dealer and say, "I want a compact car with all-weather radial tires, a stereo cassette deck, and air conditioning. I want it in black. It has to have at least a 50,000-mile guarantee on all

## THE MEDICARE PROGRAM....
## WHAT IT PAYS....WHAT YOU PAY

Program services, as well as deductibles and copayments, are subject to change on a yearly basis. For the most current information, consult the latest edition of *Your Medicare Handbook,* available at most Social Security Administration offices.

| Medicare Services | Benefit Period | Medicare Pays | You Pay |
|---|---|---|---|
| **Part A: Hospital Insurance** | | | |
| **Hospital Services\*** Semiprivate room rate Miscellaneous hospital services & supplies Dietary & meal services Special care units Diagnostic procedures, X rays, etc. Laboratory services Operating & recovery rooms Anesthesia & supplies Rehabilitation services | First 60 days | All but deductible | Deductible of $760 |
| | 61 to 90 days | All but $190/day | $190/day |
| | 91 to 150 days | All but $380/day | $380/day |
| | Beyond 150 days | Nothing | All costs |
| **Skilled Nursing Facility Care** In approved facility after a 3-day hospital stay and admitted to the facility within 30 days of discharge | First 20 days | All costs | Nothing |
| | 21 to 100 days | All but $95/day | $95/day |
| | Beyond 100 days | Nothing | All costs |
| **Home Health Care** | Unlimited as medically necessary | All costs | Nothing |
| **Hospice Care** | Two 90-day periods One 30-day period | All costs but outpatient drugs and respite care | Limited drug costs and respite care |
| **Blood Service** | As needed | All but first 3 pints | First 3 pints |

\*  Includes inpatient psychiatric care of 190 lifetime days.

| Medicare Services | Benefit Period | Medicare Pays | You Pay |
|---|---|---|---|
| **Part B: Medical Insurance** | | | |
| Physician & surgeon fees<br>Therapists (physical/speech/ occupational)<br>Diagnostic tests<br>Medical supplies<br>Ambulatory services<br>Ambulance service | As medically necessary | 80% of approved amount after $100 deductible | $100 deductible and 20% of the Medicare-approved charge (plus any cost above approved charge) |
| **Outpatient Hospital Services** | As medically necessary | 80% of approved amount after $100 deductible | 20% of approved charge after deductible |
| **Home Health Care** | As medically necessary | All costs | Nothing |
| **Immunosuppressive Drugs** | As medically necessary | One year of drugs used in immunosuppressive therapy after transplant | 20% of the cost |
| **Blood Service** | As needed | 80% of the cost after first 3 pints | First 3 pints and 20% of cost |

major parts and the body. I know cars like this can be bought for no more than $7,500. Get me the car, and I will pay you that, but no more." Chances are that you will get what you want, for no more than $7,500. The dealer will try to get a higher price, and you will have to negotiate, but you will get the car you specified.

Any insurer — including Medicare — that makes **retrospective payments** to a health care provider is in the first situation. (Retrospective payments are made after a service has been rendered. It is the main way the medical system in the United States works now, although this is changing.) In this **fee-for-service system**, in which providers render whatever services they think necessary and then bill for them, there is a danger of getting much more than is needed and paying more than is really necessary. You are also in danger of being told that you need a car when you really don't. In the second situation, you are protected: you have made the decision that you want the car, and you will not buy it at more than the agreed-upon price. This is the benefit of prospective payment, especially with appropriate controls such as second opinions on surgery and the requirement of preapproval for some operations and hospital stays. Providers argue constantly about the evils of prospective payment, but there is considerable research evidence that shows that the quality of care need not suffer and that providers can make a good profit under it.

Congress required that Medicare pay for hospital services under Medicare via a prospective payment scheme because it was convinced that this step would help avoid unnecessary hospitalization and control costs. Prospective payment protects you.

*The Diagnosis-Related Groups (DRG) System*

The DRG system is Medicare's current method of prospective payment. It was developed originally by the Yale School of Organization and Management and became law for hospitals in the state of New Jersey before Congress made it nationwide for Medicare. Using sophisticated statistical techniques, Medicare cases were analyzed to see how payments should be set to cover as many cases as possible. This research showed that the main or **primary diagnosis** of the patient, **secondary diagnoses**, age, and operations performed predicted costs for the majority of patients quite well. The billions of possible combinations of these factors were reduced to 477 **diagnosis-related groups** (**DRGs**), which are best understood as the overall condition of a patient. Congress understood that these 477 groups would not cover every case, and they made provisions for **outliers** — people who needed more days in the hospital, or more expensive hospital stays, because they had illnesses, or needed operations, that fell outside the DRGs. Hospitals can be granted payment for cases that require more hospital days than predicted by the DRG, provided the continued stay is medically necessary. Cases that do not exceed the length of stay criteria, but are more costly than predicted by a certain amount, are paid more if the hospital applies for additional payment.

*DRG, Hospitals, and You:* The DRG system was phased in over several years, and as of October 1, 1987, virtually every general, acute-care hospital in the country was paid with DRGs. The way it works is as follows: You are admitted to the hospital as a Medicare patient. Your DRG cannot be assigned when you come in, because your diagnosis may be unknown or wrong. Also, the operation(s) that you will have cannot be predicted in advance, especially if you are admitted for a **diagnostic workup.** Once everything has been done, and you are ready to be discharged (dead or alive), the hospital prepares a **face sheet** for your hospital chart which indicates your DRG. The DRG will probably have been assigned by a computer program that was purchased by the hospital and designed to pick the highest-paid DRG possible, based on your combination of age, diagnoses, operations, and other factors. The Medicare **intermediary** pays the hospital the DRG rate, after a computer review of the hospital's DRG coding.

Note that the hospital couldn't assign the DRG when you came in, and therefore could not predict the cost of your care or how much it would be paid. The result is that on some admissions the hospital will lose money and on some admissions it will make money. On the average, hospitals that are generally as "good" — measured by their use of resources on patients, not by the results they produce — as the average hospital will break even. Those that are better, in this sense, will make money, and they are allowed to keep their profits. Those that are worse will lose money, and they will have to swallow their losses.

The important point is this: *there is no guarantee from Medicare that the hospital will not lose money, or make money, on your case. Its loss or gain, under the DRG system, is supposed to have nothing to do with your care.*

Let's look at some examples:

*You are over 75 years old, have a minor heart attack, and fall down a flight of stairs as a result and break a hip. The surgeon decides that a total hip replacement is needed. You have the op-*

*eration. Much to everyone's surprise, there are no complications, and you quickly learn to walk with the artificial hip and are able to go home well before the DRG-assigned number of hospital days. The hospital makes money on your case and gets to keep it.*

*Now imagine the same circumstances, but (as might be expected given this situation) your care is long and difficult, and complications arise. You develop* **thrombophlebitis** *in your legs and have to have more surgery and additional drugs. You have a bleeding episode as a result of the drugs and need a transfusion. You are very weak and take a long time to get to the point at which you can be discharged to a* **skilled nursing facility** *to learn to walk again. Even with outlier payments, the hospital loses a great deal of money on your case.*

In both of these situations, the hospital is supposed to give you care that is medically necessary, regardless of the amount it has to spend.

Results to date suggest that *hospital profits are at their highest level in history,* based largely on profits from Medicare patients. Some types of hospitals, such as rural hospitals, inner-city hospitals with large charity care burdens, and hospitals that are the sole hospital for large areas, seem to be losing money. Congress has required Medicare to watch hospital profits carefully and to report to it, through the Prospective Payment Assessment Commission, on any adjustments that should be made. For the most part, though, DRGs have been a financial boon to hospitals.

Another point that needs to be understood is this: Since DRG payments are based on national/regional averages, it is *planned* that some hospitals will make money and some will lose money. It's part of the concept. One of the objectives of the DRG system, in fact, was the closure of the nation's least efficient hospitals. It was hoped that they would lose so much money that they would have to close. Patients would then go to the more efficient hospitals, and overall costs would be reduced. This is another reason that losses (or profits) made by the hospital under the DRG system should have nothing to do with your care. *These losses (or profits) are a result of the overall efficiency of the hospital, not your particular medical needs. No one case is going to break (or make) a hospital.*

During the early days of the DRG system, there were a number of instances of abuse. Patients were told that they had to leave the hospital "because your DRG has run out" or something similar. Discharging any patient who still needs hospital care because of financial considerations is a total violation of the hospital's contract with Medicare. The hospital has agreed to provide services to you as long as they are medically necessary.

Because of the abuses that were observed, the **People's Medical Society (PMS)** and the **American Association of Retired Persons (AARP)** joined forces to ask Medicare to require hospitals to "mirandize" Medicare patients: just as persons being arrested are told of their constitutional rights. Medicare now requires *all* hospitals to provide Medicare beneficiaries with an *Important Message from Medicare* upon admission for *any* inpatient hospital care. It appears on pages 104–106.

To sum up: the only reasons that you can be discharged from a hospital under Medicare are *medical* ones.

## Medical Necessity Determinations

Medicare does not pay for services that are not medically "reasonable and necessary."

Who makes this determination? The first one, obviously, is your doctor. If your doctor suggests that you are ready to go home, you are likely to comply. If you feel you need more time, discuss it with him or her. The real issue comes when you want to stay in the hospital and the hospital's **utilization review committee (URC)** wants you to leave, or the Peer Review Organization wants you to leave. In either case, you will receive a written notice that a decision has been made, and that you have the right to appeal it. How to appeal it is covered in chapter 8.

If you win the appeal, you stay. If you lose, you may be required to pay for up to one day of hospital stay after the original cutoff date. It's important to understand that there are two tracks here, as described in the information on requesting a review given a few pages back. If you are asking the Peer Review Organization to review the hospital's decision, you are not responsible for services received before you get the notice of the Peer Review Organization's decision. If you are asking the Peer Review Organization to rethink its own decision, the hospital may start billing you beginning with the third calendar day after you received the Notice of Noncoverage. If the Peer Review Organization does not reverse its position and you decide not to stay in the hospital, you may have to pay for the third day. If you decide to stay, you are responsible for the further cost of your care.

## AN IMPORTANT MESSAGE FROM MEDICARE

### YOUR RIGHTS WHILE YOU ARE A MEDICARE HOSPITAL PATIENT

- You have the right to receive all the hospital care that is necessary for the proper diagnosis and treatment of your illness or injury. According to Federal law, **your discharge date must be determined solely by your medical needs,** not by "DRGs" or Medicare payments.

- You have the right to be fully informed about decisions affecting your Medicare coverage and payment for your hospital stay and for any post-hospital services.

- You have the right to request a review by a Peer Review Organization of any written Notice of Noncoverage that you receive from the hospital stating that Medicare will no longer pay for your hospital care. Peer Review Organizations (PROs) are groups of doctors who are paid by the Federal Government to review medical necessity, appropriateness and quality of hospital treatment furnished to Medicare patients. The phone number and address of the PRO for your area are:

_____

_____

_____

### TALK TO YOUR DOCTOR ABOUT YOUR STAY IN THE HOSPITAL

You and your doctor know more about your condition and your health needs than anyone else. Decisions about your medical treatment should be made between you and your doctor. **If you have any questions about your medical treatment, your need for continued hospital care, your discharge, or your need for possible post-hospital care, don't hesitate to ask your doctor.** The hospital's patient representative or social worker will also help you with your questions and concerns about hospital services.

### IF YOU THINK YOU ARE BEING ASKED TO LEAVE THE HOSPITAL TOO SOON

- Ask a hospital representative for a written notice of explanation immediately, if you have not already received one. This notice is called a "Notice of Noncoverage." You must have this Notice of Noncoverage if you wish to exercise your right to request a review by the PRO.

- The Notice of Noncoverage will state either that your doctor or the PRO agrees with the hospital's decision that Medicare will no longer pay for your hospital care.

  + If the hospital and your doctor agree, the PRO does not review your case before a Notice of Noncoverage is issued. But the PRO will respond to your request for a review of your Notice of Noncoverage and seek your opinion. You cannot be made to pay for your hospital care until the PRO makes its decision, if you request the review by noon of the first work day after you receive the Notice of Noncoverage.

+ If the hospital and your doctor disagree, the hospital may request the PRO to review your case. If it does make such a request, the hospital is required to send you a notice to that effect. In this situation the PRO must agree with the hospital or the hospital cannot issue a Notice of Noncoverage. You may request that the PRO reconsider your case after you receive a Notice of Noncoverage but since the PRO has already reviewed your case once, you may have to pay for **at least one day of hospital care** before the PRO completes this reconsideration.

IF YOU **DO NOT** REQUEST A REVIEW, **THE HOSPITAL MAY BILL YOU** FOR ALL THE COSTS OF YOUR STAY BEGINNING WITH THE THIRD DAY AFTER YOU RECEIVE THE NOTICE OF NONCOVERAGE. THE HOSPITAL, HOWEVER, CANNOT CHARGE YOU FOR CARE UNLESS IT PROVIDES YOU WITH A NOTICE OF NONCOVERAGE.

## HOW TO REQUEST A REVIEW OF THE NOTICE OF NONCOVERAGE

- If the Notice of Noncoverage states that your **physician agrees** with the hospital's decision:
  + You must make your request for review to the PRO by **noon of the first work day** after you receive the Notice of Noncoverage by contacting the PRO by phone or in writing.
  + The PRO must ask for your views about your case before making its decision. The PRO will inform you by phone and in writing of its decision on the review.
  + If the PRO agrees with the Notice of Noncoverage, you may be billed for all costs of your stay beginning at noon of the day **after** you receive the PRO's decision.
  + Thus, you will **not** be responsible for the cost of hospital care before you receive the PRO's decision.

- If the Notice of Noncoverage states that the PRO agrees with the hospital's decision:
  + You should make your request for reconsideration to the PRO **immediately** upon receipt of the Notice of Noncoverage by contacting the PRO by phone or in writing.
  + The PRO can take up to three working days from receipt of your request to complete the review. The PRO will inform you in writing of its decision on the review.
  + Since the PRO has already reviewed your case once, prior to the issuance of the Notice of Noncoverage, the hospital is permitted to begin billing you for the cost of your stay beginning with the third calendar day after you receive your Notice of Noncoverage **even if the PRO has not completed its review.**
  + Thus, if the PRO continues to agree with the Notice of Noncoverage, **you may have to pay for at least one day of hospital care.**

NOTE: The process described above is called "immediate review." If you miss the deadline for this immediate review while you are in the hospital, you may still request a review of Medicare's decision to no longer pay for your care at any point during your hospital stay or after you have left the hospital. The Notice of Noncoverage will tell you how to request this review.

## POST-HOSPITAL CARE

When your doctor determines that you no longer need all the specialized services provided in a hospital, but you still require medical care, he or she may discharge you to a skilled nursing facility or home care. The discharge planner at the hospital will help arrange for the services you may need after your discharge. Medicare and supplemental insurance policies have limited coverage for skilled nursing facility care and home health care. Therefore, you should find out which services will or will not be covered and how payment will be made. Consult with your doctor, hospital discharge planner, patient representative and your family in making preparations for care after you leave the hospital. **Don't hesitate to ask questions.**

ACKNOWLEDGEMENT OF RECEIPT — My signature only acknowledges my receipt of this Message from (name of hospital) on (date) and does not waive any of my rights to request a review or make me liable for any payment.

_____

Signature of beneficiary or
person acting on behalf of beneficiary.

## Skilled Nursing Facilities

*Covered Services*

Care in a **skilled nursing facility** (SNF) is care that is less intense than that you receive in a hospital, but more intense than the custodial care provided in an intermediate care facility or custodial care nursing home. Basically, all of the services listed under hospitals are covered under skilled nursing facilities. The exceptions are services that skilled nursing facilities do not normally provide, such as operating rooms. Medicare permits hospitals with fewer than 100 beds that have empty beds to run a skilled nursing facility within their walls, using beds that have been designated as **swing beds**. Swing beds are used as skilled nursing facility beds when there is a need for skilled nursing facility services, and as hospital beds when there is a need for hospital services. In effect, the hospital uses part of its capacity as a skilled-nursing-facility-type nursing home.

Many people think that Medicare pays for long-term nursing home care. There are sometimes tragic results from confusion about this. *Medicare does not pay for "custodial" or "personal care" services in nursing homes, only for rehabilitative care. This care is limited to 100 days per benefit period.*

*Limitations on Services and Cost-Sharing*

You are entitled to 100 days of skilled nursing facility care during each benefit period. Medicare pays all costs for the first 20 days, and beginning on the 21st day you are responsible for the copayment of $95 per day. You would pay this until the 100th day, after which you are responsible for all costs. An example:

> *After a long and complicated hospital stay, Victoria Smith-Jones is sent to a skilled nursing facility. She does not improve as rapidly as everyone hoped, and has to spend 135 days there. The daily charge is $110. For the first 20 days Medicare covers all costs and she pays nothing. Beginning on the 21st day and for the next 80 days, her copayment is $95 per day for a total of $7,600. Medicare picks up the extra $15 per day during this 80-day period. For the next 35 days Victoria Smith-Jones is responsible for all costs. Her total charge for the stay in the nursing home is $14,850. Medicare contributed $3,400 toward the total cost.*

*How Payment Is Made*

The skilled nursing facility (or the hospital that provides skilled nursing facility care in a swing bed) is paid a daily amount by the intermediary, less your coinsurance.

*Medical Necessity Determinations*

Medical necessity is *the* key issue in payment for skilled nursing facility services. (The skilled nursing facility regulations go to great lengths to define what is and is not skilled nursing facility care. The key is that care complex enough to require the services of a nurse or skilled rehabilitation personnel is covered; care that you could handle by yourself is not. But complications may require skilled-nursing-facility-level care, even for situations that would normally not be covered. Basically, skilled nursing facility care is rehabilitation; if your condition cannot be expected to improve as a result of skilled nursing facility care *and* you do not need observation by skilled personnel, your care will not be covered. Obviously, what your doctor writes in the chart makes a big difference in what gets covered. If you are worried about coverage of skilled nursing facility services, discuss this with your doctor.

If you receive a written notice from the skilled nursing facility's or the hospital's utilization review committee, or from the peer review organization, that your condition no longer requires skilled nursing facility services, you can appeal. If you win the appeal, your care is paid for as long as it is medically necessary. If you lose, you pay for all care after the cutoff date. Chapter 8 explains how to appeal decisions regarding coverage related to medical necessity.

## Home Health Services

*Covered Services*

Medicare covers medical services that are needed to allow you to live at home. The scope of benefits includes part-time or intermittent nursing care; physical, occupational, or speech therapy; medical social services; part-time or intermittent services of a home health aide; medical supplies; **durable medical equipment**; and the services of interns and residents if the **home health agency (HHA)** is affiliated with a teaching hospital. If the patient needs occupational therapy alone, that is not covered, but if occupational therapy is started as part of a program of rehabilitation that includes physical or speech therapy, continuing services are paid for even after the physical or speech therapy is over.

As with skilled nursing facilities, personal care services are not covered. Housekeeping and transportation are not included. To receive home health services, you must be confined to your home or to an institution that is not a nursing home. Being able to take trips to see the doctor or to go to the hospital does not mean that you are not homebound.

Home health care (HHC) is covered under both Part A (hospital insurance) and Part B (doctor insurance) of Medicare. For coverage, all the following conditions must exist:

- You are confined to your home.
- You need part-time skilled nursing or physical or speech therapy.
- A doctor prescribes home health care.
- The **Home Health Agency** is approved by Medicare.

*Limitations on Services*

Home health care limited to 21 consecutive visits.

*Cost-Sharing*

There is no cost-sharing under home health care except for the $100 Part B deductible for services furnished under Part B, and 20 percent of the reasonable charge for durable medical equipment supplied by home health care. The home health agency will charge patients for any services provided by it that are not covered under Medicare. You should ask the doctor and the HHA if any services not covered under Medicare are provided, and ask what the charges will be. Based on what you hear, you may want to discuss your plan of care with your doctor.

*How Payment Is Made*

Home health agencies bill the Medicare intermediary directly and bill you for any noncovered services.

*Medical Necessity Determinations*

Your need for continuing home health care must be reviewed periodically by a physician. You will be notified in writing if a finding is made that home health care is no longer medically necessary, and you have appeal rights, which are discussed in chapter 8.

## Doctors' Services Under Part B of Medicare

*Covered Services*

Medicare was designed around the Blue Cross/Blue Shield model, which has one part paying for hospital services and another paying for everything else. "Everything else" is the job of Part B of Medicare, formally called supplemental medical insurance, or SMI. The scope of benefits as described in the regulations is as follows:

*Medical and other health services such as physicians' services, outpatient hospital services, diagnostic tests, outpatient physical therapy and speech pathology services, rural health clinic services and outpatient renal dialysis services . . . services furnished by ambulatory surgical centers (ASCs), Home Health Agencies, (HHAs), and comprehensive outpatient rehabilitation facilities (CORFs) . . . other medical supplies, equipment, and supplies that are not covered under Medicare Part A hospital insurance.*

Again, it's easier to talk about what is not covered than what is.

## Limitations on Services

The following is a laundry list of limited services:

- Chiropractors' services are limited to manual manipulation of subluxation of the spine demonstrated by X ray. Only twelve treatments by the chiropractor are covered, unless more are determined to be medically necessary.
- Mammograms are covered under the following conditions:
  - A patient has distinct signs and symptoms for which a mammogram is indicated;
  - A patient has a history of breast cancer; or
  - A patient is asymptomatic but, on the basis of the patient's history and other factors (the physician considers significant), the physician's judgment is that a mammogram is appropriate.
- Pap smears for early detection of cervical cancer are covered when ordered by a physician under one of the following conditions:
  - She has not had a test during the preceding three years; or
  - She is at high risk of developing cervical cancer and her physician recommends that she have the test performed more frequently than every three years.
- Optometrists' services are limited to testing and examination needed to fit artificial lenses to treat aphakia (absence of the lens of the eye, whether natural or caused by the removal of a cataract).
- Dentists' services and dental surgeons' services are covered only if they would have been covered if performed by a doctor.
- Podiatrists' services are covered only if they would have been covered if performed by a doctor.
- 50 percent copayment on outpatient psychiatric services.

## Cost-Sharing

Part B is modeled on basic Blue Cross/Blue Shield plans as they existed in the mid-1960s. You are responsible for a $100 annual deductible and 20 percent of the "reasonable cost" of all services. Your 20 percent copayment is based upon the Medicare-approved amount and may not reflect the actual charge for services provided by nonparticipating physicians. There is no cap on your out-of-pocket expenses under Medicare Part B.

*How Payment Is Made*

Now the fun begins. At one time, Medicare employed the **usual, customary, and reasonable (UCR)** process for determining doctors' payments. One of the things that doctors insisted on in the formulation of the original Blue Shield plans was that they get paid, in essence, what they wanted. This approach worked well, at least for the doctors, until the expenditures for Medicare Part B began rising at alarming rates.

In an effort to stem the rising tide of physician expenditures, Congress enacted a new payment system known as the **Resources-Based Relative Value Scale (RBRVS)**. Originally passed in the Omnibus Budget Reconciliation Act of 1989, the RBRVS system was phased in over a four-year period. This system is designed to recognize the differences in physician specialties and to reimburse physicians according to the skill and time involved in the care that they deliver. The RBRVS reimbursement system is based on the following factors:

- a nationally uniform relative value unit (RVU) for each service (primary care, surgical, nonsurgical, etc.)
- a geographical adjustment factor (recognizes different markets: urban or rural)
- a nationally uniform conversion factor for calculating payments (a certain dollar amount multiplied by the RVU)

The RVUs for each service reflect the resources involved in providing the three components of the doctor's service:

- work (skill and effort required)
- practice expenses (rent, staff salaries, supplies, etc.)
- the cost of malpractice insurance (annual premium)

For example, if a primary care physician visit for an established patient has a relative value of 1.5 units, and the conversion factor is $37, the Medicare-approved amount is $37 × 1.5 or $55.50. Medicare pays 80 percent of this amount, or $44.40, and you are responsible for your 20 percent copayment of $11.10.

Recent changes in Medicare regulations protect Medicare beneficiaries from physician charges in excess of the Medicare billing limits. This relatively new regulation applies to all physicians who do not accept Medicare assignment. Nonparticipating physicians, those who do not accept assignment, engage in a practice known as balance billing, or collecting the difference between the Medicare-approved amount and their actual charge. This means that you are responsible not only for your 20 percent copayment, but also for any balance above this amount. Balance billing costs Medicare beneficiaries billions of dollars in out-of-pocket expenses.

For example, if the approved charge for a specific procedure is $180, the most a nonparticipating physician may charge you is $196.65. Nonparticipating physicians are paid 95 percent of the Medicare-approved amount and may charge 115 percent above this amount. This means that a nonparticipating physician whose regular charge for this procedure is $275 would be allowed to collect only $196.65 ($180 × 95 percent × 115 percent). Your total out-of-pocket expense would be $52.65, which includes your copayment of $36 (20 percent of $180), plus the $16.65 in excess charge above the Medicare-approved amount ($180 + $16.65).

## Filing a Claim

Filing a Medicare Part B claim is much easier thanks to a welcome change in Medicare legislation. It is now the responsibility of your doctor or medical supplier (equipment or medical supplies) to prepare and submit your Medicare claims for you. This means that:

- Your doctor or medical supply company must file the claim even if neither of them accepts Medicare assignment.
- You cannot be charged extra for this service.
- You are responsible for paying the bill in full, if the provider does not accept assignment. You will be reimbursed by Medicare.
- You should contact the Medicare carrier for your state if any provider refuses to prepare and submit your claim.
- You will still need to submit a claim with your Medicare supplemental insurer in order to collect the 20 percent copayment that is your responsibility.

We strongly recommend that you contact the Medicare carrier for your state should you encounter a problem with this new system. See appendix A.

## Medical Necessity Determinations

Physician services under Medicare are reviewed just like other services. Actual and proposed operations are reviewed most stringently. If payment is denied to the physician on the grounds that the operation was unnecessary, you are protected from having to pay for it, because you could not have been expected to know this at the time.

## Summing Up

As you have seen, Medicare covers quite a bit. The problem is with the limitations on the amount of services you can receive, the requirements for receiving them, and the copayments and deductibles. For Part B, for example, Medicare beneficiaries pay about 43 percent of the actual bill, not the 20 percent that Congress intended. It should be clear to you that insurance to supplement Medicare would be nice to have; we'll discuss that in chapter 5.

The big exclusions, those you should be most concerned about, are as follows:

- All chiropractic services, except for treatment of **subluxation of the spine**
- Purely custodial care nursing homes
- Most dental care and dentures
- **Over-the-counter drugs**
- Most eyeglasses and eye exams
- Hearing aids and fittings
- Full-time nursing care in the home
- Routine physical exams

Also, services paid for by Worker's Compensation, automobile or other liability insurance, employer health plans (for retirees or current employees, whichever you happen to be), and other government programs are not covered to the extent that these programs pay for the services you receive. Depending on the circumstances and the service, Medicare may pay the difference between what these programs paid and what you owe, but Medicare pays nothing unless you are obligated to make a payment.

In this chapter you will learn: The role of Medicare supplemental insurance ■ How to provide for nursing home coverage that Medicare doesn't ■ How to compare supplemental policies and what to look for ■ Shopping tips to help you select the right policy ■ How and why to check the product of insurance companies ■ How health maintenance organizations may be a viable alternative

# 4. How to Pay for What Medicare Doesn't Cover

Medicare, as we've noted in other chapters, is an exercise in ambivalence. Congress wanted protection for senior citizens but did not want anything resembling national health insurance. It wanted to keep costs down and to give the **American Medical Association (AMA)** and the hospitals everything they wanted. It wanted cost-sharing by beneficiaries and wanted to sharply reduce the 15 percent of their income that the elderly were spending on health care.

If this last desire is taken as the standard, Medicare is a failure. Senior citizens once again spend 15 percent of their income on health care, and that proportion will rise sharply over the next few years, if cost trends for the under-65 population are any indication. On the other hand, Medicare has increased access to health care for the elderly and eliminated many of the abuses found in the old systems of charity care. (It all but eliminated charity care in the process, leaving us with other problems, but that's another story. . . .)

The dream of having guaranteed health care for Americans over 65, supplemented by modest amounts out of their own pockets, has not been realized. What this means, in practical terms, is that you have to buy insurance to supplement Medicare if you want the degree of protection that the original program was supposed to give you. This chapter is about how to buy the best insurance for the least money.

It's not easy. Elderly Americans will spend nearly $25 billion on Medicare supplemental insurance this year — an average of $900 each. If you've ever purchased supplemental insurance, you're well aware of the hodgepodge of policies that are on the market. Without policy standards, Medicare beneficiaries have been at the mercy of insurance companies that use unscrupulous sales tactics. This has led to beneficiaries purchasing policies with very little coverage, or committing the larger mistake of having too many policies. New supplemental policy standards were developed by the National Association of Insurance Commissioners. These standards will help you compare policies and also protect you from purchasing duplicate coverage.

## Some Insurance Concepts

Insurance is, from your angle, a gamble. Some religious groups object to it on that basis. The insurance company is betting that you will stay relatively healthy. If you do, the premiums you pay while you are insured will at least equal your actual costs of medical care, plus the costs of running the company, plus a prudent reserve for unforeseen circumstances, plus a profit. If the company is a privately held, or stock, company, the profit will be distributed to the owners or shareholders or reinvested. If it is a mutual company, the profits will be returned to the members (invisibly, in the form of low premiums, or visibly, in the form of dividends or rebates.) This is a little bit of an oversimplification, but enough to give the flavor.

You, on the other hand, are betting that you will get sick and that the company will have to pay much more to doctors and hospitals than you put in. (If you weren't making this bet and didn't believe this would happen, you would be better off just to start a savings account for future medical bills. There would be no advantage to buying insurance.)

Insurance can also be looked at as **risk pooling**, a process whereby *all* the insured cover the expenses that only a *few* of them will have in any given year. (Example: Depending on the age group, 12–20 percent of a population will have a hospital stay in a given year. This leaves the hospital insurance premiums of the other 80–88 percent to cover the costs.) In practice, there's more to it than this. Insurance companies, particularly health insurers, do a great variety of things, such as contracting with hospitals for guaranteed rates, fixing fee schedules for doctors, reviewing use of hospitalization and surgery, and so on. But what we've told you is the essence.

Insurance companies engage in awesome statistical exercises to make sure that the claims that are paid will stay in line with the premiums that are paid in. One of the insights that emerges is that protection against *all* risks is too expensive for any insurance company to offer. So all policies have *exclusions,* most have *deductibles,* many have *benefit maximums,* and a great number have a sliding scale of premiums based on the amount of risk the insured is willing to assume. Since most claims under most types of insurance are small, an insured's willingness to assume a small risk (via, say, a deductible of $200 rather than $100) is worth far more to the insurer than high-end limitations. Assuming an additional risk of $100 at the low end is worth far more to the company than a reduction of the maximum amount paid from $1,000,000 to $999,900.

So total coverage for all hazards is too expensive to offer. What happens instead is bargaining between the insured and the insurance company. This takes the form of the insured person's picking and choosing among high-option plans, low-option plans, and everything in between, adjusting the amount of risk the insured person is willing to assume versus the premium he or she has to pay until satisfied.

So goes the theory, anyway. In fact, there are pitfalls to buying insurance. The greatest of them is not knowing what it is that you want to buy in the way of protection, which is what insurance is all about.

## The Dark Side: Catastrophic Illness and Nursing Home Care

So insurance sounds like a good thing, but all is not rosy. There has been a persistent tendency in the health insurance industry to insure people against the things most can perfectly well afford — such as the $100 Medicare Part B deductible, or a copayment of more than $2 per prescription under an employer's health benefit plan — and not to insure them against what they can't afford. Since the latter is the whole purpose of insurance, something is wrong.

"Catastrophic" can be variously defined, but any illness that leaves you with medical expenses you can't pay is usually a catastrophe for you, whether the amount involved is $100 or $100,000. An illness that forces you into a nursing home for a long period of time can be a catastrophe. (Remember, Medicare pays only for **Skilled Nursing Facility (SNF)** services, not custodial care, and only at the rate of 100 days per calendar year. You may need nursing home care for the rest of your life, but Medicare will pay for a maximum of 100 SNF days per year. On the bright side, only about 5 percent of older people are in nursing homes, but this proportion is expected to grow as the overall population ages and the number of the "oldest old" (those 85 and over) grows.

Tragic stories of those who were forced to sell their homes in order to qualify for **Medicaid** payments to keep a spouse in a nursing home are all too true. The 1988 legislation eliminated the possibility of total impoverishment of the spouse, but, for a (relatively) wealthy couple, most assets over $76,000 may still go to pay for nursing home care. The new provisions are these:

- In any month in which a married person is in a nursing home, no income of the at-home spouse is to be considered available to the spouse in the nursing home.

- Income is considered the property of the person to whom it is paid. Income paid to both spouses is attributed 50 percent to each.

- The home, household goods, and personal effects of both spouses are not counted in considering Medicaid eligibility.

- All assets other than these will be counted and divided in two. If the at-home spouse has less than $15,000, the spouse in the nursing home may transfer assets to him or her to make up to $15,000 available to the at-home spouse. (States may, at their option, raise this figure to any amount less than $76,000. The $15,000 amount will be indexed to inflation.)

- The assets that remain in the name of the spouse in the nursing home are considered available to pay for his or her nursing home care. All assets in excess of $76,000 are attributed to the spouse in the nursing home and are considered available to pay for nursing home care.

- States must allow nursing home residents to retain certain sums for medical expenses not covered by Medicare or Medicaid before contributing to the expense of their nursing home care. The states may place "reasonable limits" on the amounts spent.

■ States must allow the at-home spouse sufficient income from the other spouse to bring total household income of the at-home spouse to at least 150 percent of the federal poverty level for a two-person household. States will not be required to allow more than $1,918 per month, except by court order or change in regulation.

*Outpatient Care: The Real Catastrophe*

If you are a Medicare beneficiary in reasonable health, your biggest potential for catastrophic costs in the immediate future lies with the failure of Part B of Medicare — doctor insurance — to pick up more than about 52 percent of total expenses. Doctors are doing increasingly more work outside the hospital, pressure to keep people out of the hospital is mounting, and there is a (too) slowly growing realization among doctors that hospitals are dangerous places that should be reserved for the very sick. The result is that a growing percentage of your medical expenses is being forced into the area of Medicare — Part B — that affords you the least protection. Doctors who do not participate in Medicare are free to charge more than the Medicare-approved amount for services provided. As a result of this balance billing, Medicare beneficiaries can expect to pay out additional billions in excess charges.

Medication, which Medicare does not cover at all when you are outside a hospital or skilled nursing facility, is another problem area. Dramatic progress in the development of effective drugs has been made in the last decade. Many medical problems that could be treated only poorly a few years ago now yield to new drugs. The problem is that these new drugs usually carry high research and development costs. To make matters worse, many drug patents have recently expired, which lowers their profitability and makes drug companies jack up the price of new drugs even more.

An increasing amount of care is shifting to the outpatient arena. Neither Medicare nor private insurance has caught up with the trend. Tests and treatments formerly given only to inpatients — and covered 100 percent — are being done on an outpatient basis, subject to cost-sharing. While over 1,400 procedures are now covered at 80 percent if performed on an outpatient basis, still more adjustment is needed to make Medicare reflect current realities.

The average savings account in America contains $9,733. This would cover 88 days of skilled nursing facility care at $110 per day (remember that Medicare covers only 100 days per benefit period and does not cover custodial care). Most people do not have savings to cover more than a small fraction of medical expenses.

Doctors, of course, are not required to take **assignment** — to accept Medicare's approved charge as their total payment. It is perfectly possible for the balance of your bill from a doctor who does not take assignment to exceed the Medicare-approved amount up to the full-balance billing limit. Supplemental insurance for Medicare is a good idea.

*Assignment*

What does "taking assignment" mean? It's a very important concept. A doctor who agrees to take assignment agrees to accept the payment that the Medicare carrier has decided is appropriate for the service rendered. This does not mean that the doctor has agreed to accept it as payment in full. He or she is supposed to charge you 20 percent of the Medicare price; Medicare pays the other 80 percent. The doctor handles all the paperwork with Medicare and is the recipient of the check. You just have to deal with your 20 percent of the doctor's bill and your supplemental insurance company.

## Buying Insurance to Supplement Medicare

Unfortunately, all too many insurance companies are aware of the fear of being bankrupted by health care costs that older people have. Insurance policies are not famous for being written in clear English, and when one is dealing with insurance to supplement a program as complex as Medicare, the problem gets even worse.

Our approach in this chapter is to tell you about the new Medicare supplemental insurance standards that now apply to all supplemental policies. Insurance companies are permitted to market 10 standardized supplemental policies, one of which must be a core policy with basic benefits. In addition, the companies are permitted to market up to nine other plans. This means that for the first time you will be able to make comparisons among similar policies. There's also a requirement designed to prevent duplication of coverage.

Our *first* assumption is that you want to protect your resources and stay out of debt. We also assume that you want to spend as little of your income as possible on health care. This means that you want to minimize your potential out-of-pocket expense. Our *third* assumption is that, like most older people, you are a little bit frightened of the cost of health care and want to buy some peace of mind as well as some insurance.

*Traditional Insurance Policies*

These are available in four main types; however, only one may be sold as a certified Medicare supplemental policy:

- **Service benefit policies** generally pay all the costs of a "service," such as hospitalization, surgery, outpatient care, and the like. Because of the way these policies relate to Medicare, they usually pay all of the difference between the amounts charged and what Medicare pays, leaving you with no out-of-pocket costs for the use of Medicare benefits. Generally, however, they cover nothing that Medicare does not cover. Your Medicare coverage and your insurance coverage run out together. As we've noted, this is not a real concern since most Medicare beneficiaries do not exhaust their hospital or skilled nursing facility benefits. Your real costs are likely to be on the out-patient side. These policies cover the 20 percent copayment. If the insurer uses its own fee schedule, however, the policy may not cover the difference between 100 percent of the Medicare-approved rate and what the doctor actually charged.

- **Indemnity benefit policies** provide a fixed amount per day or per service. Usually the policy states the amounts as something like "$532 per day or actual charges, whichever is lower." A policy that has high maximum payments relative to actual costs may *look* like it "covers everything," but the language of the policy, not one or two experiences with it, should be looked into.

- **"Medigap" or Medicare supplemental** policies are designed to pick up those expenses Medicare does not cover, such as Parts A and B deductibles and copayments. These policies are coordinated with Medicare and do not duplicate Medicare coverage. All insurance companies that sell supplemental policies must comply with the new federal standards for supplemental insurance. Companies are required to offer a core component of basic coverage; in addition, they may offer up to nine other plans with expanded coverage. (See appendix D.)

- **Employer retiree health insurance,** or health insurance for Medicare beneficiaries who work after 65, usually pays for all or most of a defined set of services, so they look like service benefit plans with low out-of-pocket costs to those enrolled. Since Medicare has become the *secondary* payer for plans covering employees over 65, they have gotten somewhat less generous. One of the possibilities offered by these plans may be a health maintenance organization option. (Pick up a copy of "Guide to Health Insurance for People With Medicare," HCFA publication 02110, available at any Social Security office.) Be aware that there are problems associated with rejecting your employer's health plan if you are over 65 and continue working. In that case, the employer cannot offer you a plan that is the equivalent of a Medigap policy. It can only pay for the services that Medicare does not cover at all.

The Secretary of the U.S. Department of Health and Human Services certifies insurance policies as meeting the standards for Medicare supplemental insurance. Companies may not claim that their policies are certified unless they have complied with all of the underwriting requirements. The National Association of Insurance Commissioners was responsible for developing the minimum standards that must be met by all supplemental policies. We suggest that you check with your state's insurance department if you have any questions concerning the status of a policy. For the address and telephone number of your state's insurance department, see Appendix C.

You'll recall that our criteria for Medicare supplemental insurance were as follows:

- To protect your assets and keep you out of debt
- To reduce your out-of-pocket expenses as much as possible
- To give you peace of mind

We can use these criteria to screen the types of Medicare supplemental insurance available.

The first thing that's clear is that service benefit plans are unlikely to meet your needs. They have all of the defects of Medicare itself, minus the copayments and deductibles. They provide no protection on the outpatient side, which is where you need it more and more. This leaves indemnity plans, Medigap plans, and employer plans.

Of these three, we believe *you should keep any employer plan that you have.* It may require a small contribution, but these plans were modeled after employee plans in more generous days, and companies haven't gotten around to cutting them substantially yet. With rare exceptions, they are as good as high-option Medigap policies, and possibly better. Further, a number of court cases have severely limited the right of companies to reduce benefits once you have retired, and Congress has just modified the federal bankruptcy laws so that employers' obligations to retiree medical and life insurance plans can no longer be discharged in bankruptcy proceedings. The company *must* pay. (But, obviously, it cannot do so if it genuinely has no assets left.) With your employer plan, you should, of course, make sure that you are enrolled in Part A of Medicare when you turn 65. You should also purchase Part B, doctor insurance. Why? First, if you don't purchase it during your **individual enrollment period,** you will have to wait until the next **general enrollment period** and will pay an additional 10 percent premium for every year you wait. Second, enrolling keeps the cost to your employer down and helps to preserve the benefits of your plan. Third, because premiums for Part B cover only 50 percent of the cost, enrolling gives your employer's plan a de facto injection of federal money. (For these reasons, many companies require their retirees and over-65 employees to enroll in Part B.)

If you don't have employer-provided retiree health insurance or it is a wholly unsatisfactory plan, we recommend that you purchase indemnity insurance. This is the point where we have to tell you what *not* to do:

- *Do not* purchase limited-purpose insurance, such as cancer insurance, accident insurance, and so on. Benefits in these policies are limited to certain diagnoses, they are generally full of other limitations, and many are simply fraudulent, designed never to pay off.

- *Do not* buy a policy that excludes preexisting conditions, if at all possible. If you do, make sure that the exclusion is limited to six months at most. Federal law prevents any company from calling any policy that excludes preexisting conditions for more than six months a "Medicare supplement." The fact that this is against the law doesn't mean that it won't be done, of course. What you're sick with now is what you're most likely to be sick with in the future. Buying a policy that excludes it is like buying no insurance at all.

- Do *not* buy policies that duplicate ones that you already have. The new Medicare supplemental insurance standards should reduce the amount of duplication that currently exists. Under the new regulations an insurer **may not** sell a policy that substantially duplicates existing coverage.

- *Do not,* we hate to have to say, buy a policy just because it is endorsed by a famous figure. The endorser's chief reason for endorsing the policy is the money he or she gets for doing it. Policies that are advertised this way are not necessarily bad. Neither are they necessarily good.

- *Do not* buy policies advertised with television spots and magazine ads that claim you'll face bankruptcy if you don't buy them. This is not necessarily true of insurance in general and is certainly not true of any one policy.

- *Do not* buy policies by mail if at all possible. Buy a policy through the mail *only* if you are sure that it is the best. Before you buy, call or write the company and see if there is an office or agent near you. If so, deal with that office directly.

- *Do not* buy policies that have dollar limits on total annual payments or payments over your lifetime unless those limits are *reasonably* high. Consider an annual limit of $5,000, which at least one Medigap policy has. This is *less than one shot of tissue plasminogen activator (TPA)*. It is *less than one-fourth of a bypass operation*. It is *less than one-tenth of a heart transplant*. It is probably *less than the combined helicopter and emergency room charges for a trauma center*. The ideal Medigap policy has no annual limits and a lifetime limit of at least $500,000.

- *Do not* purchase nonrenewable policies, ones that have unduly restrictive renewal clauses.

- *Do not* replace existing coverage without careful consideration of the advantages and disadvantages of both policies.

- *Do not* buy a policy just because it claims to pay for reductions in Medicare payments due to any congressionally mandated balanced budget law. The Medicare law relieves beneficiaries of responsibility for paying for the reductions in payments to providers. You'll be paying for something Medicare already provides if you fall for this one.

Some do's:

- *Do* make sure that the company that sells the policy is licensed in your state.

- *Do* check the rating of the company in *Best's Insurance Reports — Life/Health*, which is available in most public libraries. This will give you an objective rating of the merits of the company and its policies.

- *Do* make sure that you know *exactly* what your premium will be and *exactly* what it covers. Many features that companies quite honestly say they offer are available only as riders or amendments to the basic policy, and cost extra. The fact that a company offers a feature does not necessarily mean that it is included in your premium. Get a complete schedule of benefits, and ask the salesperson to mark the benefits your premium covers.

- *Do* pay by check, made out to the company, not the salesperson. This gives you proof that you paid, in the form of a canceled check, and keeps the salesperson from pocketing your payment.

- *Do* take advantage of any "free look" provisions mandated by the laws of your state. These allow you to buy a policy and cancel it with no obligation within a certain period if you decide that it is not what you want.

- *Do* ask the salesperson or agent for information on the average out-of-pocket expenses for holders of the policy. This will tell you how much protection you really are buying.

- *Do* look very carefully at the coverage offered for doctors' fees over and above the Medicare approved price. A policy that covers only your 20 percent copayment is better than nothing but you are still responsible for the fee up to the balance billing limit.

- *Do* choose a policy that has a **stop-loss provision,** if you can get it. Even if there isn't one in the policy you are considering, the agent may be able to add it in the form of a **rider,** for which there will be an additional (usually small) fee. A policy that does not protect against the small expenditures, but protects against the large ones via a stop-loss provision, makes sense.

- *Do* look for a policy that covers prescription drug charges. Prescription drug coverage is relatively expensive. Studies on older people have shown that they spend either a relatively small amount on prescription drugs or a lot.

- *Do* call your state insurance department and make sure that the policy is approved by them before you buy. (Approval to sell a policy in a state does not mean that it is a good one, simply that it violates none of the laws and conditions on insurance in that state.) A list of state insurance departments is provided in appendix C.

■ *Do* ask about typical out-of-pocket expenses. Remember that you are trying to reduce the proportion of your income that you spend on health care.

■ *Do* make sure the policy you select is automatically adjusted to cover increases in Medicare's copayments and deductibles.

You can use the form on page 126 to check your policy against our recommendations.

*The Merits of Health Maintenance Organizations*

We discussed health maintenance organizations (HMOs) competitive medical plans (CMPs), and Medicare insured groups (MIGs) in chapter 2. The big advantage of an HMO, given our assumptions about what you want, is that all but a trivial portion of care is prepaid. There are no worries about having the cash to go into the hospital. There are no service-specific charges, so there is no need to negotiate with the doctor about taking **assignment**. There are far fewer, or no, forms to fill out. One payment covers everything.

Depending on the costs of medical care in your area and the particular HMO and options you pick, the individual HMO premium may range from a few dollars to around $100 per month.

An HMO premium may seem high. But remember, you are likely to spend 15 percent or more of your income on medical care. The HMO premium, in contrast to traditional Medigap coverage, picks up many out-of-pocket expenses that you would otherwise have to pay. More important is the peace of mind achieved by knowing that this is the *only* cost, except for nominal copayments. The proper comparison of two insurance plans is always this: *Compare premiums plus out-of-pocket costs for one plan to premiums plus out-of-pocket costs for the other.*

You should get exact figures from the HMOs that you consider enrolling in. They should be able to provide you with average out-of-pocket costs for their Medicare members. Keep in mind that HMO benefit packages differ to some degree. Medicare requires the low-option plan in Medicare approved HMOs to be at least equal to Medicare benefits, *without* the Medicare copayments and deductibles. Compare these to 15 percent of your annual income. Depending on your income, the HMO may save you anywhere from nothing (a

## MEDICARE SUPPLEMENTAL
## INSURANCE COMPARISON WORKSHEET

Use the information provided by the insurance companies to complete this worksheet.

| Company Name | Policy 1 | Policy 2 | Policy 3 | Policy 4 |
|---|---|---|---|---|
| | | | | |
| Policy/Plan Name | | | | |
| **Premium:** May be affected by age and sex | | | | |
| Monthly | $ | $ | $ | $ |
| Quarterly | $ | $ | $ | $ |
| Semi-Annually | $ | $ | $ | $ |
| Annually | $ | $ | $ | $ |
| Does the Supplemental Policy cover the Deductibles and Copayments listed below? | If so, place a checkmark in the appropriate column for each policy. | | | |
| **Medicare Part A:** Hospital | | | | |
| Initial deductible*                              $ | | | | |
| 61 to 90th Day Copayment*            $      /day | | | | |
| 91 to 150th Day Copayment*          $      /day | | | | |
| 100% of Medicare approved expenses for additional 365 days | | | | |
| *Skilled Nursing Care* 21st to 100th Day Copayment*        $      /day | | | | |
| **Medicare Part B:** Physician | | | | |
| Initial deductible                              $100 | | | | |
| 20% Copayment | | | | |
| Does the Supplemental Policy provide any additional benefits? | If so, place a checkmark in the appropriate column for each policy. | | | |
| Prescription drugs | | | | |
| Private duty nursing | | | | |
| Additional physicians' fees | | | | |
| Skilled Nursing Care | | | | |
| Number of days available | _____ | _____ | _____ | _____ |
| Preventive services | | | | |
| Emergency services (travel) | | | | |

*Fill in amounts from current benefit year.

break-even situation, but with added peace of mind) to a lot. Use the forms on pages 128–130 to compare several HMOs.

Because the one big issue with HMOs is freedom of choice of doctors and hospitals, a number of alternatives that look like HMOs in some respects have emerged in recent years. **Preferred provider organizations (PPOs)** have closed panels of doctors like HMOs, but not quite: for an extra fee, you can go to the doctor or hospital of your choice; the PPO just covers less of the cost to you if you stray from the preferred providers. The extra cost can be trivial, or it can be so high that the PPO is, in effect, an HMO for all but the affluent. Generally, their benefits are not as generous as those of HMOs, but they are a little better than traditional fee-for-service plans (example: Blue Cross and Blue Shield). PPOs are just one variety of **competitive medical plans (CMPs)** with which HCFA has been experimenting. Basically, CMPs are prepaid plans that do not have to meet the very stringent (and costly) federal requirements for Medicare HMOs. They receive a set amount, based on the average cost of treating a Medicare beneficiary in the counties they serve, adjusted for local wage and price differences. For this they are supposed to offer medical care. Depending on the cost of care in the area and the options available within the CMP, they can be as generous as an HMO but should not offer less than the standard Medicare benefits. There may be a lot of advantage, or no advantage, for you in belonging to a CMP.

A major *disadvantage* of HMOs, for those who travel a good deal, is their reluctance to cover health care other than severe emergencies outside of their service area. If your HMO is in North Dakota and you are vacationing in Florida, you can expect that it will cover an emergency room visit for something serious, but not a trip to a local doctor for a cold. Many HMOs provide a toll-free number to call for preapproval of treatment. If you are committed to your HMO and want to travel, you should take note of the many storefront medical treatment offices that are opening around the country. (One wag called them "doc-in-the-boxes.") You can use them for treatment of illnesses that are not serious as you travel.

Joining an HMO is *not* forever. You have the right to drop out, and you will be covered by Medicare just as before. You can give one a try with no fear.

You may decide that the HMOs or other alternative care plans in your area are too expensive. There may be no HMO accepting Medicare patients (or no HMO) in your area. You may decide that, no matter how great the savings and the peace-of-mind factor, HMOs are

# MEDICARE HMO WORKSHEET

Use the information provided by the HMO to complete this worksheet.

| Company Name | Policy 1 | Policy 2 | Policy 3 | Policy 4 |
|---|---|---|---|---|
| | | | | |
| Policy/Plan Name | | | | |
| **Premium:** May be affected by age and sex | | | | |
| Monthly | $ | $ | $ | $ |
| Quarterly | $ | $ | $ | $ |
| Semi-Annually | $ | $ | $ | $ |
| Annually | $ | $ | $ | $ |
| Does the HMO cover the deductibles and copayments listed below? | If so, place a checkmark in the appropriate column for each policy. | | | |
| **Medicare Part A:** Hospital | | | | |
| Initial deductible*   $ | | | | |
| 61 to 90th Day Copayment*   $   /day | | | | |
| 91 to 150th Day Copayment*   $   /day | | | | |
| 100% of Medicare approved expenses for additional 365 days | | | | |
| *Skilled Nursing Care* 21st to 100th Day Copayment*   $   /day | | | | |
| **Medicare Part B:** Physician | | | | |
| Initial deductible   $100 | | | | |
| 20% Copayment | | | | |
| Does the HMO provide coverage for the following services? | If so, place a checkmark in the appropriate column for each policy. | | | |
| Prescription drugs | | | | |
| Private duty nursing | | | | |
| Additional physicians' fees | | | | |
| Skilled Nursing Care | | | | |
| Number of days available | _____ | _____ | _____ | _____ |
| Preventive services | | | | |
| Emergency services (travel) | | | | |

*Fill in amounts from current benefit year.

## MEDICARE HMO WORKSHEET, CONT'D

| Section I: Organization/Facilities | Plan 1 | Plan 2 | Plan 3 |
|---|---|---|---|
| Travel time to primary care site | | | |
| Advance time to make appointments | | | |
| Telephone access to primary care doctor | | | |
| Emergency care procedure | | | |
| Out-of-area care procedure | | | |
| Cleanliness of facility | | | |
| Modern in appearance | | | |
| Staff behavior toward patients | | | |
| Patient waiting time | | | |
| Health promotion classes (list the type available if any) | | | |
| Member grievance process | | | |
| Years in business | | | |
| Federally qualified | | | |
| Other factors: | | | |
| | | | |

| Section II: Primary Care Physician | | | |
|---|---|---|---|
| Physician's name | | | |
| Specialty board certified | | | |
| Years in practice/Years in HMO/PPO | | | |
| Partners/Back-up coverage | | | |
| Use of physicians' assistants, nurse practitioners, etc. | | | |
| Prevention oriented | | | |
| Average time spent with patients | | | |
| Prescribes generic drugs | | | |
| Uses extraordinary life-saving measures | | | |
| Admits to hospital | | | |
| Communicates well with patients | | | |
| Subscribes to PMS Code of Practice | | | |
| Other: | | | |

| Section III: Back-up System | Plan 1 | Plan 2 | Plan 3 |
|---|---|---|---|
| Additional hospitals in plan | | | |
| Travel time to each | | | |
| Second opinion surgical program | | | |
| Referrals to non-HMO/PPO specialists | | | |
| Quality assurance program | | | |
| Procedure for changing primary care doctor | | | |

just not for you.

*Medicare SELECT*

Another new product available to Medicare beneficiaries is called **Medicare SELECT.** It's a type of Medigap insurance policy that only pays full supplemental benefits if covered services are provided by selected providers and facilities (except in emergencies). Insurers, including some HMOs, offer Medicare SELECT in the same way standard Medigap insurance is offered. The policies meet federal standards for Medigap insurance and are regulated by the states in which they are approved. Medicare SELECT policies are expected to have lower premiums than comparable Medigap policies that do not have this selected-provider feature. Once a demonstration project, Medicare SELECT is now approved for sale in all 50 states; however, it may not be offered by every insurance company or HMO. Your state's insurance department can tell you if Medicare SELECT is available to you. (Pick up a copy of "Medicare and Managed Care Plans," HCFA publication number 02195, available at any Social Security office.)

*Filing Claims for Supplemental Insurance*

One of the things you have to face with traditional insurance, and occasionally with health maintenance organizations, is filing a claim. At one time Medicare beneficiaries had to complete and submit their own claims for Part B services if their physician did not accept assignment. However, that has changed for the better now that physicians are required by law to complete and submit claims for Part B services. This means less paperwork for you; however, if you want to be reimbursed for your 20 percent copayment, you still need to file a claim with your Medigap insurance carrier.

It's important that your physician file the claim within a reasonable period of time, otherwise you'll be delayed in filing your Medigap insurance claim. Some Medigap insurers require that you enclose a copy of your **Explanation of Medicare Benefits** (EOMB) before you file a claim, and you won't get an EOMB until the claim is filed and processed by the carrier. (See the sample form on page 132–133.)

There is, however, a downside to this new policy that could cause a few problems. If your physician does not accept assignment, he or she may request full payment at the time services are delivered. This may mean a rather hefty out-of-pocket expense for which you may not be reimbursed by Medicare for a number of months. In addition, without

# Explanation of Your Medicare Part B Benefits

Name of Beneficiary

Iphigenia Smith
4321 Edgar Allen Poe Drive
San Diego, CA 99110

Your Medicare number: 120-99-6789

A summary about this notice dated December 30, 1996.

| | |
|---|---|
| Total charges: | $1,755.00 |
| Total Medicare approved: | $1,339.00 |
| Medicare paid your provider: | $1,071.20 |
| You are responsible for: | $ 367.80 |

## Details about this claim (See the back of this notice for more information.)

You received these services from your provider;
Dr. Sherman T. Potter, claim-#9876-1234-2468

Midway Medical Clinic, 2552 Baskerville Rd.,
San Diego, CA 99110

This indicates amount billed and approved.

| Services and Service Codes | Dates | Charge | Medicare approved | Notes |
|---|---|---|---|---|
| 65850 surgery, incision of eye | Nov 15, 1996 | $975.00 | $780.00 | a |
| 90040 brief office visit | Nov 19, 1996 | $100.00 | $ 0 | b |
| 90070 extended office visits | Nov 17–29, 1996 | $600.00 | $516.00 | a |
| 90040 brief office visit | Nov 30, 1996 | $ 40.00 | $ 21.50 | a |
| 90040 brief office visit | Dec 15, 1996 | $ 40.00 | $ 21.50 | a |
| | Total | $1,755.00 | $1,339.00 | |

This indicates the service and date provided.

Notes:

a   We based the approved amount on the fee schedule for this service.

b   Medicare did not pay for this test. Medicare pays for this only when the laboratory is certified for this type of test.

This tells you if assignment was taken and the dollar amount billed.

Here's an explanation of this claim:

| | | |
|---|---|---|
| Of the total charges, Medicare approved | $1,339.00 | The provider accepted this amount. See #4 on the back of this notice. |
| The deductible you still owe | $   0 | You have met the $100 deductible for 1996. |
| | $1,339.00<br>× .80 | Medicare pays 80 percent of this total. |
| We are paying the provider | $1,071.20 | Your copayment is 20 percent or $267.80. |
| Of the amount approved | $1,339.00 | |
| Subtract what we pay the provider | $1,071.20 | |
| You are responsible for | $ 267.80 | |
| plus charges not covered by Medicare | $ 100.00 | |
| The total you are responsible for: | $ 367.80 | The provider may bill you for this amount. If you have other insurance, the other insurance may pay this amount. |

This indicates whether or not you have met the $100 deductible this year.

This explains what you pay.

If you have questions about this notice, call Blue Cross Blue Shield of Maryland at 410-861-2273 or toll free at 800-662-5170 or visit us at 1946 Greenspring Drive, Timonium, Maryland.
You'll need this notice when you call or visit us about this claim.
If you want to appeal this claim, see #5 on the other side. You must write us by June 30, 1997.

This is your Part B carrier. If you suspect a mistake, contact this office.

This gives you the time frame to file any appeal.

# Important Information You Should Know About Your Medicare Part B Benefits

**This part of the notice answers some common questions that people ask about collecting Medicare benefits. If you have other questions, see your copy of *The Medicare Handbook* or call us for more information.**

**1. What should I do if I have questions about this notice?**

If you have questions about this notice, call, write, or visit us and we will tell you the facts that we used to decide what and how much to pay. Turn to the front of this notice: our address and phone number are on the bottom of the page.

**2. Can I appeal how much Medicare paid for these services?**

If you do not agree with what Medicare approved for these services, you may appeal our decision. To make sure that we are fair to you, we will not allow the same people who originally processed these services to conduct this review.

However, in order to be eligible for a review, you **must** write to us within **6 months** of the date of this notice, unless you have a good reason for being late (for example, if you had an extended illness which kept you from being able to file on time).

Turn to the front of this notice: the deadline date and our address are on the bottom of the page. It may help your case if you include a note from your doctor or supplier (provider) that tells us what was done and why.

If you want help with your appeal, you can have a friend, lawyer, or someone else help you. Some lawyers do not charge unless you win your appeal. There are groups, such as lawyer referral services, that can help you find a lawyer. There are also groups, such as legal aid services, who will give you free legal services if you qualify.

**3. How much does Medicare pay?**

The details on the front of this notice explain how much Medicare paid for these services. See your copy of *The Medicare Handbook* for more information about the benefits you are entitled to as a beneficiary in the Medicare Part B program. If you need another copy of the handbook, call or visit your local Social Security office.

Medicare may make adjustments to your payment. We may reduce the amount we pay for services by a certain percentage (Balanced Budget Law). If your provider accepted assignment, you are not liable to pay the amount of this reduction. We pay interest on some claims not paid within the required time.

All Medicare payments are made on the condition that you will pay Medicare back if benefits are also paid under insurance that is primary to Medicare. Examples of other insurance are employer group health plans, automobile medical, liability, no fault, or workers' compensation. Notify us immediately if you have filed or could file a claim with insurance that is primary to Medicare.

**4. How can I reduce my medical costs?**

Many providers have agreed to be part of **Medicare's participation program.** That means that they will always accept the amount that Medicare approves as their full payment. Write or call us for the name of a participating provider or for a free list of participating providers.

A provider who accepts assignment can charge you only for the part of the annual deductible you have not met and the copayment which is the remaining 20 percent of the approved amount.

If you are treated by one of these doctors you can save money. See *The Medicare Handbook* for more information about how you can reduce your medical costs.

**5. How can I use this notice?**

You can use this notice to:

- Contact us immediately if you think Medicare paid for a service you did not receive

- Show your provider how much of your deductible you have met

- Claim benefits with another insurance company. If you send this notice to them, make a copy of it for your records.

**Keep this notice for your records.**
*Health Care Financing Administration*

PLEASE
DO NOT
STAPLE
IN THIS
AREA

**CARRIER**

| | PICA | | | | | | **HEALTH INSURANCE CLAIM FORM** | | PICA | | |

| 1. MEDICARE MEDICAID CHAMPUS CHAMPVA GROUP HEALTH PLAN FECA BLK LUNG OTHER | 1a. INSURED'S I.D. NUMBER (FOR PROGRAM IN ITEM 1) |
|---|---|
| (Medicare #) (Medicaid #) (Sponsor's SSN) (VA File #) (SSN or ID) (SSN) (ID) | |

| 2. PATIENT'S NAME (Last Name, First Name, Middle Initial) | 3. PATIENT'S BIRTH DATE MM DD YY SEX M F | 4. INSURED'S NAME (Last Name, First Name, Middle Initial) |
|---|---|---|

| 5. PATIENT'S ADDRESS (No., Street) | 6. PATIENT RELATIONSHIP TO INSURED Self Spouse Child Other | 7. INSURED'S ADDRESS (No., Street) |
|---|---|---|
| CITY  STATE | 8. PATIENT STATUS Single Married Other | CITY  STATE |
| ZIP CODE  TELEPHONE (Include Area Code) ( ) | Employed Full-Time Student Part-Time Student | ZIP CODE  TELEPHONE (INCLUDE AREA CODE) ( ) |

**PATIENT AND INSURED INFORMATION**

| 9. OTHER INSURED'S NAME (Last Name, First Name, Middle Initial) | 10. IS PATIENT'S CONDITION RELATED TO: | 11. INSURED'S POLICY GROUP OR FECA NUMBER |
|---|---|---|
| a. OTHER INSURED'S POLICY OR GROUP NUMBER | a. EMPLOYMENT? (CURRENT OR PREVIOUS) YES NO | a. INSURED'S DATE OF BIRTH MM DD YY SEX M F |
| b. OTHER INSURED'S DATE OF BIRTH MM DD YY SEX M F | b. AUTO ACCIDENT? PLACE (State) YES NO | b. EMPLOYER'S NAME OR SCHOOL NAME |
| c. EMPLOYER'S NAME OR SCHOOL NAME | c. OTHER ACCIDENT? YES NO | c. INSURANCE PLAN NAME OR PROGRAM NAME |
| d. INSURANCE PLAN NAME OR PROGRAM NAME | 10d. RESERVED FOR LOCAL USE | d. IS THERE ANOTHER HEALTH BENEFIT PLAN? YES NO If yes, return to and complete item 9 a-d. |

**READ BACK OF FORM BEFORE COMPLETING & SIGNING THIS FORM.**

| 12. PATIENT'S OR AUTHORIZED PERSON'S SIGNATURE I authorize the release of any medical or other information necessary to process this claim. I also request payment of government benefits either to myself or to the party who accepts assignment below. | 13. INSURED'S OR AUTHORIZED PERSON'S SIGNATURE I authorize payment of medical benefits to the undersigned physician or supplier for services described below. |
|---|---|
| SIGNED _____ DATE _____ | SIGNED _____ |

| 14. DATE OF CURRENT: MM DD YY ILLNESS (First symptom) OR INJURY (Accident) OR PREGNANCY(LMP) | 15. IF PATIENT HAS HAD SAME OR SIMILAR ILLNESS. GIVE FIRST DATE MM DD YY | 16. DATES PATIENT UNABLE TO WORK IN CURRENT OCCUPATION MM DD YY MM DD YY FROM TO |
|---|---|---|
| 17. NAME OF REFERRING PHYSICIAN OR OTHER SOURCE | 17a. I.D. NUMBER OF REFERRING PHYSICIAN | 18. HOSPITALIZATION DATES RELATED TO CURRENT SERVICES MM DD YY MM DD YY FROM TO |
| 19. RESERVED FOR LOCAL USE | | 20. OUTSIDE LAB? $ CHARGES YES NO |

| 21. DIAGNOSIS OR NATURE OF ILLNESS OR INJURY. (RELATE ITEMS 1,2,3 OR 4 TO ITEM 24E BY LINE) | 22. MEDICAID RESUBMISSION CODE  ORIGINAL REF. NO. |
|---|---|
| 1. ____ . __ 3. ____ . __ | |
| 2. ____ . __ 4. ____ . __ | 23. PRIOR AUTHORIZATION NUMBER |

**PHYSICIAN OR SUPPLIER INFORMATION**

| 24. A DATE(S) OF SERVICE From To MM DD YY MM DD YY | B Place of Service | C Type of Service | D PROCEDURES, SERVICES, OR SUPPLIES (Explain Unusual Circumstances) CPT/HCPCS MODIFIER | E DIAGNOSIS CODE | F $ CHARGES | G DAYS OR UNITS | H EPSDT Family Plan | I EMG | J COB | K RESERVED FOR LOCAL USE |
|---|---|---|---|---|---|---|---|---|---|---|
| 1 | | | | | | | | | | |
| 2 | | | | | | | | | | |
| 3 | | | | | | | | | | |
| 4 | | | | | | | | | | |
| 5 | | | | | | | | | | |
| 6 | | | | | | | | | | |

| 25. FEDERAL TAX I.D. NUMBER SSN EIN | 26. PATIENT'S ACCOUNT NO. | 27. ACCEPT ASSIGNMENT? (For govt. claims, see back) YES NO | 28. TOTAL CHARGE $ | 29. AMOUNT PAID $ | 30. BALANCE DUE $ |
|---|---|---|---|---|---|
| 31. SIGNATURE OF PHYSICIAN OR SUPPLIER INCLUDING DEGREES OR CREDENTIALS (I certify that the statements on the reverse apply to this bill and are made a part thereof.) SIGNED DATE | 32. NAME AND ADDRESS OF FACILITY WHERE SERVICES WERE RENDERED (If other than home or office) | 33. PHYSICIAN'S, SUPPLIER'S BILLING NAME, ADDRESS, ZIP CODE & PHONE # PIN# GRP# |

790-0115 (12/90) (OCR) 1 pt.

(APPROVED BY AMA COUNCIL ON MEDICAL SERVICE 8/88)   *PLEASE PRINT OR TYPE*   FORM HCFA-1500 (12-90)
FORM OWCP-1500   FORM RRB-1500

**134**

**BECAUSE THIS FORM IS USED BY VARIOUS GOVERNMENT AND PRIVATE HEALTH PROGRAMS, SEE SEPARATE INSTRUCTIONS ISSUED BY APPLICABLE PROGRAMS.**

**NOTICE: Any person who knowingly files a statement of claim containing any misrepresentation or any false, incomplete or misleading information may be guilty of a criminal act punishable under law and may be subject to civil penalties.**

an EOMB you won't be able to file a claim with your Medigap insurance, which means a further delay in getting your money.

Your physician should have an ample supply of claim forms on hand: if not, suggest that he/she contact Medicare to obtain a supply of the forms shown on pages 134–135.

Your Medigap insurer's claim form will tell you if you are required to submit a copy of the EOMB with a claim. It's convenient just to send the EOMB, but we recommend that you *never* do this. First, the EOMB is official correspondence between an agency acting for the U.S. government and you. Second, you will need it to make sure that your insurer has paid the difference between the provider's charge and the Medicare payment. Third, you won't be able to keep your claims log straight without it. Fourth, if you are still working, you'll need it to keep your medical expense deduction right if you itemize.

A typical supplemental insurance claim form asks for a lot of standard information: your name, your policy number, your Social Security number, the number from your Medicare insurance card, whether or not you have Part B (doctor insurance), your address, your telephone number, and so on. You should make a note in your claims log (appendix B) that you have filed a claim *before* you mail it. Don't rely on memory.

If you do not get the amount you believe the policy should pay or if the insurer rejects the claim, see chapter 8, which is a troubleshooting kit for all sorts of situations. The one thing you should know before you go into a full-scale effort is that insurers often reject claims *because they're duplicates.* Your claims log will help you avoid being thrown by this. We believe that insurers would be well advised simply to notify you that the claim is a duplicate, and that processing of the original is still going on, rather than telling you it has been rejected, but that day has not arrived yet.

In this chapter you will learn: Why it's important to negotiate with your doctor ▪ When to negotiate with your doctor ▪ How assignment can save you money ▪ How the balance billing limits can save you money ▪ What is meant by fully informing a patient ▪ How to get the right diagnosis ▪ When to get a second opinion

---

# 5. Negotiating with Your Doctor

The images that comes to mind when people think of negotiating are usually confrontational: strikes and diplomatic encounters. They also think that the term implies that something has gone wrong, and the negotiating is being done to set it right. People also think in terms of winners and losers. The word — at least as defined by good ol' *Webster's* — doesn't have the connotations of confrontation, things going awry, and wins and losses. "Negotiations" can simply mean "the carrying on of business" or "dealing with some matter that requires ability for its successful handling."

It's fair to say that there is a confrontation of sorts going on between many members of the medical profession and American society, that it's happening because things have gone wrong, and that there will be winners and losers. But that doesn't have to be the case in your dealings with doctors. We make no secret of the fact that if it does come down to a win/loss situation, we prefer the consumer, the patient — you — to be the winner. But often the discussions that we suggest in this chapter can be carried out so that you *and* the doctor win.

Of course, a win-win situation depends on what each party views as a successful outcome. Let's use accepting **assignment** as an example. If you use a doctor who does not currently accept assignment, and you persuade him to accept it in your case (the best outcome) or at least for the treatment of the moment (better than nothing), he is giving up the right to charge you more than 20 percent of the Medicare approved price. He is also required by law to file your Part B claim for you. He may consider this a loss; that is fine. How he looks at it is up to him. In any case, negotiating shouldn't be an exercise in doctor-bashing. Think of it, rather, as helping your doctor to help you as much as he can, and educating him about the medical marketplace. Negotiating is getting the best service for the best price.

It has been said that "the man (or woman) who asks for nothing is quite likely to get it." To negotiate successfully, you have to know what you're trying to get. We specify some goals for you in this chapter. You should aim for this:

- Paying no more than the Medicare approved charge for the services you receive
- Getting the best possible treatment to produce what you consider the best overall outcome
- Staying in control of your treatment — being able to make and enforce the choices that you think best for you and avoiding unnecessary risk and expense — at all times, even if you are unable to communicate your wishes

For each of these issues, we give you the background you need to deal with the issue, some suggestions for dealing with the general situation, and some examples (or scenarios) of successful negotiations.

## Why It's Hard to Negotiate with Doctors

Nurses (among others) have a longstanding joke that the initials "M.D." stand for "mostly divine." With divine beings, one does not negotiate. One prays. It is therefore not surprising that the idea of negotiating with your doctor is foreign to most people.

It should not be foreign. It should be standard practice. There are a number of reasons why it isn't. At a time when doctors were among the few educated people in society — when only about 4 percent of the population had a college education and most adults had not finished high school — it was unrealistic to expect that the patient could understand matters well enough to negotiate treatment without a crash course in biology. Rather than provide it, doctors relied on intimidation, furthered by their extremely rare level of learning and high social position to get patients to cooperate. This has always been the style of physicians in largely unlettered societies. In the late nineteenth century, the style of medicine practiced today was struggling to establish itself as the only "scientific" kind of medicine, and to end legislative control of medicine and establish control by the profession. This effort reinforced the tendency to treat the patient as a child — a sick child, at that.

Another reason has its roots in the history of American medicine. In the nineteenth century, the group of medical practitioners who had the M.D. degree — only one of the kinds of degrees, or certificates of study, issued to the various types of medical practitioners — made a move to take over all of medical practice through the legislatures. This was done at a time when those with the M.D. degree, who practiced a kind of medicine that is called "allopathic," had no greater claim to a scientific foundation for their practices that any of the other schools did. (Those other schools, for example, practiced osteopathic, chiropractic, naturopathic, and homeopathic brands of medicine. They still survive.)

Part of the strategy for taking over the whole medical field was a conscious, long-range effort to place holders of the M.D. degree (as opposed to other kinds of doctors such as osteopaths) on a pedestal. The strategy required a "mythology of medicine" — a presentation of M.D.-style medicine as far more scientific, far more founded in careful, controlled experiments, than it really was (or, for that matter, far more scientific than it is today). Doctors are still trained in the mythology. The game still goes on. A federal court recently concluded that the **American Medical Association** had deliberately engaged in an attempt to restrain the practices of chiropractors.

In fact, medicine still has much in common with engineering. The engineer solves problems by trying out solutions, based on general knowledge of a problem, until something works. If she's good, it works on the first try. If not, she keeps trying. Medicine still has little in common with the hard sciences, such as physics, where the classic experiments work all of the time.

Finally, doctors consciously and unconsciously cultivate an aloofness, an above-the fray attitude and a hypercompetent appearance. To some extent, this is a matter of emotional survival. But this attitude is acknowledged by many to get in the way of sympathizing with patients' personal concerns about illness, growing old, and death.

With these factors still dominant in medical training and practice, it's up to the patient — you — to educate doctors to treat you as you wish to be treated.

*Why It's Important*

Medicare beneficiaries — whether over 65 or disabled — need to negotiate more than most people. There are several reasons for this:

- Most Americans experience their first serious illnesses only when they are about 50 or older. Yuppies may have heart attacks in their 30s, but serious illness, for most people, comes with age.
- Because of this, the most expensive illnesses come when people have reduced incomes, are not fully employed, and are dependent on Medicare for health coverage.
- Medicare pays most of the hospital expenses of the elderly, but the proportion of nonhospital expenses covered is falling rapidly. This is happening at a time when care is increasingly being shifted out of the hospital into other settings. Medicare was designed largely as hospital insurance and has not caught up with the reality of current medical practice.
- Almost no form of supplemental insurance covers everything that the elderly need.
- The cost of treatment, the physical and psychological burdens of treatment, and the effect on relatives are all determined mostly by the doctor.
- The doctor, in large measure, determines how and when people die.

If you want to have *any* influence on the cost of your treatment, how much (or little) you benefit from it, and how and when you go, you have to negotiate with doctors. There's no other option.

There are three more reasons to take this business of negotiating seriously. First, doctors in many areas are hungry for patients right now, and getting hungrier. The United States is heading toward a ratio of 2 doctors per 1,000 population, while there is good evidence that 1.2–1.4 per 1,000 is what is really needed. From the patient's side, the doctor glut shows up in increased exposure to treatments designed to augment the doctor's income rather than the patient's health. From the doctor's side, it means a scramble for a static pool of patients. It means that the loss of a single patient is more serious, and more effort needs to be made to keep patients happy. There are still regions of the country where one or two doctors monopolize a specialty, but they are growing fewer.

Second, the new breed of doctors — the most recent graduates of medical school — are much more inclined to involve patients in treatment decisions than are their older colleagues. Part of the reason for this is dissatisfaction with the traditional style of practice. Another reason is the knowledge that fully informing patients (or doing what they *think* is fully informing patients) protects them to some degree from malpractice suits — they can blame a poor outcome partly on the patient's dumb choice. You can take advantage of their sincere desire to inform you to get better care at a better price.

Third, when one enters a large hospital with lots of departments and lots of specialties — particularly a teaching hospital — several doctors are likely to be involved in the patient's care. The admitting physician may shrink into the background as surgeons, radiologists, nuclear medicine specialists, internists, cardiologists, pulmonary medicine specialists, intensivists, and a corps of residents and doctors gets into the act. Often, no one person is clearly in charge. Some doctors and hospitals realize the danger (to patients and to their malpractice insurer) in this situation and are trying to do something about it, but those efforts are in their infancy. It may well be that if you want anyone to be in charge, it will have to be you. Thus it is essential that you and someone you trust be prepared to negotiate your care.

## The First Big Issue: Prices

We said that throughout this book we give you bits of the history of the Medicare program and just enough technical detail to make you an empowered consumer, but not enough to overwhelm you. The first big issue is prices. Talking about prices in Medicare requires, first and foremost, that we talk about **assignment.** Assignment is defined as the transfer of benefits of a policy to another party; for example, telling your insurance company to send the check directly to your doctor or hospital, rather than to you.

Assignment in Medicare means this: a doctor who "takes assignment" on all or part of your treatment accepts what Medicare pays, less the deductibles and your 20 percent copayment. You only have to deal with the paperwork that relates to your insurance company (if you have supplemental insurance for Medicare).

Assignment is one of those topics that has a long, complicated history and deserves a bit of background information. When a doctor agrees to take assignment, she agrees to accept the payment that the Medicare carrier has decided is appropriate for the service she rendered. This does *not* mean that she has agreed to accept it as payment in full. She is supposed to charge you 20 percent of the Medicare price; Medicare pays the other 80 percent. The Medicare check goes to her. You have to deal only with your portion of the bill and with your insurance company. If you have insurance that covers the 20 percent that Medicare doesn't pay (called the copayment), you pay nothing. If you don't have supplemental insurance, then the 20 percent copayment would be an out-of-pocket expense for you. That is why it's important to carry supplemental insurance.

Until recently, doctors could pick and choose whether or not to take assignment on a service-by-service basis. Now they are either participating doctors — which means that they take assignment on all services they render — or nonparticipating, which means that they can still pick and choose among patients and services, taking assignment on some but not on others.

*Doctors and Their Prices: History Past and Present*

The Code of Hammurabi, a compilation of Babylonian law that dates to 1750 B.C. — almost forty centuries ago — sets limits on how much doctors may charge. (It also prescribes strict punishment for bad results of treatment.) Some 140 years before the American Revolution, the colony of Virginia set maximum allowable prices for doctors' services. As you can imagine, control of doctors' fees has been a big issue with the medical profession from the time it first recognized itself as such.

Doctors in the United States argued strongly with everyone who has tried to limit fees some way. When health insurance became generally available because of employer funding after World War II, health insurers faced a dilemma. They had to get doctors to accept enough payment from them to convince the insured that expenses really were covered. They had to make the amount small enough that policies were affordable. The result was the **usual, customary, and reasonable (UCR)** reimbursement system.

*Why Assignment and Participation Are Important Issues for You*

The importance of assignment and participation can best be explained by examples. Suppose you have a cardiac catheterization. (This is a procedure in which a small tube is inserted into the arteries of the heart, or into the heart itself, for diagnosis and sometimes treatment. Dye can be injected to show the arteries and detect blockages, arteries can be dilated with a balloon, drugs can be injected to abort heart attacks.) The doctor charges $3,000. He is free to pull this number out of his hat; there are no set prices. It may be much more, or much less, than his colleagues charge. Most studies show that at least a 2-to-1 ratio can be found in a given community — that is, the highest-charging doctor will charge at least twice as much as the lowest-charging. (Remember, however, that price has nothing to do with quality. High prices do not necessarily mean better care.)

If he is a participating doctor, he has agreed to accept assignment — which, again, means accepting the Medicare-approved payment as payment in full — for all services he renders to Medicare beneficiaries.

(Again, this does not mean you pay nothing; Medicare pays 80 percent, and you [or your insurance company] pay 20 percent.) Does this mean that Medicare will pay 80 percent of the $3,000? No. It means that Medicare pays 80 percent of the Medicare-approved amount, based on the new **RBRVS** fee schedule payment system.

Unlike the old usual, customary, and reasonable payment system, which rewarded doctors for constantly raising their prices, the RBRVS system considers the skills and resources required to deliver medical services. The RBRVS reimbursement system is based on the following factors:

- a nationally uniform relative value unit (RVU) for each service (primary care, surgical, nonsurgical, etc.)
- a geographical adjustment factor (recognizes different markets: urban or rural)
- a nationally uniform conversion factor for calculating payments (a certain dollar amount multiplied by the RVU)

The RVUs for each service reflect the resources involved in providing the three components of the doctor's service:

- work (skill and effort required)
- practice expenses (rent, staff salaries, supplies, etc.)
- the cost of malpractice insurance (annual premium)

Let's say the approved charge is $2,000. Medicare pays the doctor 80 percent of that — $1,600 — and you or your insurance company pay the remaining 20 percent — $400. Your doctor files the claim, the check goes to him, and he bills you for the remaining $400. You pay it or file a claim with your supplemental insurance company. If you have not met your $100 annual deductible, it will be subtracted from the amount that Medicare pays. You and your insurance company pay it, depending on your policy. Both situations are illustrated in the following chart:

| Example 1: Doctor Accepts Assignment | |
| --- | ---: |
| Actual charge: | $3,000 |
| Medicare-approved charge: | $2,000 |
| Medicare pays: 80% of $2,000 = | $1,600 |
| You pay: $2,000 − $1,600 = | $ 400 |
| If $100 Medicare Part B deductible not met: | |
| Medicare-approved charge: | $2,000 |
| Less: Part B deductible | $ 100 |

```
Medicare pays: 80% of $2,000 ( = $1,600),
                      less $100 =                    $1,500
                      You pay:                       $  500
```

By becoming a **Medicare-participating physician,** your doctor has agreed to eat the other $1,000. It's no great loss. He knew that he wasn't going to get it anyway. That's because his charge of $3,000 is greater than the Medicare-approved amount based on the RBRVS fee schedule system. As a participating physician, he knows that his reimbursement is based on the fee schedule, and he is willing to accept this amount as payment in full.

But what happens if you go to a nonparticipating doctor? In addition to the 20 percent copayment, you are also responsible for any excess charge up to the balance billing limit. This means that a nonparticipating doctor may charge you no more than 115 percent of the Medicare-approved amount. Using the figures from our previous example, the doctor's charge is $3,000, the Medicare-approved amount is $1,900 ($2,000 × 95 percent), and the balance billing limit is $2,185 ($1,900 × 115 percent). Medicare pays $1,520 ($1,900 × 80 percent), which leaves a balance of $665 for you and your supplemental insurance. *You are not responsible for the remaining $815.*

The doctor files the claim with Medicare, and you file a claim with your supplemental insurance carrier to collect your 20 percent. You are responsible for the difference between the Medicare-approved amount and the balance billing limit. Here's the arithmetic again:

```
             Example 2: Doctor Does Not Accept Assignment
Actual charge:                                               $3,000
Medicare-approved charge: 95% of $2,000 =                    $1,900
Balance billing limit: 115% of $1,900 =                      $2,185
Medicare pays: 80% of $1,900 =                               $1,520
You pay: $2,185 − $1,520 =                                    $  665
```

If $100 Medicare Part B deductible not met:
Medicare pays: 80% of $1,900                          $1,520
Less Part B deductible:                                $  100
Medicare pays doctor:                                  $1,420
You pay: $2,185 − 1,420 =                              $  765
Total payment to doctor:                               $2,185

## Example 3: Comparison of an Assigned Versus a Non-Assigned Claim

|  | Doctor takes assignment | Doctor does not take assignment |
|---|---|---|
| Actual charge: | $3,000 | $3,000 |
| Medicare-approved charge: | $2,000 | $1,900 |
| Balance billing limit: | — | $2,185 |
| Medicare pays: | $1,600 | $1,520 |
| You pay: | $  400 | $  665 |
| If Part B $100 deductible not met: Medicare-approved charge: | $1,600 | $1,520 |
| Less Part B deductible: | $  100 | $  100 |
| Medicare pays: | $1,500 | $1,420 |
| You pay: | $  500 | $  765 |

The limits on balance billing will definitely save you money when you must use a nonparticipating doctor.

Medicare has developed a rather complicated formula for determining how much a doctor may charge for his/her services. By law, nonparticipating doctors are limited in the amount they may charge you above the Medicare-approved amount. The balance billing limit is determined by multiplying the Medicare-approved amount by 95 percent and then by 115 percent. The immediate effect of this is to save you money when you must use a doctor who does not accept assignment.

If your doctor's charges exceed the maximum charges permitted by law, neither you nor your insurance company has to pay the difference between the maximum charge and the doctor's actual charge. However, you will be responsible for the difference between the approved charge and the balance billing limit. Follow the example shown below.

| Example 4: Comparison of Out-of-Pocket Expenses with Balance Billing Limits on Nonparticipating Doctors | |
| --- | --- |
| Actual charge: | $3,000 |
| Medicare-approved charge: | $1,900 |
| Balance billing limit: | $2,185 |
| Medicare pays: | $1,520 |
| You pay without limits: | $1,480 |
| You pay with limits: | $ 665 |
| You save: | $ 815 |

It should be obvious that persuading your doctor to take assignment on all your bills — or going to a doctor who accepts assignment — can save you large sums of money. Since most people over 65 are not particularly wealthy, the potential savings really count. You should not feel that you are cheating your doctor by asking him to accept assignment. The charge that Medicare has determined as "reasonable," in most cases, takes into account what other doctors charge. Remember, too, that the relationship of real costs to charges in all of American medicine is not tight. It is unlikely that whatever Medicare pays is below what it cost your doctor to provide the service, plus a reasonable profit. Your doctor may *feel* that the Medicare payment is too low. Unless he presents you with hard evidence that Medicare is not covering his real costs, don't worry. Point out to him that other doctors who accept assignment seem to do well.

*Some New Incentives for Doctors to Accept Assignment*

**The States:** Medical licenses are still granted by states, not by the federal government, even though proposals for a national medical license are growing more frequent. (The reasons for these demands range from evidence that many states handle the licensing of doctors in a haphazard way to the desire to have uniform disciplining of incompetent practitioners).

Because the states have the licensing power, they can attach requirements to the license. The Commonwealth of Massachusetts became the first state to require mandatory assignment as a condition of licensure. Rhode Island recently passed a mandatory assignment law; however, it was not linked to licensure. Other states taking action to encourage Medicare assignment are: Connecticut, Minnesota, New York, Ohio, Pennsylvania and Vermont. Pennsylvania's law bans balance billing (charging the difference between the Medicare-approved amount and what the doctor usually charges), while Connecticut and Vermont laws have eligibility requirements based on income.

**The Federal Government:** The federal government has not yet attempted to require that doctors accept assignment as a condition of being in the Medicare program. Instead, from 1980 through 1988, the Reagan administration attempted to use free-market incentives to encourage greater physician participation. Some of the incentives actually do have a chance of encouraging more doctors to participate.

Some of the incentives are of direct benefit to you:

- The *Directory of Participating Doctors in Your Area* is available to you free of charge. You should receive a notice of the availability of this directory annually, and you can obtain one at any time by writing to the Medicare carrier for your state. Copies are available for review at Social Security offices. Medicare-participating doctors also can display emblems or certificates that show they accept assignment on all Medicare claims. The directory shows the specialties of the doctors as well. (A list of Medicare carriers is contained in appendix A.)

- If your hospital refers you to a doctor for outpatient care, the hospital must *inform you if the doctor is a nonparticipating doctor and must identify at least one participating doctor from whom you can obtain the same services,* "if practicable."

- If a nonparticipating physician is preparing to perform **elective surgery** on you and will not take assignment, and if the charge for surgery will exceed $500, *you must be provided with written notice of the estimated actual charge, the estimated approved charge, and the estimated expense to you* (or your insurance plan). This will give you time to seek the same services from a participating doctor or to negotiate with your doctor to provide the services on assignment.

There are a few additional incentives for doctors. Each **Explanation of Medicare Benefits** (the paper that the Medicare carrier sends to tell you what it paid for [see a copy in appendix E]) that contains unassigned charges will include a message reminding you that you would have fared better if you had obtained the services from a participating doctor. In addition, claims that do not require investigation by the Medicare carrier to resolve a discrepancy are paid for participating doctors about a week earlier than those for nonparticipating doctors. If a doctor has cash flow problems, this can make a big difference and be a real incentive to become a participating doctor.

*Negotiating with Your Doctor About Fees*

The most effective way to negotiate fees with your doctor is with your feet: Attempt to find a doctor who is a Medicare participant. Doctors need customers these days, and the need will grow. It will be very easy, as time goes by, to find a participating doctor — even if you don't live in Connecticut, Massachusetts, Minnesota, New York, Ohio, Pennsylvania, or Rhode Island.

But there may be reasons for not using a participating doctor:

- You may not be able to find one.
- You may have been getting genuinely good service from your family doctor, who for whatever reason does not participate.
- A specialist your family doctor refers you to may be the only one in town, or a good one, and may not participate.

Whether or not the doctor participates, you have a reason to negotiate fees. You especially have a reason if the doctor doesn't participate, because in that situation the amount you wind up paying out of pocket — or that has to be covered by your insurance — will be up to the balance billing limit. You may also decide not to use this doctor again unless he agrees to accept assignment. In other words, it is just good business to bargain.

There are other reasons for negotiating. Many doctors' prices are pulled out of thin air. They are not set by any market forces the way the prices for other services are. For most services, prices are publicly available and advertised. With doctors, it doesn't work that way, if only because the prices aren't published. The previous Medicare system of "prevailing charges" — inherited from Blue Cross and Blue Shield, which were set up by hospitals and doctors — is as good a price-fixing mechanism as any ever invented. Medicare's new **Resources-Based Relative Value Scale** is the first real attempt at placing a reasonable dollar value on the services provided by doctors.

Finally, the strongest reason to negotiate fees is that, for your doctor, medicine is (whatever else he thinks it is) a business. It is subject to far less regulation than other businesses that involve far smaller portions of the American economy and have far smaller potential for harm.

## The Second Big Issue: Treatment

Now let's discuss negotiating with your doctor about treatment. The basic questions you should ask and discuss with your doctor are these:

- Does she recognize her obligation to inform you fully?
- What are her criteria for the success or failure of a treatment?
- How sure is she of your diagnosis? How did she establish it? What alternatives did she consider?
- If she has recommended surgery, is there a medical treatment option? If she recommended a medical treatment, is there a surgical option? How long should you stay with the medical option before looking at surgery?
- If she has recommended surgery, where can you get a second opinion? What are the various surgical options?
- If she has recommended medical treatment, what are the various medical options?
- Is she willing to accept your prior instructions concerning your treatment in the event that you become incapacitated?

- If (when) she calls in specialists, how will you and she maintain control of the team treating you?
- What steps will be taken to control potentially harmful diagnostic tests?

## The Doctor's Obligation to Inform You Fully

The number of situations in which it is legally permissible for a doctor *not* to inform you fully about your condition and the treatment options available has shrunk dramatically over the last two decades. It is safe to say that in most states the only situations in which a full explanation of your situation can legally be withheld from you are those in which your mental competence is in doubt. Standards for finding you incompetent are becoming stricter. However, this does *not* mean that you will, in fact, be fully informed.

Ideally, your doctor should sign the **People's Medical Society (PMS)** Code of Practice, which is included in this book as appendix F. This is the most detailed attempt we know of to define what informed consent *ought* to mean from the patient's point of view. Unfortunately, if the number who have agreed to sign the code is any indication, most doctors don't agree with the PMS view of informed consent; you have to be on your guard. This does not mean refusing to trust your doctor. It does mean recognizing that she may have not one but several blinders on. Below we show the PMS Code of Practice in the form of questions you should ask your doctor:

- Does he post a printed schedule of fees for office visits, procedures, testing, and surgery?
- Does he provide itemized bills?
- Is he available for nonemergency telephone consultation during certain hours each week?
- Does he schedule appointments to allow the time necessary to see you, with minimal waiting time? Will he promptly return phone calls and report test results to you?
- Will he allow and encourage you to bring a friend or relative into the examining room with you?
- Will he facilitate getting your medical and hospital records to you and provide you with copies of your test results?
- Will he let you know your prognosis, including whether or not your condition is terminal or will cause disability or pain?
- Will he explain why further diagnostic activity or treatment is necessary?
- Will he discuss diagnostic, treatment, and medication options for

your particular problem with you (including the option of no treatment) and describe in understandable terms the risk of each alternative, the possibility of pain, the effect on your functioning, the number of visits each alternative would entail, and the cost of each?

- Will he discuss his qualifications to perform the proposed diagnostic measures or treatments?
- Will he let you know of organizations, support groups, and medical and lay publications that will assist you in understanding, monitoring, and treating your problem?
- Will he agree not to proceed until you are satisfied that you understand the risks and benefits of each alternative and he has your agreement on a particular course of action?

If you ask the doctor these questions, you'll be pretty well informed about your treatment and the doctor's style of practice. But to get a serious response, you still have to work around some obstacles that impede communication.

First, a general prejudice exists in our society against the aged (and the disabled). There is a general prejudice against people who appear less than middle-class in social status. Nothing in the education of a doctor necessarily removes either of these prejudices. As a Medicare beneficiary, you are (automatically) either aged or disabled. As a recipient of Social Security, you may be poor. (The average Social Security payment in the United States is $8,640 for an individual, $14,580 for a couple.)

Second, doctors are told that they must arrange treatment according to your best interest, but that means *the doctor's* view of your best interest. Nothing in the training of doctors prepares them to be more sympathetic to your view of your own best interest than to their own. They are raised in the tradition of "doctor knows best." If you want them to treat you according to your view of your best interest, you have to tell them. Loudly. Clearly. Especially loudly.

Third, doctors in general and American doctors in particular don't like to treat chronic conditions. (Chronic conditions are those that are marked by long duration and frequent recurrence and are hard or impossible to cure once and for all.) Doctors want a clear victory over disease, and they want it quickly.

Fourth, you may have difficulty in seeing, hearing, or speaking. This will make communicating with you more difficult. On top of your chronic conditions, this will make you even more frustrating to the doctor, and you more frustrated with him.

Fifth, you may have dementia — the general label for a condition in which your brain is not working as well as it did at one time. It may be mild to severe, acute or chronic. It may or may not be caused by, or made worse by, drugs the doctor has prescribed for you. The problem is that once there is any sign of it, you are likely to be treated as though you had no brains (and no free will) at all. The doctor will see his job as curing you in spite of yourself. All your protests, reasonable or not, will be discounted. There is also a medical prejudice in the belief that anyone who is not a perfectly functioning adult either has a diminished pain response or doesn't mind pain. (It is only now being recognized that very small children *do* need anesthetics for surgery.) If you're uncomfortable or in pain, you will be less likely to make yourself heard, and so . . .

It's up to you to make sure that you are informed enough to give consent to whatever the doctor has in mind for you. Trust in him is not enough. Liking him is not enough. Both are good, but they don't add up to *knowing* what he plans for your treatment, what alternatives are available, and what might go wrong with each. *You can't count on him to overcome all the prejudices about the elderly and the disabled in our society.*

You'll note that the PMS Code of Practice requires the doctor to allow someone else to be with you when you are examined. Having a friend or relative assist you in dealing with the doctor will help with the fourth and fifth points we've just made. But more important, having someone with you will keep the doctor on his toes. That means you get better care. In fact, if you feel that you are functioning at less than full capacity, or if there is some sign that the doctor believes so, we recommend that you insist on having someone with you. (Some of us may never attain what the medical profession considers "full capacity.")

With all the hurdles that have to be jumped to get to the point where you feel fully informed, some criteria are needed. We believe you can feel fully informed if (and *only* if)

- You understand what is wrong with you, what the doctor thought was wrong with you before he arrived at the current diagnosis, and how he arrived at the current diagnosis.
- You understand the medical and surgical treatments available, and the risks and benefits of each; the doctor should have given you some objective measure of the risks.

Let's look at an example. For a while, you've been feeling run down and have had a vague, dull pain in your abdomen. Lately, it has become much sharper, and you are having diarrhea. Going to the bathroom relieves the pain, but only for a short time. You've been taking some medicine you bought off the shelf at the drugstore, but lately it isn't working. You have started to lose weight and to have soaking sweats at night. You've been putting off going to the doctor because you're afraid he'll find cancer. But you now feel so bad that you want something done. Wisely, you decide to go to the doctor.

He examines you and discovers that you are bleeding slowly from somewhere in your digestive tract. He draws blood for tests and asks the laboratory (which is fortunately in the same building as his office) to get the results back to him "stat" (medicalese for "right now!"). You sit in the waiting room for about an hour, with time out for a few trips to the bathroom. The nurse calls you back to the examining room. The doctor says, "You definitely have a bleeding problem somewhere inside. You're anemic, which could account for the tiredness. I was worried that you might have a tumor in the colon, but the blood tests show signs of something called inflammatory bowel disease."

He continues, "I want to do a colonoscopy on you. It's a simple procedure I can do here in the office. We place a small tube with a light and a lens into your colon through the rectum. I can take biopsies to confirm my guess, and also look for tumors. If you have polyps, which could cause the bleeding, I can remove any I see. We'll sedate you lightly. All you'll have is a few cramps, and you won't remember much."

You ask what he suspects — a tumor, inflammatory bowel disease, or something else. He tells you that you might have a tumor, or inflamed bowel, or both, or possibly a parasite causing diarrhea. You ask why he can't use X rays and tell him that you don't like the sound of the colonoscopy.

"I could take a large bowel series," the doctor replies, "which involves an enema of barium. It's nearly as uncomfortable as the colonoscopy and doesn't differentiate between some of the conditions I think you might have. We might still wind up with a colonoscopy after the X rays if we find polyps. I want to examine a stool specimen for parasites, but I'm pretty sure you don't have them. The other symptoms don't fit." You ask if there are any other tests that might be used. The doctor says no. It's X rays or the colonoscopy. You ask about the risks.

The doctor says, "It's possible that I will accidentally perforate your bowel; that happens about once for every 450 colonoscopies done in the United States. My record is better. I've done two thousand of these and only perforated somebody's bowel twice. If this happens, I will have to put you in the hospital. It's almost certain that surgery will be needed. Survival for major perforations of the bowel without surgery is poor."

You ask what will happen with each of the conditions the doctor suspects. He tells you that with a benign tumor, you'll continue to be miserable; with a cancerous one, you might die. A parasitic infection might clear up, or leave you growing weaker and weaker. It could be treated with drugs, but these would have no effect if there were no parasites. An attack of inflammatory bowel disease could subside on its own, or it could ultimately lead to serious surgery to remove a large part of the intestines. There are fairly good drugs to treat it.

You reluctantly agree to the colonoscopy, which is a bit more unpleasant than the doctor made it sound, but not as bad as you feared. The biopsy shows that you have a mild case of inflammatory bowel disease. The doctor prescribes medicine for the cramps and diarrhea and tells you that he is putting you on steroids.

"Like a weightlifter?" you ask in some puzzlement. The doctor tells you no, there is another kind of steroid. You ask about side effects. He tells you that there are some serious ones, but they are only associated with long-term use. He suspects that you will be off them in a month or two. You ask about short-term side effects. He tells you that these include weight gain, a puffy face, and lowered resistance to infection. You ask if there are any others. The doctor tells you that there is something called "steroid psychosis" and that he usually puts patients who are on high doses in the hospital. He tells you that the dose he proposes for you is not high enough to worry about.

You go home, take the drug, and almost immediately feel better. The diarrhea stops, the cramps go away, you stop soaking the sheets with sweat at night, and you feel even better. In fact, you feel wonderful. Then you clearly feel your heart missing beats. You call the doctor in a panic. He tells you to come to the office right away. He orders an electrocardiogram, which shows nothing seriously out of order except missed beats, and more blood tests, again "stat."

"Steroids can cause increased potassium loss in the urine," the doctor tells you. " Potassium is an element in the blood that helps control heartbeat and muscle contraction. Yours is very low. Apparently your body reacts more strongly to that effect than most. I'll prescribe a potassium supplement for you."

You point out, with a bit of embarrassment, that the doctor mentioned nothing about heart problems when he prescribed the drug. You also ask if feeling abnormally good is another side effect. The doctor admits that these are side effects he didn't tell you about because he did not think them likely in your case. He tells you that he will reduce the dosage of steroid in a few days, and he devotes a lot of time to warning you about stomach irritation from the potassium supplement.

The point of the story is this: you'll have to *work* to get this much; your doctor should be able to give it to you. If he doesn't know, make him look it up. With in-office computer services for doctors now readily available, he can get the answer within seconds. Making him look up the answer will contribute to his continuing professional education, raise the general level of medical practice in the United States, and possibly save your life.

Let's continue with our list of criteria for being a more informed consumer. We believe you can feel fully informed if (and only if)

- You have a clear understanding of the doctor's criteria for the success or failure of a treatment — whether or not he expects a complete recovery, and if he does not, what improvement he hopes for. (More on this later.)

- You know the best that can be expected from the treatment you are receiving for a person of your age, sex, and general condition. Sometimes cures aren't possible, but it may be possible to make you much more comfortable. Doctors call treating a condition that can't be cured in order to make the patient more comfortable and better able to function "palliation." If you *both* understand what he's after, you will control your treatment much more effectively.

- You understand who will be in charge (you) if you are referred to a specialist and you've had a chance to make your own choice.

- If surgery is recommended, you have received a second opinion from someone who is not professionally or financially associated with the doctor who recommended the surgery.

- The doctor has disclosed any financial benefit he will receive from recommending a treatment or prescribing a drug. (The AMA code of ethics requires this, and state laws should.)

- You have made arrangements to ensure that your wishes are carried out if you are unable to remain in charge of your treatment.

- If you brought a friend to the visit with the doctor, does your friend feel comfortable on the above points.

Let's look at a hypothetical example. You have had arthritis for several years but have been taking aspirin and exercising as prescribed. You have been doing well in general, and you have been free of pain and stiffness most of the time. Now, suddenly, your right knee is almost too painful to move. You increase the dosage of aspirin as your doctor instructed you, but that doesn't seem to help. You call him, and he tells you to come to the office the next day. He looks at the knee, which is hot, red, and swollen.

He takes some blood for a test, suggests that you rest the knee as much as possible and splint it at night, and gives you a prescription for a nonsteroidal antiinflammatory drug (these drugs are like aspirin but much more powerful). The test results come back and show that you have rheumatoid arthritis on top of the osteoarthritis that was already damaging the knee. (Both forms of arthritis can damage joints. Rheumatoid arthritis is generally much more severe.) Various drugs for both forms of arthritis are tried without success. You develop stomach bleeding with one of the antiinflammatory drugs and have to be put on steroids for a short while. This produces a good deal of relief, but your doctor does not want to use steroids for any length of time. Finally, he recommends replacement of the knee with an artificial one. You ask why.

"You've effectively lost use of the knee," he says. "If we could get it quieted down for a while, we could work on some physical therapy and try to preserve enough function to let you at least walk. But we just can't do it. I think surgery is the only alternative." He gives you the name of an orthopedic surgeon, Dr. Konrad Kowboi, who has done numerous knee replacements.

You go to see the surgeon. He examines the knee and says he agrees that surgery is needed. He can do it on Wednesday, and he starts to ask his nurse to reserve a room for you at the hospital. You ask him to wait a minute. Doesn't he want to look at your X rays? Your medical record?

"No," he replies, "I trust Howard Fassnacht [your doctor] implicitly. If he says you need surgery, I'm ready to do it." You say that replacing a knee sounds like an awfully drastic step. What's involved?

"We just cut the old knee out, and put the new one in." You ask if you will be able to walk, to climb stairs, to ride your bike as you used to like to do.

"Sure. I'll make sure that you'll have no limitations." You are worried by the surgeon's offhand manner and tell him that you want a second opinion. He scowls. "My schedule fills up pretty fast, and that knee is deteriorating further every second. I might not be able to get you in when you absolutely have to have it." You stand firm and tell him that you will call him when you get a second opinion. You make some calls and get the names of doctors who will give second opinions. One of them is Vanessa Virtuevessel, an orthopedic surgeon in a group practice with three other surgeons at a local clinic. You call for a second opinion appointment. The nurse tells you that she will mail you a form to sign so that Dr. Fassnacht can release your records and X rays. When you go to the clinic, you discover that Dr. Virtuevessel has your chart spread out on her desk and X rays up on the light box. Even you can see that the knee doesn't look good. As she examines you, you explain that you were uncomfortable with the surgeon's breezy approach and too-deft answers.

Dr. Virtuevessel says, "I'm sorry that Dr. Kowboi made you feel uneasy. He's a bit like that sometimes. We surgeons sometimes cut first and ask questions later. But I think both Dr. Fassnacht and Dr. Kowboi are right. You've had reasonable trials of all the drugs you can tolerate. Your rheumatoid factor (a measure of how severe the disease is) is quite high. I think we ought to replace the knee."

You are immediately calmed by Dr. Virtuevessel's manner. You ask if she can do the surgery. She replies that as the source of the second opinion, she can't ethically do it. You ask her to recommend someone else. She tells you that any of the other two orthopedic surgeons in the group can handle knee replacements.

"You should understand," she adds, "that we're a partnership, and I will receive some of the surgery fee in the form of profits at the end of the year. We also rent space to a physical therapist. If you use him, I will receive some of the rent. If this makes you uncomfortable, I can recommend someone outside our group." You're impressed with her honesty and tell her that someone from the group will be fine — if they're good.

"Both of them are board-certified. We have their résumés on file with the nurse, if you want to see them." You ask if there are any statistics on their results. Dr. Virtuevessel makes a face. "The state just made us start keeping numbers on that. The nurse has the file." You ask about the usefulness of the new knee. Dr. Virtuevessel says that with good healing, you will eventually be able to walk and climb stairs and ride the bike, but you will have to set the seat high to avoid too much bending of the artificial knee.

You look at the statistics on her two partners. You notice that, even though both have good results, Dr. Norman Noscrub has had many more patients with postoperative infections than the other, Dr. Stanley Sterildrape. You decide on Dr. Sterildrape.

You ask Dr. Fassnacht to be in charge of your overall care in the hospital. You have filed a living will and want to make sure that your wishes are carried out if anything goes wrong. Since Dr. Fassnacht has agreed to your wishes, you want him in control of the team of doctors treating you. The hospital records him as the "physician in charge" on your case. Everything goes well, and after a few months of rehabilitation, you are back on the bike.

This is an idealized picture to some degree, but it represents what *should* happen when the patient and the patient's chosen doctor are in control, and nothing happens without their approval. If you don't feel that your situation meets these criteria, do not allow the doctor to pass go. Negotiate and, if you can't win, seek another doctor.

## The Doctor's Criteria for Success and Failure (and Yours)

This may seem to be a strange subject to raise. Don't doctors know when a treatment has succeeded or failed? Generally, yes. Aren't the criteria — what to look for — to determine success or failure set by the medical profession? Not at all.

We've all seen at least one television movie in which the life (or appearance, or sanity) of a patient was saved because one doctor kept on pushing after all his colleagues had given up. There is much truth in this fiction. Doctors are people, and they differ. Some of them will try any new thing that they read about in the medical journal that arrived yesterday afternoon. Others will not adopt new treatments until they feel that the treatment is completely proven and most other doctors have adopted them.

Some pore over the medical journals like pirates in search of buried treasure. Others have read nothing in years, choose their continuing education courses by the quality of the resort at which they are held, and sleep through the classes. Some prescribe with abandon, believing that "there's a pill for everything." Others are so afraid of the negative side effects of drugs in the elderly that they neglect drugs that could be useful. Surgeons think internists are unduly cerebral, and cautious to a fault. Internists think surgeons live by the motto "If it moves, cut it." One cardiologist may prescribe stopping smoking, losing weight, a walking program, and nitroglycerin tablets. Another may prescribe the same, plus a triple bypass.

Some strive to treat the whole person, and are satisfied with a patient who has avoided the risks of surgery and is handling his condition well on medical therapy. Others see no irony in the claim that "the operation was a success, but the patient died."

This wide variety of approaches is not necessarily bad (it gives you the option of shopping around), and it does not mean that doctors know nothing. It simply indicates that medicine is, as Lewis Thomas, M.D. wrote, "the youngest science." Various experts have estimated that it was not until somewhere between 1920 and 1950 that one had an equal chance of being helped or harmed by an encounter with a doctor. Before that, one was more likely to be harmed.

Medicine has also evolved (some would disagree about the choice of verb) into a bewildering variety of specialties and subspecialties. Most assume that if a patient has been referred to them (or has called for an appointment), choosing them was obviously the right thing to do, and they will plow ahead until it becomes obvious that they are not helping. "If you go to Midas, you get a muffler," is the way one doctor has put it.

Doctors respond to peer pressure (as do all people) and tend to practice like their colleagues. The gang at the hospital across town may have a completely different approach.

The upshot is that you have to find out what it is the doctor is trying to do for you, and tell him whether or not that is what you want. We can't stress one point strongly enough: *Nothing in a doctor's training equips him to make the choice for you. Nothing in his training makes him better able to make the choice than you can.* Doctors don't share their standards of success and failure with patients because they have never realized that you have your own standards. They are a parent, you are a child. The prejudices we described above get in the way, too. It's up to you to find out two things:

- What outcome does the doctor expect and accept?
- What are the alternatives?

A patient may feel that what the doctor has recommended — say, medical treatment and use of a portable oxygen tank — is a fine outcome, and preferable to the 20 percent risk of death, and the 15 percent risk of a worsened condition, attached to surgery. But the *doctor* may well have recommended this because success, for him, is keeping the patient out of the operating room. Another patient may decide that anything is preferable to being attached to an oxygen tank for the rest of his life, and will accept the doctor's recommendation for surgery. The *doctor* may have recommended this because, for him, success is avoiding dependence on oxygen. The reasons the doctor recommends a treatment may have nothing to do with the way *you* look at it.

People tend to think that because a doctor recommends something, he must know how to balance medical considerations with considerations of the "quality of life," based on some more or less objective set of values shared with the patient. Nothing could be further from the truth.

A doctor's education is usually exclusively in medicine or the sciences that make up the foundation for medicine, unless his undergraduate professors or the medical school has decided to help him be a more broadly educated human being somewhere along the line. The doctor may have no acquaintance with the humanities, with philosophy, with values, with literature, art, music, or history. The typical doctor is probably less well equipped to deal with issues of value and choice than the typical English major. The upshot: Find out what your doctor is thinking, and why — then make your own choices.

## How Sure of the Diagnosis Is the Doctor? How Did He Get to It?

Some diagnoses are obvious. Many are not. The diagnosis recorded at hospital admission is wrong about 40 percent of the time.[1] A portion of this admission diagnosis error rate reflects the current state of medicine and not necessarily a failing on the part of the doctor. (Even the suspicion of some diagnoses, such as a heart attack or a ruptured appendix, is a good reason to send someone to the hospital; tests done in the hospital may establish some other diagnosis as correct, but the decision to hospitalize, based on the knowledge the doctor had at the time, was correct.) Another portion is simply error, sometimes fatal error.

## Is Overtesting or Undertesting the Problem?

Autopsy results show that there is always a certain percentage of cases in which a diagnosis of an incurable, fatal disease is made when the correct diagnosis is a disease that is not fatal if treated. Since the diagnosis led to no treatment or only palliative treatment, the patients in these cases died unnecessarily. The few studies that have been done on this issue show that *the percentage of these types of cases has probably been rising over the last three decades.* It reached 10 percent of cases in a study done in the early 1980s. To put it in the most forceful terms possible: Misdiagnosis accounts for 10 percent of all deaths in which the patient died in the hospital. At least as measured by this

---

[1] Alan Brewster, M.D., personal oral communication. Other studies have shown diagnosis error rates of 10 percent to 81 percent, depending on study methods. See, for example, the studies cited in Charles B. Inlander, Lowell Levin, and Ed Weiner, *Medicine on Trial* (New York: Prentice-Hall, 1988), pp. 67–80.

kind of fatal mistake, the problem of misdiagnosis is getting worse, not better.[2]

What can you do to protect yourself and ensure that you get the best (and right) treatment? You need to get your doctor to share her diagnostic thinking with you. What else did she think you might have? What is in favor of the diagnosis she chose? How sure is she? What test results — if any — tipped the scales in favor of one diagnosis over another? How does the diagnosis affect the treatment? What else can she do to make the diagnosis more certain?

You can help deal with the problem of misdiagnosis by keeping several points in mind: First, symptoms may be real and troubling to you, but they do not necessarily indicate something that can be, or should be, medically treated. The labor that accompanies the birth of a child is painful, but pregnancy is not a disease. Many people have a tendency to "somatize" — to express problems in their lives as physical symptoms. The symptom can be reduced by drugs, but it will not go away until the problem is solved. An understanding friend may be better equipped to help than a doctor. Sometimes even talking to a pet may be of more value than everything in the pharmacy. It's ultimately up to each individual to know the difference. The doctor can only help, by communicating what the tests show.

The second point is this: Doctors talk about the "sensitivity" and the "specificity" of tests. "Sensitivity" refers to the ability of the test to detect *something*, regardless of what it is. "Specificity" refers to how accurately the test distinguishes between the various somethings that might be there. The ideal test is 100 percent sensitive — it detects something every time something is present — and specific to only one something. Every test in existence falls short of this ideal. Many, in addition to being less than 100 percent sensitive — that is, they miss something that is really there — give "false positives," — indicating that something is wrong when it isn't. Most are less than specific — they narrow the possibilities to a few things, assuming something is really there, but they don't tell which one. Example: Elevated amounts of enzymes produced by the liver can indicate that one has liver damage, or that one is taking one of the many drugs that harmlessly elevate the level of these enzymes.

Since perfect tests don't exist, doctors have to use the ones they have.

---

[2] H. H. R. Friederici and M. Sebastian, *Archives of Pathology Laboratory Medicine*, (June 1984): 521, cited in Inlander et al., *Medicine on Trial*, p. 72.

Almost all tests have some risk associated with them. So the dilemma arises: "For $200 worth of tests, and a small amount of risk, I am 97 percent sure of what this patient has. For $2,000 more, and more risk, I can be 99 percent sure. Is it worth it?"

Worth it for whom? You? The doctor? Her malpractice insurer? Many doctors say that they do more testing than they feel is wise simply to protect themselves from malpractice suits. Taken at face value, this means that *doctors think they are doing too many tests now. If they considered only their patients' welfare, they would do fewer.*

This suggests that the problem you face, as a patient, is not under-testing that may miss a diagnosis — even though the results from the autopsy studies we mentioned are disturbing. The danger you face is *overtesting.* Pennsylvania Blue Cross and Blue Shield apparently agree; they have decided to pay for some tests only in special situations.

What can you do to protect yourself?

- At each step of the process, ask your doctor why she is doing each test and what information she expects to gain from it.
- Ask her about the risks associated with it.
- Ask her how sure she is of the diagnosis now, and ask her to express it *in percentage terms.* If she says she is more than 50 percent sure, ask how sure she expects to be as a result of the test. If she indicates less than 85 percent certainty, ask *how* the test will narrow the diagnostic range.
- Most important, ask her why she can't make the diagnosis from your history alone.

Don't let her proceed until you're satisfied.

*Surgery and the Medical Alternatives; Medicine and the Surgical Alternatives*

Surgery is serious business. But so is medicine. Drs. Paul Gertman and Knight Steele did a study of **iatrogenesis** — doctor-induced illness — on a medical service (a division of a hospital that primarily offers one branch of medicine, such as internal medicine, cardiac care, or surgery) at the Boston University Hospital. They found that more than one-third of the patients had some doctor-caused illness, the severity ranging from mild to fatal. Nine percent had doctor-caused illnesses that were either disfiguring or life threatening. Two percent died. Gertman and Steele used very strict criteria for iatrogenesis and noted that their results probably underestimated the actual occurrence.

So medical treatment and surgery are both risky. Avoiding the danger is not a simple matter of staying out of the operating room. In negotiating the risks and benefits of both surgery and medical treatment, you need to figure out your doctor's reasoning, just as you had to do with the matter of diagnosis. Again, there are no right and wrong answers here that the doctor learned in medical school. Balancing the risks and benefits is ultimately your decision.

First you need to find out what your doctor thinks a good outcome is. You may be surprised at how little she will be satisfied with. (Example: Parkinson's disease, a disorder in which uncontrollable trembling and twitching of the hands and loss of coordination develops, is primarily a disease of those over 60. It can often be controlled with drugs, but these have significant side effects. With constant monitoring, and surgical therapy if necessary, most patients can achieve a high degree of control of symptoms. But they won't if the doctor considers reduction of hand tremors as the best possible outcome and does not work at balancing the drugs used, or consider surgery.)

After you've squared expectations with the doctor, you need to find out how beneficial, and how risky, the various medical and surgical alternatives are likely to be. This is your decision, not the doctor's. His job is to give you the facts. Even so, it's important to recognize that, overall, surgery is generally riskier than medical treatment. There is another virtue to the conservative approach that many internists take: it is usually, although not always, possible to proceed with surgery after a trial of medical therapy. The reverse may not be possible — the offending organ may have been removed.

You should understand the one big exception to this advice is **cancer**. For some **tumors**, medical therapy may be the best approach, but in general, it is best to remove suspected **malignancies** surgically as soon as possible. The primary reason is that cancers can **metastasize**, or spread throughout the body. Cancers that have metastasized are much harder to treat. The secondary reason is that tumors grow, and what can be a small operation that leaves an inconspicuous scar for a small tumor may turn into a major, disfiguring one if it is allowed to grow. Even here, the approaches taken by various experts may differ. What you need to know are the risks and benefits of each.

Let's say that you need surgery. The first thing you should do is find out all you can about the type of operation that will probably be used in your case. The books in appendix G, which are usually available in public libraries, will help.

The second thing you should do is obtain a second opinion for nonurgent, or **elective**, procedures. You should get this second opinion from someone other than the surgeon who will do the surgery and who is not connected financially with the doctor who recommended it. This is something you should ask about, even though the doctor should disclose any financial connection he has with the one who recommended surgery. You should obtain from the second physician the same sort of information you received (or tried to get) from the first: risks and benefits of the various courses of treatment.

You should seek a third opinion if the second opinion does not concur with the first. Find out why there is disagreement. Most often, there will be disagreement because the medical profession hasn't agreed on a right (or wrong) approach. But there may be doubt about the diagnosis. (Example: An internist feels a lump in your breast and suggests that you see a surgeon for a needle biopsy, an in-office procedure in which a fine, hollow needle is used to remove a tiny bit of tissue for examination. The surgeon can't feel the lump and suggests that you have a mammogram. The mammogram, as is usually the case with older women, shows all sorts of changes, none of them particularly benign and none of them clearly suggestive of cancer. The surgeon refers you back to the internist, who can feel no lump this time. Nothing has been established, you're worried, and both doctors are concerned and embarrassed. A third opinion, perhaps from an oncologist [a specialist in the treatment of cancer] could help.)

Suppose you decide on surgery. The job is still not finished. You should insist on seeing the **anesthesiologist** or **anesthetist** who will give the anesthesia. You should ask what he will do if the first approach, for some reason, does not work. (Example: The anesthetist decides on spinal anesthesia but can't get the needle into the spinal canal, so a general anesthetic is used instead.)

You should ask about preoperative sedation (a shot or pill to relax you before you go to surgery) and plans for repeating it if you do not get to the operating room on time. (Example: You are scheduled for removal of a portion of an enlarged prostate gland via a cystoscope [a hollow tube that can be inserted into the bladder through the penis, and through which an instrument can be used to remove diseased prostate and bladder tissue.] You have been very worried about this ever since the urologist [a surgeon specializing in operations on the kidneys, bladder, and urinary tract] described the procedure to you. You're told that you will be heavily sedated for this, and possibly out completely if you respond to the drug that way. You're given a shot and you spend a pleasant, dreamy hour lying on the gurney. An emergency case bollixes the operating room schedule and you are taken in two hours late — more awake than you've ever been in your life.)

The anesthesiologist or anesthetist will usually be happy to write an order for repeating the preop sedation *if* you remind him.

You should, of course, make him aware of any drug allergies that you may have. Sometimes an allergy to one drug means potential problems with a whole class of drugs.

The preoperative consent form that you will be asked to sign may have a clause in it allowing the surgeon to perform any procedure he deems necessary, after he gets "inside." Signing an operative consent this broad completely defeats all the careful effort that you have devoted to making sure that you stay in control of your treatment. Your surgeon has a pretty good idea of what he will find when he starts; if you discuss limiting the operative consent to those things *when you agree to surgery* (not when the consent form is handed to you in the hospital), he may be willing to eliminate the overbroad clause.

To sum up:


- Make sure you know what outcome from the surgery is expected and what can go wrong.
- Ask for the possible results in numerical terms — 85 percent chance of a good result, 15 percent chance of a bad one, and the like. Don't accept general reassurances like "everything will be fine."
- Don't sign a blanket operative consent.
- Insist on seeing the anesthesiologist. Let him know about allergies, make arrangements for repeating preoperative sedation, and make sure you understand what arrangements have been made for alternative anesthesia.


## Specialists

Today more doctors are specialists rather than generalists. The all-purpose doctor of yore is today a minority. There are at least two reasons for this: first, the specialties are far more lucrative than internal medicine, general practice, and family practice. Second, because the general fields are so broad, and an internist's training in particular overlaps those of other specialties, **residencies** in these fields are very demanding. (A residency is a period of time, usually three to five years, spent in training at a hospital before a doctor obtains certification from one of the numerous national medical boards that she is adequately trained in her field.) So is practice, once the doctor is into it. The fact is that one has much more control over one's time if one is an eye surgeon, limited to one type of treatment for one organ, than if one is an internist, whose purview is any nonsurgical treatment of anything.

As we noted earlier, the **fee-for-service system** is heavily biased in favor of procedures, discrete and well-defined things that a doctor can do, usually of a surgical nature. Cognitive skills, such as making the diagnosis that may avoid an unnecessary operation costing tens of thousands, are far less well rewarded. So the United States has too many surgeons and not enough generalists. The medical students go where the livin' is easiest.

You face different situations when you are referred to a specialist as an outpatient, and when you are hospitalized.

*Outpatient Referrals:* Some abuses of referrals have taken place under Medicare (and other insurance systems). The most common is called "Ping-Ponging," when a specialist and a generalist refer a patient back and forth between them, getting a fee at each visit while the patient flies across town like a Ping-Pong ball across the table. Generally, referral to a specialist on an outpatient basis should be for a *limited* term, and for either diagnostic testing treatment the generalist is not qualified to give or doesn't have the equipment for, or a consultation.

You can save yourself needless repeat testing, exposure to multiple X rays, and the like if you make sure that a copy of your medical record and test results (including X-ray films) is either mailed to the specialist in advance or given to you to take with you to the appointment. This is simple common sense, but it rarely happens. The specialist may have no more to go on than what was said in the initial phone call from your doctor. Insist that your records and test results get to the specialist no later than you do.

The simple answer is for you to obtain a *current* copy of your medical record. This is yet another case where patients have to do something the doctors should be doing in order to make sure it gets done at all. You have a definite right to your medical record in only a few states, and even then there are restrictions. We suggest that you find a consumer-oriented doctor who will request the records and then give you a copy. It's the simplest, cheapest, and fastest way.

If you are referred more than once to the same specialist, or to another specialist for what seems to be the same reason, stop your doctor and ask why the referrals are going on. Don't accept another one unless you are satisfied with the reasons. If your doctor is referring you because she genuinely does not feel competent to perform the service the specialist is providing, fine; a doctor who knows her limits is a wonderful thing. But if these are not the reasons, each referral is costing you unnecessarily, even if all the doctors involved take assignment. Again, you should be the judge and decide for yourself whether or not to see the specialist you're referred to.

*Specialists in the Hospital:* Your situation in the hospital is different. There are services and departments within hospitals, such as medicine, surgery, intensive care, trauma, geriatrics, and so on. Let's say that your doctor admits you for medical treatment of a problem. You are admitted under her care to the medical service, the part of the hospital that handles general problems that don't fall under some specialty such as obstetrics or psychiatry. If it is a teaching hospital, a corps of **residents**, senior medical students, and nurses in training will descend upon you. Many of them will be charged with some aspect of your care and will be reading your chart to carry out orders or writing more orders in your chart for others to carry out. If you don't have a personal physician in the area and have been admitted under the care of the house staff, you are fair game for all of the residents and all of the **attending physicians** on the service.

Additional testing reveals that you need surgery. You are transferred to the surgical service. Let's say that you have medical problems that are complicated enough to require continuing care by an internist, even as preparations for surgery go on. You will now have the residents and senior students of the surgical service on the case as well. An attending physician who is called in as a consultant and becomes interested in your case ("good teaching material") will stay on it, and bill for the visits that satisfy her curiosity, unless she is told to stay away by whoever's in charge (who may be hard to identify). The medical myth working here is that since every doctor works to the highest standard, and the hospital oversees them all, you are safe even if no one is obviously in charge, and the pharmacy computer is the only defense against incompatible and contradictory treatments.

Some hospitals have recognized that the situation we have described is fraught with risk. They are designating a "physician in charge" of each case who is supposed to coordinate everything done by everybody. If you, or someone who has your **power of attorney** (a legal document giving him or her the power to act for you in certain situations) in the event you are too ill to exercise control, are not in charge, *no one* may be.

Another reason one person should be in charge is to make sure that all of your doctors accept assignment; otherwise, you could find yourself responsible for additional out-of-pocket expenses up to the balance billing limit. In the earlier example on pages 143 and 144, you avoided an additional $265 out-of-pocket expense when the doctor accepted assignment and did not charge you the balance billing limit.

Without an advocate to negotiate assignment with your doctors, you could be responsible for thousands of dollars in additional out-of-pocket expenses.

## Advance Directives

Death and dying have always been major human preoccupations; many psychologists have noted that people (at least in developed Western countries, in the late twentieth century) spend the first half of their lives trying to deal with their adolescence and the last half trying to come to terms with death.

One of the more dubious achievements of late-twentieth-century medicine has been the development of the ability to delay death almost inevitably. It can be delayed long after a person has entered a **permanent vegetative state** and will never exercise any of the faculties that make him or her human again. Even after the **brain stem** has lost the ability to control breathing, even after the heart has lost the ability to beat on its own, "life" of a sort can be continued with **respirators and pacemakers**. The **artificial heart**, which may someday be used to keep potential organ donors "alive" indefinitely, can be called in if these fail. Some people resist all the technology and die anyway; one cynical physician has expressed it as "You die, but you die with your **electrolytes in balance**."

Doctors, who are often so ready to inject their value judgments into treatment decisions with no formal training to do so, have shrunk from it here. They have forced most decisions in this area into the courts, and the case law that is developing is quite clear: You *always* have a right to refuse treatment — of any sort — if you are mentally competent and have not fallen into the clutches of a hospital. This principle, at least, is well established: The competent individual can refuse to *begin* treatment. The cases that have garnered so much attention recently have been about stopping treatments already begun.

The evolving case law suggests that even "treatments" such as supplying food or water, which one or more of your doctors may regard as merely humane measures designed to comfort you, are not part of medical practice per se. If you are not mentally competent, the recent cases suggest, the wishes you expressed while alive must be respected. (Of course, expressing those wishes in a formal way via a **living will** or **durable power of attorney** can avoid a host of problems.)

*Quality of Life: Is It Worth the Living?*

Deciding how you want to be treated at the end of your life requires some imagination and rather fearless self-analysis. First, recognize that experience of illness and the medical world, for most people, is rather limited. One should not judge one's ability to accept pain on the basis of a visit to the dentist, with Novocain and nitrous oxide. Pain has heights that most people will never scale. (Ask anyone who has passed a kidney stone.) Relief for pain is limited to what the doctor feels he can prescribe without killing you. Whatever that dose is, the nurses will give less, because they are afraid of addiction, even if you have two weeks to live. An *extremely* painful condition is unlikely to be given adequate relief in a hospital. (A hospice is another matter. See chapter 7, page 221.)

Even if you are not in real pain, you may be acutely uncomfortable. A **nasogastric tube** that moves constantly and irritates the throat with each swallow, a dry mouth and cracked lips from being denied any more fluid than ice chips, a catheter that creates the sensation of having to urinate desperately even while it drains urine, and **intravenous lines** that prevent you from using your hands or bending your arms, plus the sensation of whatever incision you've had, even if there's no pain until you move, are triple-distilled misery. Add the pain of cancer and nausea from chemotherapy to the mix, and one has a "quality of life" that many would argue is not worth living unless there is the hope of a cure.

*Your Rights Right Now*

A 28-year-old **quadriplegic** woman suffering from severe cerebral palsy and arthritis sufficiently painful to require morphine, Elizabeth Bouvia, was in almost this same situation (substitute the pain of severe arthritis for the cancer), and she petitioned a California court to let her die. She was being kept alive by feedings through a **nasogastric tube**. She asked to have the tube removed, which would eventually lead to death by starvation. The hospital and her doctors refused. The California Second Circuit Court of Appeals ruled that, as an article in the *New England Journal of Medicine* paraphrased it, "a patient need not be comatose or terminally ill to refuse medical treatment, even when the treatment may be lifesaving and even when its absence may lead to an earlier death. The court added that the right to refuse medical treatment was virtually absolute and the patient's motives were not a matter for debate or decision by others" (*New England Journal of Medicine* 318 [1988]: 288).

The *Bouvia* case is important because it is the only one to date in which a conscious, coherent individual requested the withdrawal of medical treatment solely on quality of life grounds and was upheld in court. Other cases having to do with artificial feeding and **hydration** are important because they are rapidly establishing a judicial/medical consensus that, as the same article put it,

> *The focus of discussion should be the patient's wishes, not the type of treatment or the patient's **prognosis**. Artificial feeding can be viewed on a level with other medical interventions — **cardiopulmonary resuscitation**, mechanical ventilation, **dialysis**, and antibiotic therapy. It should not be considered a part of "ordinary care" or the routine provision of nursing care and comfort. Competent patients have the right to refuse this treatment after assessing for themselves the benefits and burdens. This right is not limited to comatose or terminally ill patients. For incompetent patients, feeding, like other treatments, can be stopped in accordance with the patient's previously expressed wishes.* (New England Journal of Medicine *318 [1988]: 288*)

This consensus is, however, an *emerging* one, not firmly fixed in law, and will probably be subject to much attempted cutting and trimming. For the moment, however, what these cases establish — after much needless suffering and expense on the part of the persons and families involved — is that courts in several states are inclined to view patients' own assessments of their quality of life as the deciding factor in refusing or stopping treatment. The Supreme Court's refusal to review one of these cases, *Brophy v. New England Sinai Hospital*, indicates that it would be inclined to agree. The *New England Journal of Medicine* paraphrased the court's decision this way:

> *The state had no duty to preserve life when the patient would feel that the means of doing so demeaned his or her humanity. Only Brophy could make decisions about the quality of his life — not physicians or third parties, including the court. . . . Even though he was not terminally ill, he had the right to refuse life-sustaining treatments, including artificial feeding . . . the discontinuation of Brophy's feeding would not represent suicide or direct killing, the court ruled, nor would it subject him to a painful death by starvation. Instead, it would merely allow the underlying disease to*

*take its natural course.* (New England Journal of Medicine *318* [1988]: 287)

Again, what applies to artificial feeding applies even more strongly to respirators and artificial hearts. *You have a constitutional right to refuse any medical treatment.*

Having the right does not mean that others will honor it. It is probably safe to assume that, in the current state of the law, you or your family will have to bear at least some legal expenses and needless anguish, if you do not take definite steps to make sure that your doctor knows your wishes and is willing to honor them.

Thanks to organizations such as Choice in Dying, every state now has legislation recognizing **advance directives** (living wills and durable powers of attorney for health care). These documents allow people to prepare for their future health care should they become unable to make their own medical decisions. Appendix H includes samples of the forms used in California, Florida, and New York. We suggest that you contact Choice in Dying at 800-989-WILL to obtain a free advance directives packet that complies with your state's law.

Given the current state of the law, we believe that you should both establish a living will and execute a durable power of attorney, giving control of decisions about your health care to a trusted friend or relative in the event you are no longer able to make them. The living will allows you to specify exactly what you mean, and doing both covers all bases. Phrases such as "no heroic measures" and "no artificial life support" are too vague to be enforceable on your doctors and the hospital and will in all likelihood land the matter back in court, which is what you want to avoid.

There is one area where you, the doctor, and the hospital will wind up talking the same language without much effort: "no code" orders. This means "Do no attempt cardiopulmonary resuscitation" — if your heart stops, let it stay stopped. You can specify to your doctor that you do or do not want a no-code order written. Perhaps the most relevant (and well-hidden) fact here is that only about 4 percent of patients who have cardiopulmonary resuscitation are discharged from the hospital alive. In that sense, contrary to what we see on television, it's a procedure that has a 96 percent failure rate.

In this chapter you will learn: How review agencies can get you into or keep you out of the hospital ▪ How to contact the Peer Review Organization in your area ▪ How to make an ally of your doctor ▪ How to request reconsiderations and appeals ▪ When to file a request for an expedited review ▪ How to request a hearing before an Administrative Law Judge

# 6. Medicare and Hospitals

The purpose of this chapter is to explain how to make sure you get what you are entitled to under Medicare from hospitals. Chapter 2 explained the diagnosis-related groups (DRG) system, which is the way Medicare currently makes payments to hospitals. Chapter 5 explained how to negotiate with your doctor and the hospital about your treatment. This chapter is a legalistic one, designed to show you how to make sure Medicare pays for the care you need.

## PROs and URCs

There is a lot of variation between regions of the country in the rate at which people of all ages are admitted to hospitals and in what they are admitted for. Research has shown that this has little to do with the demographics of the populations being served — with how old people are, how sick they are, and so on. It has much more to do with the practice patterns of the doctors in a community. It is also affected to some extent by the availability of hospital beds. For this and other related reasons, Medicare and the various providers of health insurance have been concerned to make sure that people stay out of the hospital if they don't really need to be there. They are also concerned with getting people out as soon as they are ready to go, either home or to a **skilled nursing facility (SNF)**.

The most recent study done on this subject, conducted by the RAND Corporation and reported in April 1988, showed that Medicare spends over $2 billion every year on unnecessary hospital care.

The mechanisms that Medicare uses to deal with this problem have accumulated over the years, the **Joint Commission on the Accreditation of Healthcare Organizations (JCAHO)** has added others, and the DRG system brought the **peer review organizations (PROs)** with it. These are layered on top of one another. For the first time in Medicare's history, the Peer Review Organizations are involved in deciding whether or not you can get into the hospital, as well as when you have to leave. And, of course, your doctor has a lot to do with whether or not you go into the hospital. We'll discuss the roles of each of these in turn.

*Your Doctor*
The medical profession is losing its control over American health care. Experts differ over whether this is a good or bad thing and about the extent of the loss. Most agree that it has happened because the medical profession is seen by many opinion leaders as having broken the "social contract" with society that gave it that control in exchange for selfless dedication to people's health. At the same time, technology has made it possible to render in the doctor's office or an **ambulatory surgery** center much care that formerly could be given only in a hospital. This has meant that there are new income opportunities for doctors. For example, they can operate on you in an ambulatory surgery center in which they have part ownership and receive fees for the use of the facilities that formerly would have gone to the hospital. Your doctor is being pulled in many different directions.

Generally, a doctor who wants to keep you out of the hospital is a good thing. What is important for you is that you understand what your options are and why the doctor is proposing to treat you outside the hospital.

According to the **American Medical Association's (AMA's)** code of ethics, the doctor is obliged to inform you if he is referring you to a facility that he partly owns or from which he derives a profit. This does not apply, of course, to treatment in his own office but to referral to an **ambulatory surgery** center, outpatient **radiotherapy** center, or **outpatient rehabilitation center.**

If he is performing surgery in his office or in an ambulatory surgery center, be sure to ask what you need to do to prepare for the operation and what you can do for pain relief afterward. One of the biggest complaints that patients have about ambulatory surgery concerns pain relief afterward. (The **procedure** itself is often more pleasant than it would be in the hospital.) You will usually be advised not to eat anything for several hours before the procedure and to have someone drive you home afterward if you will be given **sedation** or a **general anesthetic** of some sort. The most important thing to discuss is any reason why you think you should be treated in the hospital; make sure you understand his reasons and agree with them. You are always free to seek another doctor, even in a **health maintenance organization (HMO)** or **competitive medical plan (CMP)**.

In some cases, the peer review organization decides that a patient's surgery must be performed outside the hospital. We'll tell you what to do about that a little later.

The latest source of pressure affecting your doctor is the hospital's response to the DRG system. Remember that the hospital gets to keep any profit it makes on a case and must "eat" any loss. This has led to pressure on doctors from hospitals to admit as many patients as possible and, then, to get them out of the hospital as soon as possible. The result of these pressures is that Medicare patients are being discharged "quicker and sicker." There are a number of reasons to think that this is a good trend and that it might actually protect patients from the potential harm resulting from long hospital stays. It does represent a change from past practice and an additional pressure on your doctor.

## *Peer Review Organizations*

Medicare's latest attempt to control the costs and monitor the quality of health care for Medicare beneficiaries are the **peer review organizations (PROs)**. PROs are groups of doctors who have contracts with Medicare to review various aspects of treatment Medicare pays for. Usually, one PRO covers an entire state or a large portion of it. The idea is that the medical profession will remain self-policing, since the reviewers are doctors; at the same time, Medicare can obligate them to focus on what it considers to be problem areas through contracts. The PROs are supposed to work toward targets, such as: "Unnecessary hospital admissions should be reduced by 35 percent over the next two years." The key term for Medicare is "35 percent"; the key word for the doctors is "unnecessary." How the two perspectives work together determines what the PRO in a particular area is concentrating on at any given time. The areas currently under review around the nation include the following:

- Reviews of proposed hospital admissions for various procedures
- Reviews of lengthy hospital or skilled nursing facility stays
- Reviews of discharges, readmissions, and deaths

- Reviews of charts after discharge, to measure the appropriateness of admissions and the quality of care given

The **Health Care Financing Administration (HCFA),** which runs Medicare, is basically free to add review functions to PRO contracts whenever it sees a need to review some aspect of the quality of care paid for by HCFA programs, including Medicare. Depending on your diagnosis, the previous performance of your doctor and hospital, and the operations or procedures that are proposed for you, the PRO may be reviewing your care before, during, or after your treatment. We'll explain what to do in each situation.

*The Hospital Utilization Review Committee*

One of the requirements for hospitals to be accredited is to have a committee of doctors that looks at utilization of services, called (generically) **utilization review committees (URCs).** (Some hospitals give them slightly different names.) According to JCAHO rules, these committees are supposed to operate in the same manner regardless of who is paying for your care. To make matters even more confusing, the PRO can elect to delegate some or all of its review responsibilities for individual cases to the URC of a hospital, if it believes that the URC is performing well. So you may get a notice regarding your care, before or after you enter the hospital, from the URC, from the PRO, or from the UCR-acting-as-PRO. (The stationery the notice is on will be different.)

There are good reasons to have hospital URCs looking at care in addition to PROs. They are much better structured to deal with problems of individual doctors than the PROs, are closer to the scene, and can act more quickly. (Whether this makes a bit of difference depends on the internal politics of the hospital and how freely the URC is allowed to operate. In some institutions, it's a paper tiger.)

*Medicare Intermediaries and Carriers*

Medicare's **intermediaries** and **carriers** have review responsibilities, too, basically related to oddities that show up during their processing of claims. These functions overlap those of the PROs and the URCs to some extent.

*Your Retiree or Employee Insurance Plan*

Several years ago Congress made Medicare the *secondary* payer for Medicare beneficiaries who are still working and have health insurance through their employer or who have employer-provided retiree health insurance. This change made employers sit up and take notice of retiree health costs. Many have established preadmission and postadmission review procedures or hired firms to review the cost and quality of care they pay for. These may affect your hospital stay.

## Getting In: The First Hurdle

The various review bodies making decisions about whether or not you can go to the hospital at all are the following:

- Your doctor
- A reviewer for your employee or retiree health plan
- The hospital's utilization review committee
- The carrier or intermediary
- The peer review organization

In reading the rest of this section, it is important to remember that *only your doctor or the hospital utilization review committee, acting in accordance with medical staff bylaws, can deny your admission to the hospital.* The only thing the others can decide is whether they will pay for the hospital stay or the procedure. *You are always free to seek admission to the hospital if you think you need it.*

*Your Doctor*

If your doctor decides that you do not need hospital care, you can discuss it with him or find another doctor. There are no avenues of appeal that result in someone's giving your doctor an order to admit you against his will. You probably would not want to be treated by a doctor who is being forced to do something against his better judgment anyway. You can, of course, ask for a second opinion, and the doctor rendering it may be able to convince your doctor that you do need hospitalization. But remember — for most conditions, you're safer outside the hospital than in.

*Your Retirement or Employee Health Plan Reviewer*

If your employee or retiree health plan reviewer decides that the plan will not pay for hospital care, Medicare will still pay for what the employer plan does not cover as long as the services you need are Medicare-covered and medically necessary. *The employee or retiree health plan review has no effect on Medicare's decisions.* If this situation arises, we suggest that you contact your employer and your doctor. Your employee or retiree health plan will have some procedures for appeals, and you should pursue this channel first if your situation is not an emergency. The first rejection may have come from a computer, a nurse reviewer, a doctor, or a combination of all three. In cases that are appealed, most of the review entities make use of expert physician consultants to decide cases, in order to protect themselves from liability. A rejection of an appeal from one of these services generally is solid evidence that you do not need hospitalization. You should ask your doctor about the medical necessity for the treatment he proposes.

If your appeal is denied, you or your doctor should contact the Medicare **intermediary** or **carrier** and ask if there is a problem with the admission, given your (current or former) employer's refusal to pay. Generally, you will be told that Medicare will cover the treatment and that the carrier and your employer will fight it out later. This is a tricky area that is not exactly the responsibility of any one of Medicare's review agents right now. You should document all your contacts with your employer and the reviewer in writing. A suggested appeal letter is shown below.

**Sample Appeal Letter for Rejection of Admission Request by an Employee or Retiree Health Plan Reviewer**

Your name
Your street address
Your city, state and ZIP code

The date [Important!]
Office to which appeals are addressed
Street address
City, state, and ZIP code
ATTN: Proper person, if any

REFERENCE: Your employer/retiree medical plan number
Your medicare number

Dear Madam or Sir:

I have been advised that you have rejected my doctor's plans to hospitalize me for (name of condition, or operation, or both).

My physician, Dr. _____, feels strongly that I should be treated in the fashion he has suggested. I am attaching a letter from him, plus additional medical evidence (if any), in support of my request for a reconsideration of your decision.

I look forward to hearing from you.

Sincerely yours,
Your signature

Your doctor will usually handle such appeals for you, but you can strengthen the case for review and add pressure to the reviewers by acting on your own.

*The Hospital's Utilization Review Committee*

It is unlikely, but not impossible, that you will be informed that your admission to the hospital will not be accepted by the hospital's URC. There are really only two instances: In the first, the PRO has delegated review of proposed admissions and procedures to the hospital's URC. In the second, the URC will be reviewing your doctor's cases for admission because of some problems he has had with unnecessary admissions in the past, or — more rarely still — if the hospital's URC is reviewing all nonemergency admissions because of problems in the past or a PRO mandate. Hospitals are so hungry for bed-filling patients now that any hospital-initiated preadmission review is unlikely.

Two different situations need to be carefully distinguished here: if the hospital's URC is acting on its own, you essentially have no appeal. Your doctor's right to admit you is limited by the hospital's bylaws and the conditions of his membership in the medical staff. Generally these do not allow him to admit cases the URC says should not be admitted.

If the URC is acting as the agent of the PRO, things are different. *You have a right to appeal the PRO's decision.* We'll cover how in an upcoming section on PROs.

*Carriers and Intermediaries*

Carriers are insurance companies who have a contract with the Health Care Financing Administration to process Part B Medicare claims. Carriers also determine when a beneficiary has met the $100 Part B deductible. In addition, Carriers conduct reviews and hold hearings when claims are questioned by beneficiaries.

Intermediaries perform essentially the same function for hospital based services, and they also conduct reviews and hearings on Part A benefits.

*The Peer Review Organization*

As explained earlier, the PROs have been set up to measure, preserve, and, one hopes, improve the quality of care under Medicare. They can do anything within their contracts in this field that the Medicare law permits. The law permits them to deny you admission under the following circumstances:

- There is a problem with unnecessary admissions in your area and Medicare has contracted with them for a preadmission review service.
- You are scheduled to have one of the procedures for which second opinions, preadmission review, or outpatient surgery is required, and one or more conditions have not been met.

They can do nothing, in regard to Medicare patients, that their contracts do not call for.

If you are denied admission by a PRO preadmission review or by a decision that your operation must be done in an outpatient facility, you can request a reconsideration. The instructions at the end of this chapter explain how.

## Staying In: The Second Hurdle

People have the idea that they are supposed to stay in the hospital until they are completely well. The simple fact is that Medicare never intended this, and it isn't a good idea anyway. Medicare intended to pay for hospitalization only as long as it is **medically necessary** — that is, as long as the hospital is the only place you could receive the needed care. Most hospital patients are able to be discharged to a **skilled nursing facility (SNF)**, to **home health care,** or to their homes, after relatively short stays. Medicare will not pay for the nonmedical care of people who have limited ability to care for themselves, unless their conditions can be expected to improve with further medical treatment.

Only about 5 percent of older citizens are in an SNF or under custodial care in a nursing home at any one time. This figure reflects two facts: First, most older citizens are at least healthy enough to care for themselves, and second, most don't have the money for nursing homes, which can cost anywhere from $27,500 per year up to more than $50,000. Nursing homes are, in many cases, not the ideal solution for care of the chronically ill.

Not needing hospital care does not mean that you are completely well. It is likely that you will go home from the hospital needing some further recuperation. As we discussed in chapter 5, it is important to find out how well you can be and to make realistic plans within those limits. Being told that you are ready to be discharged should not be a crisis if you have discussed your situation with your doctor or have asked relatives to make provisions for your postdischarge care.

## The Effect of the Diagnosis-Related Groups System

As stated earlier, the only limit on your hospital stay is its **medical necessity.** You *cannot* be discharged for any of the following reasons:

- Because your care has cost more than the money amount of your DRG
- Because you have been in the hospital more days than the number of days assigned to your DRG

- Because your hospital has not requested **outlier** payments
- Because your hospital has not received outlier payments

*Only medical necessity* should govern your length of stay. When you go into the hospital, you are supposed to receive a notice telling you that you cannot be discharged "because your DRG has run out." A copy is shown on pages 181–182.

The same logic and the same procedures that we discussed above under *getting in* apply to *staying in*. We'll discuss the few differences for each of the following:

- Your doctor
- A reviewer for your employee or retiree health plan
- The hospital's utilization review committee
- The carrier or intermediary
- The peer review organization

*Your Doctor*

Discuss discharge plans with your doctor before you go into the hospital or as soon as possible after admission in an **emergency** or **urgent** situation. You should ask what course your care is likely to take, what might go wrong, what limitations on your ability to care for yourself you can expect after your hospitalization, and what plans you should be making for discharge. Asking these questions *now* puts you in control of the process to some extent.

*Your Employee or Retiree Health Plan Reviewer*

Just as is the case with admission, a decision by your employer or retiree health plan reviewer that hospital care is not needed has no effect on Medicare, as long as the care you need is covered by Medicare and is medically necessary. A finding by your employer health plan reviewer should alert you to the possibility that the PRO or the hospital's URC may find that your continued stay in the hospital is not medically necessary. Again, you should discuss the situation with your doctor and make plans for discharge if he does not seriously disagree with the reviewer.

*The Hospital's Utilization Review Committee*

The hospital's URC review of your case has no effect on Medicare *unless* the PRO has delegated review of continued hospital stays to it. If you receive a notice that your continued stay in the hospital is no longer needed, you have the right to request a reconsideration and to appeal if the reconsideration is not favorable. The last part of this chapter explains how.

## AN IMPORTANT MESSAGE FROM MEDICARE

### YOUR RIGHTS WHILE YOU ARE A MEDICARE HOSPITAL PATIENT

- You have the right to receive all the hospital care that is necessary for the proper diagnosis and treatment of your illness or injury. According to Federal law, your discharge date must be determined solely by your medical needs, not by "DRGs" or Medicare payments.

- You have the right to be fully informed about decisions affecting your Medicare coverage and payment for your hospital stay and for any post-hospital services.

- You have the right to request a review by a Peer Review Organization of any written Notice of Noncoverage that you receive from the hospital stating that Medicare will no longer pay for your hospital care. Peer Review Organizations (PROs) are groups of doctors who are paid by the Federal Government to review medical necessity, appropriateness and quality of hospital treatment furnished to Medicare patients. The phone number and address of the PRO for your area are:

_____

_____

_____

### TALK TO YOUR DOCTOR ABOUT YOUR STAY IN THE HOSPITAL

You and your doctor know more about your condition and your health needs than anyone else. Decisions about your medical treatment should be made between you and your doctor. If you have any questions about your medical treatment, your need for continued hospital care, your discharge, or your need for possible post-hospital care, don't hesitate to ask your doctor. The hospital's patient representative or social worker will also help you with your questions and concerns about hospital services.

### IF YOU THINK YOU ARE BEING ASKED TO LEAVE THE HOSPITAL TOO SOON

- Ask a hospital representative for a written notice of explanation immediately, if you have not already received one. This notice is called a "Notice of Noncoverage." You must have this Notice of Noncoverage if you wish to exercise your right to request a review by the PRO.

- The Notice of Noncoverage will state either that your doctor or the PRO agrees with the hospital's decision that Medicare will no longer pay for your hospital care.

   + If the hospital and your doctor agree, the PRO does not review your case before a Notice of Noncoverage is issued. But the PRO will respond to your request for a review of your Notice of Noncoverage and seek your opinion. You cannot be made to pay for your hospital care until the PRO makes its decision, if you request the review by noon of the first work day after you receive the Notice of Noncoverage.

   + If the hospital and your doctor disagree, the hospital may request the PRO to review your case. If it does make such a request, the hospital is required to send you a notice to that effect. In this situation the PRO must agree with the hospital or the hospital cannot issue a Notice of Noncoverage. You may request that the PRO reconsider your case after you receive a Notice of Noncoverage but since the PRO has already reviewed your case once, you may have to pay for at least one day of hospital care before the PRO completes this reconsideration.

**IF YOU DO NOT REQUEST A REVIEW, THE HOSPITAL MAY BILL YOU FOR ALL THE COSTS OF YOUR STAY BEGINNING WITH THE THIRD DAY AFTER YOU RECEIVE THE NOTICE OF NONCOVERAGE. THE HOSPITAL, HOWEVER, CANNOT CHARGE YOU FOR CARE UNLESS IT PROVIDES YOU WITH A NOTICE OF NONCOVERAGE.**

## HOW TO REQUEST A REVIEW OF THE NOTICE OF NONCOVERAGE

- If the Notice of Noncoverage states that your **physician agrees** with the hospital's decision:
  - + You must make your request for review to the PRO by **noon of the first work day** after you receive the Notice of Noncoverage by contacting the PRO by phone or in writing.
  - + The PRO must ask for your views about your case before making its decision. The PRO will inform you by phone or in writing of its decision on the review.
  - + If the PRO agrees with the Notice of Noncoverage, you may be billed for all costs of your stay beginning at noon of the day **after** you receive the PRO's decision.
  - + Thus, you will **not** be responsible for the cost of hospital care before you receive the PRO's decision.

- If the Notice of Noncoverage states that the PRO agrees with the hospital's decision:
  - + You should make your request for reconsideration to the PRO **immediately** upon receipt of the Notice of Noncoverage by contacting the PRO by phone or in writing.
  - + The PRO can take up to three working days from receipt of your request to complete the review. The PRO will inform you in writing of its decision on the review.
  - + Since the PRO has already reviewed your case once, prior to the issuance of the Notice of Noncoverage, the hospital is permitted to begin billing you for the cost of your stay beginning with the third calendar day after you receive your Notice of Noncoverage **even if the PRO has not completed its review.**
  - + Thus, if the PRO continues to agree with the Notice of Noncoverage, **you may have to pay for at least one day of hospital care.**

NOTE: The process described above is called "immediate review." If you miss the deadline for this immediate review while you are in the hospital, you may still request a review of Medicare's decision to no longer pay for your care at any point during your hospital stay or after you have left the hospital. The Notice of Noncoverage will tell you how to request this review.

## POST–HOSPITAL CARE

When your doctor determines that you no longer need all the specialized services provided in a hospital, but you still require medical care, he or she may discharge you to a skilled nursing facility or home care. The discharge planner at the hospital will help arrange for the services you may need after your discharge. Medicare and supplemental insurance policies have limited coverage for skilled nursing facility care and home health care. Therefore, you should find out which services will or will not be covered and how payment will be made. Consult with your doctor, hospital discharge planner, patient representative and your family in making preparations for care after you leave the hospital. **Don't hesitate to ask questions.**

ACKNOWLEDGMENT OF RECEIPT — My signature only acknowledges my receipt of this Message from (name of hospital) on (date) and does not waive any of my rights to request a review or make me liable for any payment.

_____              _____
Signature of beneficiary or                                                    (Date of receipt)
person acting on behalf of beneficiary.

*Patient
Self-
Determination
Act*

You must be advised of your right to make patient care decisions under the following circumstances:

- All adult individuals must be provided with written information about their rights under State law to make health care decisions, including the right to accept or refuse treatment and the right to execute advance directives.

- The descriptions of State law will be developed at the State level, through State agencies, associations, or other private not-for-profit entities. The federal law also does not override any State law which would allow a health care provider to object on the basis of conscience to implementing an advance directive.

- Hospitals, nursing facilities, and hospices must provide written information at the time of the individual's admission.

- Home health or personal care services must provide the information prior to providing care.

- Medicare- and Medicaid-certified prepaid health plans such as HMOs must provide the information upon enrollment.

- Document in patient's medical record whether he/she has signed the advance directive.

- Not discriminate against an individual based on whether he/she has executed an advanced directive.

- Provide staff and community education on advance directives.

For more information on advance directives, contact any Social Security office and request a copy of "Medicare and Advance Directives," HCFA publication 02175.

*The Peer Review Organization*

One of the jobs of the PRO is to review cases that have extended hospital stays. This review can be triggered in a number of ways. See the end of this chapter for instructions on how to appeal a decision not to pay for more time in the hospital.

The PRO's decision affects Medicare's payment for your hospital stay in the following way: you can stay in the hospital until the third day following the date you received the notice that your continued stay was no longer necessary. If you do not request a reconsideration, Medicare will cease payment on the third day following the notice. If you do request reconsideration and get a favorable ruling at any stage of the process, Medicare will pay for time spent in the hospital up until you are discharged or die. If you lose the appeal, you or your insurer must pay for these days.

There is an oddity in the law on this that you should be aware of. If you request an *expedited* reconsideration of the PRO's decision, it *may* come before the two days to which you would otherwise be entitled have passed. Some Medicare experts believe that this is not the result Congress intended. The moral of the story is that you should not request an expedited reconsideration unless you are unable to make reasonable plans for posthospital care in the event you lose.

## Making Sure Your Care Is Adequate

Making sure that you receive adequate care in the hospital is a subject that is beyond the scope of this book. There is, in fact, a book devoted exclusively to this subject: *Take This Book to the Hospital With You,* by Charles B. Inlander and Ed Weiner. We suggest that you read it. It contains valuable advice for any hospital stay, whether or not Medicare pays for it.

There is a temptation for hospitals to provide less than adequate care to Medicare beneficiaries. First, they are afraid that your care will cost more than the DRG for your condition(s) will pay. Second, they are afraid that they will not be able to maximize the profit they could make on the DRG. Right now, economic reality for hospitals is that they can make the most money by admitting you unnecessarily and then giving as little care as possible. This is the situation the PROs were set up to police. There are **perverse incentives** in any payment system, and the DRG system is better, from a number of angles, than the pay-for-each-day system that preceded it.

The key point to remember is that your status as a Medicare patient should make no difference. Hospitals make about 50 percent of their revenues from Medicare patients. The hospital needs you as much as you need it.

All this assumes, of course, that you know what good care is. This is something about which lay opinions have been disregarded in the past. The Hospital Patient's Bill of Rights (see appendix I) gives you an indication of what the hospital industry thinks you should think good care is. This document has no legal standing. We think that the PMS Code of Practice, located in appendix F, is better. Both should serve to give you some idea of an ideal you should expect your hospital care to live up to. We've discussed how to negotiate for the kind of hospital care you want in chapter 5.

## Controlling the Doctors

All the controversy about hospitals and Medicare makes us forget that it is ultimately the doctors who control the hospital, at least as far as medical care is concerned. There is a good deal of self-doubt in the profession about the way things are done now. You can see a wide sampling in *Medicine on Trial*, by Charles B. Inlander, Lowell Levin, and Ed Weiner. The material covered in that book is beyond the scope of this one.

We do want to mention one thing to watch out for, something that doctors regret but feel they can't control: the clinical "cascade." What happens is this: You go in for a relatively simple treatment, and you have a bad reaction to the dye used in a test, or something else goes not exactly according to your doctor's original plan. She asks a specialist to look at you. The specialist treats you for the bad reaction to the dye, but thinks he spots something else, so he orders some tests. They show a possible abnormality, you're in the hospital, so it might as well be checked out now, and . . .

All too soon you are the recipient of as much medical attention as the hospital can muster, being treated for reactions to treatments that were given because you had reactions to other treatments, with your admitting doctor somewhere in the background, peering over the shoulders of the specialists and house staff who have you surrounded.

The only one who can stop this is *you*, sad to say. You should question every treatment, and insist on knowing, at every moment, which doctor is primarily responsible for your care. You should negotiate for assignment with every doctor who treats you. If you need to ask whether or not you will be billed for a service, do so. Refuse it if the doctor will not take assignment, and ask whoever is in charge of your case to find someone who will.

If you are too ill to deal with this, we suggest that you give someone you trust, and who is willing to steer your care, a **durable power of attorney**. This was discussed at considerable length in chapter 5. A durable power of attorney will enable him or her to handle these matters for you.

Remember:

- You have a right to the same quality medical care as anyone else the hospital serves.
- You have the right to refuse services you do not want.
- You have the right to leave the hospital, even against medical advice.

## Reconsiderations and Appeals

This section covers how to obtain reconsideration of the following:

- Decisions about hospital care by the peer review organizations
- Decisions about payment for hospital care
- Decisions about payment of doctor's bills

*Peer Review Organization Decisions*

The PRO is involved in determining the following:

- Whether or not Medicare will pay for your hospital admission
- Whether or not Medicare will pay for your continued stay in the hospital
- Whether or not Medicare will pay for your admission to a skilled nursing facility
- Whether or not Medicare will pay for your continued stay in a skilled nursing facility
- Whether or not Medicare will pay for an outpatient procedure to be done in the hospital
- Whether or not Medicare will require a second opinion before paying for surgery

*Key Points:*
- In all your dealings with the peer review organizations, there is one issue only: the *medical necessity* of your being cared for at all, or the *medical necessity* of your being cared for *in the way your doctor wants to do it*. All other issues are extraneous. Stay focused on this point.

- There is a great deal of uncertainty in medicine. It is unlikely that what your doctor wants to do is totally unreasonable. You and he should emphasize *why* it is acceptable as good medical care.

- Keep copies of everything you send to the PRO. It is advisable to send materials *certified mail, return receipt requested.* This gives you proof of the date you mailed material and the date on which the PRO (or other recipient of your papers, such as your Social Security district office) received it.

- If you are dealing with a decision that your continued stay is no longer medically necessary, make sure you understand when Medicare will no longer pay for your hospital stay.

- A PRO review of care that you have already had *never* requires you to pay for it. You cannot retroactively be required to pay for care you've already received, unless you can reasonably be expected to have known that it wasn't covered. (See chapter 2 for more information on this.)

*Procedure*

The procedure that follows is *generic.* It applies to all actions by the PROs. Only the evidence submitted would differ.

*Notices:* Your denial is called a Notice of Noncoverage, and it will explain why something is being denied.

If you receive such a notice *while you are in the hospital,* it's important to understand that there are two tracks possible. If you are asking the *PRO* to review the hospital's decision, you are not responsible for services received before you get the notice of the PRO's decision. If you are asking the PRO to rethink its own decision, the hospital may start billing you beginning with the third calendar day after you received the Notice of Noncoverage. If the PRO does not reverse its position and you decide not to stay in the hospital, you may have to pay for the third day. If you decide to stay, you are responsible for the further cost of your care.

*How to Appeal (Request a Reconsideration) of a Peer Review Organization Decision:* You can appeal the decision of the PRO by filing a request for reconsideration with the PRO itself, at the address for the PRO shown on the notice you received; at any **Social Security office**: or at a Railroad Retirement Board office, if you are a railroad retirement beneficiary.

Your doctor and the hospital also have the right to file an appeal. They do *not* have the right to an "expedited reconsideration" that you have.

*Time to File the Request for Reconsideration:* You must file your request for reconsideration within sixty days of the date you receive the notice of denial. Unless you can prove otherwise, the notice is deemed to have been received by you five days after the date on it. (Example: The notice is dated January 5. You are deemed to have received it on January 10, unless you can prove you received it later. Your sixty-day period for appeal started on January 10. The last day you can file an appeal is March 10, the sixtieth day after the deemed receipt of the notice.) Some more examples of how the dates run are provided below.

| Time Periods for Filing Requests for Reconsideration | | |
| --- | --- | --- |
| NOTICE OF NONCOVERAGE MAILED | DEEMED RECEIVED | LAST DAY TO FILE REQUEST |
| January 2 | January 7 | March 7 |
| March 15 | March 20 | April 17 |
| November 27 | December 1 | January 29 (of next year) |

*"Good Cause" for Late Filing:* Generally, you will be allowed to file late if there is what the PRO considers to be "good cause" for it. The regulations are very broad, and it is hard to see what exactly might count. The regulations give examples such as serious illness, a death in the family, failure to receive information you had requested before the sixty-day limit, a misunderstanding of what the PRO notice told you, and so on.

*Obtaining Information:* Both you and your doctor have a right to see the information on which the PRO based its decision. You should ask for this when you file your request for reconsideration. You may add to the information anything you or your doctor want to add.

*Expedited Reconsideration and Time Limits:* You can request that the PRO make an expedited review or reconsideration of the denial. How fast "expedited" has to be depends on the circumstances:

- Within three working days if you are still a patient in the hospital (this doesn't really apply here, of course, since you're trying to get in)
- Within three days if the initial determination was a denial of hospital admission and you are still in the hospital

- Within ten working days if you are in a skilled nursing facility
- Within thirty working days in all other situations, and in every situation where someone other than you files the appeal. Having expedited redetermination available is a very important reason for *you* to file the appeal and have the doctor or hospital submit information as part of an appeal.

***What to Include:*** You should file your claim using HCFA Form 2649, which is shown on page 190. Other forms for other situations are also shown:

- HCFA HA501.1 — Request for a Hearing on Part A Claims. This form is used to request a hearing if you are not satisfied with the results of your request for reconsideration.
- HCFA 1964 — Request for Reconsideration on Part B Claims. This is used initially to request a reconsideration of a denial for services under Part B, doctor insurance. It is analogous to the 2649.
- HCFA 1965 — Request for Hearing on Part B Claims. Like the HA501.1, this is used to request a hearing if you are not satisfied with the results of your request for reconsideration.

You never have to use these forms, but using them will help you record all the information you need. You can supplement them with a letter if you wish.

You can request an appeal with just a letter, but using the form will ensure that you include everything that is needed. You should ask your doctor to provide medical documentation. It is important for both you and your doctor to focus on the issue at hand, and not editorialize. The general issue you will be dealing with in PRO denials of admission is the *medical necessity* for you to be hospitalized at all, to have a procedure done in the hospital, or to have it done at all. Keep the focus on these issues. They will boil down to appropriate medical judgment. Your doctor will probably want to submit information regarding your condition, plus evidence from the medical literature indicating that what the PRO wants done is unwise.

***Notices and Appeals:*** When the PRO provides you with its reconsidered decision, it must do so *in writing* and inform you of the following:

- The decision
- The reasons for it

DEPARTMENT OF HEALTH, EDUCATION, AND WELFARE
HEALTH CARE FINANCING ADMINISTRATION

Form Approved.
OMB No. 066-R-0067

# REQUEST FOR RECONSIDERATION OF PART A HEALTH INSURANCE BENEFITS

INSTRUCTIONS: *Please type or print firmly.* Leave the block empty if you cannot answer it. Take or mail the WHOLE form to your Social Security office which will be glad to help you. Please read the statement on the reverse side of page 2.

| 1. BENEFICIARY'S NAME | 2. HEALTH INSURANCE CLAIM NUMBER |
|---|---|
| | |

3. REPRESENTATIVE'S NAME, IF APPLICABLE

(☐ RELATIVE  ☐ ATTORNEY  ☐ OTHER PERSON)  ☐ PROVIDER FILING

## 4. PLEASE ATTACH A COPY OF THE NOTICE(S) YOU RECEIVED ABOUT YOUR CLAIM TO THIS FORM.

5. THIS CLAIM IS FOR
☐ INPATIENT HOSPITAL  ☐ SKILLED NURSING FACILITY (SNF)  ☐ HEALTH MAINTENANCE ORGANIZATION (HMO)
☐ EMERGENCY HOSPITAL  ☐ HOME HEALTH AGENCY (HHA)

| 6. NAME AND ADDRESS OF PROVIDER *(Hospital, SNF, HHA, HMO)* | CITY AND STATE | PROVIDER NUMBER |
|---|---|---|
| | | |
| 7. NAME OF INTERMEDIARY | CITY AND STATE | INTERMEDIARY NUMBER |
| | | |

| 8. DATE OF ADMISSION OR START OF SERVICES | 9. DATE(S) OF THE NOTICE(S) YOU RECEIVED |
|---|---|
| | |

10. I DO NOT AGREE WITH THE DETERMINATION ON MY CLAIM. PLEASE RECONSIDER MY CLAIM BECAUSE

_____

_____

_____

_____

_____

11. YOU MUST OBTAIN ANY EVIDENCE *(For example, a letter from a doctor)* YOU WISH TO SUBMIT.

☐ I HAVE ATTACHED THE FOLLOWING EVIDENCE:
_____

☐ I WILL SEND THIS EVIDENCE WITHIN 10 DAYS:
_____

☐ I HAVE NO ADDITIONAL EVIDENCE OR OTHER INFORMATION TO SUBMIT WITH MY CLAIM.

13. ONLY ONE SIGNATURE IS NEEDED. THIS FORM IS SIGNED BY:
☐ BENEFICIARY  ☐ REPRESENTATIVE  ☐ PROVIDER REP.

SIGN HERE ▶

14. STREET ADDRESS

12. IS THIS REQUEST FILED WITHIN 60 DAYS OF THE DATE OF YOUR NOTICE?
☐ YES  ☐ NO

IF YOU CHECKED "NO" ATTACH AN EXPLANATION OF THE REASON FOR THE DELAY TO THIS FORM.

CITY, STATE, ZIP CODE

| TELEPHONE | DATE |
|---|---|
| | |

15. If this request is signed by mark (X), TWO WITNESSES who know the person requesting reconsideration must sign in the space provided on the reverse side of this page of the form.

## DO NOT FILL IN BELOW THIS LINE — FOR SOCIAL SECURITY USE — THANK YOU

16. ROUTING
☐ INTERMEDIARY
☐ HCFA, RO-MEDICARE
☐ BSS, ODR

18. SSA OR INTERMEDIARY DATE STAMP

17. ADDITIONAL INFORMATION

FORM **HCFA-2649** (8-79  FORMERLY SSA-2649)
DESTROY PRIOR EDITIONS

INTERMEDIARY

Page 1 of 4

# REQUEST FOR HEARING
## PART A HEALTH INSURANCE BENEFITS

### Take or mail original and all copies to your local Social Security office.

| | |
|---|---|
| CLAIMANT'S NAME | CLAIM FOR<br>☐ Hospital Services<br>☐ Extended Care Facility Services<br>☐ Home Health Agency Services<br>☐ Emergency Services |
| WAGE EARNER'S NAME (Leave blank if same as above) | |
| HI CLAIM NUMBER | PERIOD IN QUESTION<br>FROM:       TO: |
| NAME AND ADDRESS OF INTERMEDIARY | NAME AND ADDRESS OF PROVIDER |

I disagree with the determination made on the above claim and request a hearing before a hearing examiner of the Bureau of Hearings and Appeals. My reasons for disagreement are: (additional pages may be added if necessary.)

Check one of the following:

☐ I have additional evidence to submit.
(Attach such evidence to this form or forward to the Social Security Office within 10 days.)

☐ I have **no** additional evidence to submit.

Check <u>ONLY ONE</u> of the statements below.

☐ I wish to appear in person before the hearing examiner.

☐ I waive my right to appear and give evidence, and hereby request a decision on the evidence before the hearing examiner.

Signed by: (Either the claimant or representative should sign-Enter addresses for both. If claimant's representative is not an attorney, complete Form SSA-1696)

| | |
|---|---|
| SIGNATURE OR NAME OF CLAIMANT'S REPRESENTATIVE<br>☐ ATTORNEY ☐ NON-ATTORNEY | CLAIMANT'S SIGNATURE |
| ADDRESS | ADDRESS |
| CITY, STATE, AND ZIP CODE | CITY, STATE, AND ZIP CODE |
| TELEPHONE NUMBER | DATE: | TELEPHONE NUMBER |

Claimant should not fill in below this line

Is this request filed within 6 months of the reconsideration determination?  ☐ Yes    ☐ No

If "No" is checked: (1) attach claimant's explanation for delay, (2) attach any pertinent letter, material, or information in the Social Security Office.

## ACKNOWLEDGMENT OF REQUEST FOR HEARING

Your request for a hearing was filed on_____at_____

The hearing examiner will notify you of the time and place of the hearing at least 10 days prior to the date which will be set for the hearing.

| | | |
|---|---|---|
| Hearing Examiner Copy | TO:<br>☐ Hearing Examiner _____ (Location) | For the Social Security Administration |
| Claim File Copy | TO:<br>☐ BHI, Reconsideration Branch<br><br>☐ BHI, Regional Office _____<br>(Only emergency services in other than Federal Hospitals) | By:_____<br>(Signature)    (Title)<br><br>_____<br>(Street Address)<br><br>_____<br>(City)  (State)  (ZIP Code) |
| | Interpreter Needed_____ (Language) | _____Servicing District Office Code_____ |

Form HA 501.1
(2-72)

HEARING EXAMINER

DEPARTMENT OF HEALTH AND HUMAN SERVICES
HEALTH CARE FINANCING ADMINISTRATION

Form Approved
OMB No. 0938-0033

## REQUEST FOR REVIEW OF PART B MEDICARE CLAIM
### Medical Insurance Benefits - Social Security Act

NOTICE—Anyone who misrepresents or falsifies essential information requested by this form may upon conviction be subject to fine and imprisonment under Federal Law.

**Carrier's Name and Address**

The name and address of the
Carrier for your state will
be listed in this space.

**1** Name of Patient

**2** Health Insurance Claim Number

**3** I do not agree with the determination you made on my claim as described on my Explanation of Medicare

Benefits dated:

**4** MY REASONS ARE: *(Attach a copy of the Explanation of Medicare Benefits, or describe the service, date of service, and physician's name—NOTE.—If the date on the Notice of Benefits mentioned in item 3 is more than six months ago, include your reason for not making this request earlier.)*

_____

_____

_____

_____

_____

_____

_____

**5** ☐ I have additional evidence to submit. *(Attach such evidence to this form)*

☐ I do not have additional evidence.

COMPLETE ALL OF THE INFORMATION REQUESTED. SIGN AND RETURN THE FIRST COPY AND ANY ATTACHMENTS TO THE CARRIER NAMED ABOVE. IF YOU NEED HELP, TAKE THIS AND YOUR NOTICE FROM THE CARRIER TO A SOCIAL SECURITY OFFICE, OR TO THE CARRIER. KEEP THE DUPLICATE COPY OF THIS FORM FOR YOUR RECORDS.

**6**                    SIGNATURE OF **EITHER** THE CLAIMANT **OR** HIS REPRESENTATIVE

| Representative | Claimant |
|---|---|
| ➡ | ➡ |
| Address | Address |
| City, State, and ZIP Code | City, State, and ZIP Code |
| Telephone Number | Date | Telephone Number | Date |

Form **HCFA-1964** (1-78) (Formerly SSA-1964)          **CARRIER'S COPY**                    (over)

DEPARTMENT OF HEALTH AND HUMAN SERVICES
HEALTH CARE FINANCING ADMINISTRATION

Form Approved
OMB No. 0938-0034

## REQUEST FOR HEARING - PART B MEDICARE CLAIM
### Medical Insurance Benefits - Social Security Act

NOTICE—Anyone who misrepresents or falsifies essential information requested by this form may upon conviction be subject to fine and imprisonment under Federal Law.

| Carrier's Name and Address | **1** Name of Patient |
|---|---|
| The name and address of the Carrier for your state will be listed in this space. | |
| | **2** Health Insurance Claim Number |

**3** I disagree with the review determination on my claim, and request a hearing before a hearing officer of the insurance carrier named above.

MY REASONS ARE: *(Attach a copy of the Review Notice. NOTE.—If the review decision was made more than 6 months ago include your reason for not making this request earlier)*

**4** Check one of the Following:

☐ I have additional evidence to submit. *(Attach such evidence to this form or forward it to the carrier within 10 days.)*

☐ I do not have additional evidence.

Check <u>Only One</u> of the Statements Below:

☐ I wish to appear in person before the Hearing Officer.

☐ I do not wish to appear and hereby request a decision on the evidence before the Hearing Officer.

**5** EITHER THE CLAIMANT OR REPRESENTATIVE SHOULD SIGN IN THE APPROPRIATE SPACE BELOW:

| Signature or Name of Claimant's Representative ➡ | Claimant's Signature ➡ |
|---|---|
| Address | Address |
| City, State, and ZIP Code | City, State, and ZIP Code |
| Telephone Number | Date | Telephone Number | Date |

*(Claimant should not write below this line)*

### ACKNOWLEDGMENT OF REQUEST FOR HEARING

Your request for a hearing was received on _____. You will be notified of the time and place of the hearing at least 10 days before the date of the hearing.

| Signed | Date |
|---|---|

Form **HCFA-1965** (8-79) (Formerly SSA-1965)

**CARRIERS COPY**

- A statement of the effect the decision has on what Medicare will pay for or has paid for
- A statement of your appeal rights, with complete instructions for filing the appeal

When you receive a notice of a reconsidered decision that is not in your favor, consider whether you want to request a hearing. A hearing is more formal than a reconsideration, and it entitles you to appear before an **administrative law judge (ALJ)**. If you do request a hearing, it is wise to have a lawyer involved. Hearings can involve subpoenaing witnesses and other legal steps. It is less formal than a court case, but far more formal than a request for reconsideration. Medicare is emphasizing doing all business possible, including hearings, over the phone. Although a hearing can be conducted over the phone, you should carefully consider appearing in person. It is sometimes easier to make your case in person, depending on the circumstances.

Only you, not your doctor or the hospital, have this right. The rules for filing an appeal are exactly the same as for filing for reconsideration with the PRO — sixty days, counted from five days after the date of the notice, and all that. You should file your appeal on HCFA HA-501-US, unless the information you received with the PRO's Notice of Reconsideration tells you to do something else.

The first thing the ALJ will attempt to determine is whether or not the controversy involves at least $200 (with the price of health care these days, it almost surely will). If the ALJ determines that the amount is less than $200, he will notify you and any other concerned parties that he has determined this and that they have fifteen days to show why he is wrong. If no evidence is submitted within fifteen days, the request for a hearing is dismissed. (You will not have to worry about this if you don't receive such a notice.)

You will be notified by the ALJ of the date of the hearing at least ten days before it is filed.

If the ALJ's decision is unfavorable, you can appeal to the Social Security Appeals Council. Your attorney can tell you how to do this. The Appeals Council does not take all the appeals addressed to it. If $2,000 or more is at issue, you can appeal an Appeals Council decision, or the ALJ's decision if the Appeals Council refused a hearing, to the federal courts. This must be done within sixty days of the date of the Appeals Council decision on your case, or its decision not to hear it.

*Requesting Reconsiderations on Payment*

The procedures in this section apply to denial of payment for all services, other than doctors' services, after you have left the hospital. They also apply to notices regarding hospital care that you receive from the Medicare intermediary while you are in the hospital.

*Notices:* Your notice of denial will come either in the form of an **Explanation of Medicare Benefits (EOMB)** or in the form of a letter. In any case, it must be in writing. It will explain the reason that something is being denied. A typical EOMB is shown on pages 132–133.

*How to Appeal (Request a Reconsideration) of a Payment Denial or Intermediary Determination that Care Is Not Medically Necessary:* You can appeal the PRO decision by filing a request for reconsideration with the intermediary itself, at the address shown on the EOMB, at any Social Security office, or at a Railroad Retirement Board office, if you are a railroad retirement beneficiary, or at any office of the **Health Care Financing Administration.**

Your doctor and the hospital have the right to file an appeal only if you do not plan to do so and you certify this in writing on a form they will provide. They do *not* have the right to an "expedited reconsideration" that you have.

*Time to File the Request for Reconsideration:* You must file your request for reconsideration within sixty days of the date you receive the notice of denial. Unless you can prove otherwise, the notice is deemed to have been received by you five days after the date on it. (Example: The notice is dated January 5. You are deemed to have received it on January 10, unless you can prove you received it later. Your sixty-day period for appeal started on January 10. The last day you can file an appeal is March 10, the sixtieth day after the deemed receipt of the notice.)

*Request for Extension of Time to File:* If you need more than sixty days to file your appeal, you can request more time at any Social Security office, Medicare office, or the Railroad Retirement Board. You cannot file an extension request with an intermediary. You will be notified in writing of the time granted you.

*"Good Cause" for Granting a Time Extension:* Generally, you will be allowed to file late if there is what the PRO considers to be "good cause" for it. The regulations are very broad, and it is hard to see what

exactly might count. The regulations give examples such as serious illness, a death in the family, failure to receive information you had requested before the sixty-day limit, a misunderstanding of what the PRO notice told you, and so on.

*Obtaining Information:* Both you and your doctor have a right to see the information on which the PRO based its decision. You should ask for this when you file your request for reconsideration. You may add to the information anything you or your doctor want to add.

*Expedited Reconsideration:* There is a procedure for expedited appeals under Part A (hospital insurance), but it may be used only if both the person appealing and the secretary of Health and Human Services (HHS) agree that the only issue is a constitutional one. This is a rare situation.

*What to Include:* You should file your claim using HCFA Form 2649. You can request an appeal with just a letter, but using the form will ensure that you include everything that is needed. You should ask your doctor to provide medical documentation. It is important for both you and your doctor to focus on the issue at hand, and not editorialize. The general issues you will be dealing with are as follows:

- The medical necessity of the service
- Whether or not Medicare covers it
- Whether or not you are entitled to it
- Whether or not the amount paid is what ought to have been paid

Medical necessity issues will boil down to appropriate medical judgment. Your doctor will probably want to submit information regarding your condition, plus evidence from the medical literature that indicates that the decision is unwise.

*Time Limits:* The regulations provide no time limit for a decision on a Part A request for reconsideration.

*Notices and Appeals:* When you are provided with the reconsidered decision, it will include, in writing, the following:

- The decision
- The reasons for it

- A statement of the effect the decision has on what Medicare will pay for, or has paid for
- A statement of your appeal rights, with complete instructions for filing the appeal

When you receive a notice of a reconsidered decision that is not in your favor, consider whether you want to request a hearing. A hearing is more formal than a reconsideration, and entitles you to appear before an ALJ. If you do request a hearing, it is wise to have a lawyer involved. Hearings can involve subpoenaing witnesses and other legal steps. It is less formal than a court case, but far more formal than a request for reconsideration.

Only you, not your doctor or the hospital, have this right. The rules for filing an appeal are exactly the same as for filing for reconsideration — sixty days, counted from five days after the date of the notice, and all that. You should file your appeal on HCFA HA-501-US, unless the information you received with the Notice of Reconsideration tells you to do something else.

You may request a hearing only if the amount in controversy is $100 or more.

You should also note that your request for a hearing will be deemed received *five days* after the date on it, unless you can show that it was received earlier. If you are within five days of the sixty-day limit, send it *certified mail, return receipt requested,* so you will have proof of the date it was actually received.

The first thing the ALJ will attempt to determine is whether or not the controversy involves at least $100 (with the price of health care these days, it almost surely will). If the ALJ determines that the amount is less than $100, he will notify you and any other concerned parties that he has determined this and that they have fifteen days to show why he is wrong. If no evidence is submitted within fifteen days, the request for a hearing is dismissed. (You will not have to worry about this if you don't receive such a notice.)

You will be notified by the ALJ of the date of the hearing at least ten days before it is filed.

If the ALJ's decision is unfavorable, you can appeal to the Social Security Appeals Council. Your attorney can tell you how to do this. The Appeals Council does not take all the appeals addressed to it. If $1,000 or more is at issue, you can appeal an Appeals Council decision, or the ALJ's decision if the Appeals Council refused a hearing, to the federal courts. This must be done within sixty days of the date of the Appeals Council decision on your case, or its decision not to hear it.

If you receive a favorable determination, Medicare will pay its usual amounts for the services rendered. If you do not receive a favorable determination, you pay.

In this chapter you will learn: What Medicare covers under skilled nursing care ▪ How Medicaid can help pay for nursing home care ▪ What to look for when selecting long-term-care insurance ▪ How to evaluate a nursing home ▪ What home health care services are covered

# 7. Nursing Homes, Home Health Care, and Medicare

The nursing home business is a $60-billion-per-year industry. Of the nation's 36 million citizens aged 65 and above, 2.3 million (6.5 percent) live in nursing homes. The average cost of a year's stay is $27,500. The average stay, 465 days, costs $34,875. The average charge is around $75 per day. The Brookings Institution, a Washington think tank, estimates that by the year 2018, almost 8 percent of the elderly will live in nursing homes, at an annual cost of $55,000.

We explained in chapter 3 that Medicare does not, as many people think, pay for nursing homes. It does pay for **skilled nursing facilities** (**SNFs**) care, but only for 100 days per calendar year. What follows is a brief summary of the explanation of coverage in chapter 3.

Care in a SNF is less intense than that you received in a hospital, but more intense than that provided in **intermediate care facilities** (**ICFs**) or custodial care. ("Custodial care" is defined as the provision of room, board, and personal services, generally on a long-term basis, without additional medical services such as those provided by SNFs and ICFs. Some facilities provide all three levels of care — skilled, intermediate, and custodial — in the same building or in different buildings on the same grounds.)

Many of the services listed under hospitals are covered under SNFs.

The exceptions are services that SNFs do not normally provide, such as operating rooms. Medicare permits small hospitals (fewer than 100 beds) that have empty beds to run a SNF within their walls, using beds that have been designated as **swing beds**. Swing beds are used as SNF beds or as hospital beds, depending on which are needed.

You are entitled to 100 days of SNF care during each benefit period. Medicare pays all costs for the first 20 days; however, you are responsible for the copayment of $95 per day, beginning on the 21st through the 100th day. Medicare also picks up any additional charge above the $95. From the 101st day on you are responsible for all costs.

Medical necessity is *the* key issue in payment for SNF services. The SNF regulations go to great lengths to define what is and is not SNF care. The key is that care complex enough to require the services of a nurse or skilled rehabilitation personnel is covered; care that you could do yourself is not. But complications may require SNF-level care, even for situations that would normally not be covered. Basically, SNF care is rehabilitation; if your condition cannot be expected to improve as a result of SNF care *and* you do not need observation by skilled personnel, your care will not be covered. Obviously, what your doctor writes in the chart makes a big difference in what gets covered. If you are worried about coverage of SNF services, discuss this with your doctor.

## Do You Really Need a Nursing Home?

Nursing homes can cost anywhere from $27,500 per year up to more than $50,000. Medicaid, another state/federal program that provides health care, does pay for nursing homes, but the price may be the loss of substantial amounts of assets and income. The old law virtually guaranteed that the spouse who stayed at home would have to impoverish him- or herself to pay for the care of the spouse in the nursing home. Legislation passed in 1988 greatly reduces the burden but can still lead to a substantial loss of assets.

- In any month in which a married person is in a nursing home, no income of the at-home spouse is to be considered available to the spouse in the nursing home.

- Income is considered the property of the person to whom it is paid. Income paid to both spouses is attributed 50 percent to each.

- The home, household goods, and personal effects of both spouses are not counted in considering Medicaid eligibility.

- All assets other than these will be counted and divided in two. If the at-home spouse has less than $15,000, the spouse in the nursing home may transfer assets to him or her to make up to $15,000 available to the at-home spouse. (States may, at their option, raise this figure to any amount less than $76,000. The $15,000 amount will be indexed to inflation.)

- The assets that remain in the name of the spouse in the nursing home are considered available to pay for his or her nursing home care. All assets in excess of $76,000 are attributed to the spouse in the nursing home and are considered available to pay for nursing home care.

- States must allow nursing home residents to retain certain sums for medical expenses not covered by Medicare or Medicaid before contributing to the expense of their nursing home care. The states may place "reasonable limits" on the amounts spent.

- States must allow the at-home spouse sufficient income from the other spouse to bring total household income of the at-home spouse to at least 150 percent of the federal poverty level for a two-person household. States will not be required to allow more than $1,918 per month, except by court order or change in regulation.

These changes greatly ease the situation of the spouse who remains at home, but if assets and income are substantial, one may be forced to use most of them to pay for a nursing home before becoming eligible for Medicaid. Even after one is eligible, the income of the spouse who remains at home is limited.

Purchasing long-term-care insurance may be an option; however, always investigate fully before you purchase any policy. Make sure it covers the type of care you are most likely to require. Before discussing how to choose a nursing home, we want to raise a question that is rarely asked: *Do you really need a nursing home?* It is true, of course, that some older people are crippled by arthritis, have Alzheimer's disease, or have another form of senile dementia that makes it impossible for them to live without constant supervision; others have another problem that requires constant, round-the-clock custodial care. These people are only about 5 percent of the elderly. (There are, of  ourse, others who are cared for by a spouse or other relative.) The majority of the over-65 population seems to do quite well without nursing home care.

In our experience, many older people think they need nursing home care because they are no longer able to do one or a few of the things they did when they were young. If you are no longer able to drive, this does not mean  ou need a nursing home — it means you need transportation. If you are unable to cook, this does not mean you need a nursing home — it means you need someone to prepare meals for you. Most of the elderly face difficulties that are no more severe than those faced by younger handicapped people who are able to live independently.

Part of the reason many older people think they need a nursing home if they are no longer able to do everything they used to do is that they share society's prejudice against the aged. A problem that is a handicap heroically overcome in a 35-year-old is an infirmity that demands that a 65-year-old be tucked away in a nursing home — or so people think. We discussed some of these prejudices as they affect your dealings with your doctor in  hapter 5. We suggest you read that section "The Doctor's Obligation to Inform You Fully" again. Are you, perhaps, prejudiced against the elderly yourself?

The Health Status Checklist on page 203 will help you assess the level of care that you (or an aged relative) need. In using it, think very carefully about the person's level of functioning. If you're not sure, put a question mark. On items with a question mark, you may want to seek some professional advice in evaluating the person's capabilities.

Caring for a bedridden, elderly person can be a full-time job. The caregiver must be on the lookout for the development of pressure sores (decubitus ulcers), incontinence, dehydration, malnutrition, development of contractures from too little limb movement, and the unusual drug reactions that are common in the elderly.

For those who are not bedridden, adult day care, home health care, homemaker services, sharing a home with other elderly people, Meals on Wheels, shopping services, and adult foster care may be alternatives that will avoid a nursing home stay. For the availability of these services, you can check with your local agency on aging, the medical social services office of the hospital (if the person is in the hospital awaiting discharge), and departments of social services. Many are listed in the telephone book under the names we've used above, for example, "shopping services."

## Health Status Checklist*

Read each statement *very carefully* before deciding if it applies to the person in question, then place a check mark in front of those that describe the person's condition. Think in terms of *"Does this person have difficulty with"*:

_____ 1. *Bathing* — Requires assistance from another person

_____ 2. *Continence* — Difficulty in controlling either the bladder or bowels

_____ 3. *Dressing* — Either requires assistance or does not dress at all

_____ 4. *Eating* — Requires assistance, either from a person or via tube or intravenously

_____ 5. *Mobility* — Either requires the assistance of a person to walk or is confined to chair/bed

_____ 6. *Using toilet room* — Either requires assistance from another person or does not use one at all

_____ 7. *Speech* — Either completely lost or is so severely impaired that it can be understood only with difficulty (person cannot carry on a normal conversation)

_____ 8. *Hearing* — Either completely lost or so impaired that only a few words a person says or loud noises can be heard

_____ 9. *Vision* — Either blindness or so severely impaired that television cannot be seen eight to twelve feet away (features of a familiar person can be recognized within two to three feet)

_____ 10. *Mental status* — Cannot understand (or remember) simple instructions, requires constant supervision or restraints for his or her own safety

*Suggested by the Department of Health and Human Services, Long-term Care Survey.

## Paying for Custodial Care in a Nursing Home

As we have seen, Medicare does not cover care in a nursing home that is custodial, or nonmedical, in nature. Two alternatives may help you pay for custodial care if you really need it: Medicaid and private nursing home insurance.

*Medicaid*

The Medicaid program provides medical care for the poor. It was tacked onto the Medicare bill at the last possible second, and its passage by Congress, together with Medicare, amazed it advocates. The program still shows the features of its hasty design.

Medicaid is intended for the very poor who have nowhere else to turn, but not all of the very poor are covered. It is a state-run program that receives federal funds. States make many of the rules, and the trend in recent years has been to make Medicaid requirement more stringent. Congress recently liberalized them for persons who need nursing home care.

- In any month in which a married person is in a nursing home, no income of the at-home spouse is to be considered available to the spouse in the nursing home.

- Income is considered the property of the person to whom it is paid. Income paid to both spouses is attributed 50 percent to each.

- The home, household goods, and personal effects of both spouses are not counted in considering Medicaid eligibility.

- All assets other than these will be counted and divided in two. If the at-home spouse has less than $15,000, the spouse in the nursing home may transfer assets to him or her to make up to $15,000 available to the at-home spouse. (States may, at their option, raise this figure to any amount less than $76,000. The $15,000 amount will be indexed to inflation.)

- The assets that remain in the name of the spouse in the nursing home are considered available to pay for his or her nursing home care. All assets in excess of $76,000 are attributed to the spouse in the nursing home and are considered available to pay for nursing home care.

- States must allow nursing home residents to retain certain sums for medical expenses not covered by Medicare or Medicaid before contributing to the expense of their nursing home care. The states may place "reasonable limits" on the amounts spent.

- States must allow the at-home spouse sufficient income from the other spouse to bring total household income of the at-home spouse to at least 150 percent of the federal poverty level for a two-person household. States will not be required to allow more than $1,918 per month, except by court order or change in regulation.

The current regulations require that the assets and income of *your* spouse and your parents be considered in determining your eligibility for Medicaid, with few exceptions. This is a very important point: Your spouse and parents do not *actually* have to give anything toward the cost of your care, but your *eligibility* is determined as though they do. The exact requirements, as well as the amount of assets and income you may retain and still be eligible, vary from state to state, because of the latitude allowed by the federal government in setting some of the income and assets limits. Check the list of Medicaid state offices in appendix N to find out where to call to determine the exact eligibility requirements for your state.

You are automatically eligible for Medicaid if you are eligible for, or receiving, **Supplemental Security Income (SSI)** payments for aged, blind, and disabled, but you must apply at a state welfare office. If you meet the requirements for SSI, there is little chance that you would have to give up additional income or assets to qualify for Medicaid.

If your income, less certain deductions and medical bills, is within certain (low) limits, you may be eligible for Medicaid as medically needy. You must "spend down" to pay medical bills to the point at which you are eligible; after that, Medicaid pays for medical bills as long as you are eligible.

Medicaid services in some states are more restrictive than Medicare services. If the service you are receiving is covered under Medicare and not Medicaid, Medicaid will not pay the Medicare copayments and deductibles applicable to that service. Otherwise, it will, although there may be additional limits. To find out if you are eligible for Medicaid, apply at any state welfare office. The welfare office is required to take your application and make a formal determination of eligibility even if you are told that you are not eligible.

When you apply, you should bring proof of age, financial status, and any disability you may have. The proof of financial status should include bank statements for checking and savings accounts, rent or mortgage payment receipts, loan papers for your car or the title to it, any documents relating to stock or bond ownership, and check stubs for any regular payments you receive. You should also have the amount of your Social Security check, if you receive Social Security payments. You should always have your Social Security number. Bring your medical bills, or copies of them, for the last year.

When you call the welfare office for your appointment, ask what is needed. This will save you a delay in getting your eligibility determined and perhaps avoid another trip.

You can transfer your assets to someone other than your spouse (for example, to a child) in order to become eligible for Medicaid, but you must have done so before you become eligible for Medicaid (time frames vary by state). The exception to this is the division-of-assets provision designed to protect the financial interests of the at-home spouse. Under it, the spouse who is entering the nursing home can transfer assets up to $15,000 (or higher, if a state elects, with a limit of $76,000) to the spouse who is staying at home. Outside this provision, if you want to transfer your assets in order to become eligible for nursing home coverage under Medicaid, *you should do so only with the services of a lawyer who understands the Medicaid program.* This is both to protect you and to ensure that you actually will be found eligible for Medicaid, based on the action you took. There is no point in transferring assets only to find that you are still not eligible.

This translates into what we've said before: *You should explore all other alternatives before deciding to enter a nursing home.*

*Private Insurance for Nursing Home Care*

In early 1987 there were only two companies offering nursing home insurance. Today there are more than one hundred. Now for the bad news: *Many of them exclude so much that you may be paying more than $100 per month for unusable coverage.*

The May 1988 issue of *Consumer Reports,* a highly respected magazine that rates various products and accepts no advertising, cut through a great deal of confusion by offering a set of features that should be found in a good policy. These are as follows:

- The policy should provide a daily nursing-home benefit of at least *$80.*
- The waiting period before benefits begin should be no more than *20 days.*
- The maximum benefit period should be at least four years for one stay. If no time period is given, the dollar ceiling per benefit period should be at least 1,460 (365 days × 4) times the daily benefit.

- The maximum benefit period for all stays should be *unlimited.*
- It should pay full benefits for **skilled nursing facilities (SNF), intermediate care facilities (ICFs)**, and custodial care.
- If there is a rule requiring that you be in a hospital before entering the nursing home, *coverage should begin within thirty days after a hospital stay of three days or more.*
- It should pay *home care benefits.*
- These should be paid *without* requiring a prior nursing home or hospital stay.
- It should have *waiver of premium,* which means that you need not pay premiums while you are in a hospital or nursing home. (You may have to pay extra for waiver of premium, but it should be available at least as an option.)
- It should be *guaranteed renewable for life.*
- The policy should specifically state that *Alzheimer's disease is covered.*
- The premium should stay *level for life.*
- The *Best's rating* of the company should be *A* or *A+.* (Best's is a service that, among other things, assesses the financial health of insurance companies.)

*Consumer Reports* did not recommend a premium, which varies with the age of the policyholder. The magazine recommends that if the insurance salesperson does not provide adequate answers, ask for a specimen policy. If he or she will not provide one, write the company, ask for one, and give the salesperson's name and address. If they will not send one, look for another company.

Some other points to watch out for:

- The policy may say that the premium is level for life but actually permit increases if the company applies for one covering all the insured, or all the insured in one state. Ask about this.

- Find out if the company can decide whether or not you qualify for payments (usually on the basis of medical necessity). If so, what are your appeal rights?

- Find out how many nursing homes in your state the policy will pay for. Some policies pay only for selected homes.

- Find out whether or not a need for nursing home care caused by a pre-existing condition is covered. It almost surely will not be covered in full. The question is, how bad are the restrictions? A waiting period during which Medicare will pay for the nursing home (remember, **skilled nursing facility** only), after which the policy picks it up, is not bad. A two-year exclusion is too much; nursing home stays last an average of 465 days, or 1.3 years.

Finally, resign yourself to the fact that no policy currently offered has adequate inflation coverage. No policy *Consumer Reports* reviewed had an unlimited daily benefit. The Brookings Institution has estimated that private insurance will cover only 7–12 percent of nursing home expenses in the year 2018, and that, at best, no more than half of the elderly will buy nursing home coverage.

*Consumer Reports* advises that no one under 60 buy a nursing home policy unless it offers some definite way to cover cost increases due to inflation. For those over 60, policies should be bought only by those who have more than modest assets. The rest of us should rely on Medicaid for nursing home coverage.

## Selecting a Nursing Home

You can begin the process of selecting a nursing home by eliminating those you know you don't want to use. Don't consider nursing homes that are as follows:

- Too far away to allow visiting by relatives and friends
- Too expensive
- Not properly certified or licensed
- Not offering the medical or other services needed
- Unsuitable for some other reason, such as being owned by a religious denomination with which you do not want to associate

You can find out whether or not a home is properly certified or licensed by contacting the state agencies regulating nursing homes that are listed in appendix K at the back of this book.

Pages 209–214 contain a checklist for use in reviewing up to four nursing homes at one time. We suggest that you copy it (on a photocopying machine) for use on a clipboard as you review homes in your area.

When you examine the checklist closely, you will note that some of the questions are starred. These questions can be answered only by your own observations.

Remember that you don't necessarily have to answer every single question on this checklist. You should try very hard to answer the ones that are important to you. If you forget to ask something important during your visit, you can always call later and try to get the answer.

However, if you find that you didn't observe something important, the only way to get the answer is to schedule another visit. The best thing to do is to look over the checklist carefully before you end each interview you have during your visit, to make sure you have asked and answered all the relevant starred questions. Then look over the rest of the questions before you end your tour, to make sure that you have seen everything you need to see to answer them. *We suggest that you don't rely on memory. Circle the answer to each question as you observe/ask it.*

## NURSING HOME CHECKLIST

| THE BUILDING AND GROUNDS | NURSING HOMES | | | |
|---|---|---|---|---|
| | A: | B: | C: | D: |
| **Outside** | | | | |
| 1. Is the building neat and well maintained? | Y N | Y N | Y N | Y N |
| 2. Does it appear fireproof? (Wood-framed buildings can be dangerous.) | Y N | Y N | Y N | Y N |
| 3. Are the sidewalks clean and well maintained? | Y N | Y N | Y N | Y N |
| 4. Do the sidewalks have wheelchair ramps? | Y N | Y N | Y N | Y N |
| 5. Does the entrance have handrails and wheelchair ramps? | Y N | Y N | Y N | Y N |
| 6. Is the home located within easy walking distance of public transportation? | Y N | Y N | Y N | Y N |
| 7. Are the grounds spacious? | Y N | Y N | Y N | Y N |
| 8. Are they well maintained? | Y N | Y N | Y N | Y N |
| 9. Is there an area where patients can sit? | Y N | Y N | Y N | Y N |
| 10. Do they sit outside (weather permitting) or otherwise use the outside area? | Y N | Y N | Y N | Y N |
| **Inside** | | | | |
| 11. Is the lobby clean and well furnished? | Y N | Y N | Y N | Y N |
| 12. Do residents use the lobby? | Y N | Y N | Y N | Y N |
| 13. Are the corridors well lighted and wide enough for two wheelchairs to pass easily? | Y N | Y N | Y N | Y N |
| 14. Does there seem to be enough room in general for the residents? | Y N | Y N | Y N | Y N |
| 15. Are emergency exits well marked? | Y N | Y N | Y N | Y N |
| 16. Is there an emergency lighting system? | Y N | Y N | Y N | Y N |
| 17. Is there an actively functioning safety committee? | Y N | Y N | Y N | Y N |
| 18. Is fire-fighting equipment (such as fire extinguishers) prominent? | Y N | Y N | Y N | Y N |
| 19. Are there sufficient smoke detectors? | Y N | Y N | Y N | Y N |

| THE BUILDING AND GROUNDS | NURSING HOMES | | | |
| | A: | B: | C: | D: |
|---|---|---|---|---|
| **Rooms** | | | | |
| 1. Are the rooms neat and clean? | Y  N | Y  N | Y  N | Y  N |
| 2. Is there sufficient light? | Y  N | Y  N | Y  N | Y  N |
| 3. Are there curtains on the windows? | Y  N | Y  N | Y  N | Y  N |
| 4. Do all the rooms open on a hallway? | Y  N | Y  N | Y  N | Y  N |
| 5. Do residents hang their own pictures? | Y  N | Y  N | Y  N | Y  N |
| 6. Is there sufficient closet space? | Y  N | Y  N | Y  N | Y  N |
| 7. Does each resident have a sink and mirror? | Y  N | Y  N | Y  N | Y  N |
| 8. Is there counter space for personal objects? | Y  N | Y  N | Y  N | Y  N |
| 9. Is the room nicely furnished? | Y  N | Y  N | Y  N | Y  N |
| *10. Is the room air conditioned? | Y  N | Y  N | Y  N | Y  N |
| *11. Do the rooms have individual thermostats? | Y  N | Y  N | Y  N | Y  N |
| *12. Is there an adjoining bathroom? | Y  N | Y  N | Y  N | Y  N |
| *13. Are the bathrooms shared by no more than four residents? | Y  N | Y  N | Y  N | Y  N |
| *14. Do residents have a choice between single and jointly shared rooms? | Y  N | Y  N | Y  N | Y  N |
| 15. In general, do residents have enough personal space? | Y  N | Y  N | Y  N | Y  N |
| *16. Are procedures for changing roommates liberal and clearly spelled out? | Y  N | Y  N | Y  N | Y  N |
| *17. If the rooms have television sets, are they equipped with earphones? | Y  N | Y  N | Y  N | Y  N |
| 18. Do the beds have bedspreads? | Y  N | Y  N | Y  N | Y  N |
| 19. Are there grab bars on the toilet and bathtub? | Y  N | Y  N | Y  N | Y  N |
| 20. Do the tubs have nonslip surfaces? | Y  N | Y  N | Y  N | Y  N |
| 21. Do bathrooms and toilet areas have sufficient privacy? | Y  N | Y  N | Y  N | Y  N |
| 22. Do the rooms have private telephones? | Y  N | Y  N | Y  N | Y  N |
| **Personnel** | | | | |
| * 1. Does the home's administrator have a current license? | Y  N | Y  N | Y  N | Y  N |
| 2. Was the administrator or his or her representative courteous to you? | Y  N | Y  N | Y  N | Y  N |
| 3. Did he or she see you promptly? | Y  N | Y  N | Y  N | Y  N |
| 4. Were the home's administrative policies well explained? | Y  N | Y  N | Y  N | Y  N |
| 5. Was the administrator open to your questions? | Y  N | Y  N | Y  N | Y  N |
| * 6. Does the home employ: | | | | |
| a. a physical therapist? | Y  N | Y  N | Y  N | Y  N |
| b. an occupational therapist? | Y  N | Y  N | Y  N | Y  N |
| c. a speech pathologist? | Y  N | Y  N | Y  N | Y  N |

| THE BUILDING AND GROUNDS | NURSING HOMES | | | |
|---|---|---|---|---|
| | A: | B: | C: | D: |
| d. a dietitian? | Y  N | Y  N | Y  N | Y  N |
| e. a nurse practitioner? | Y  N | Y  N | Y  N | Y  N |
| * 7. Is the nursing supervisor an R.N.? | Y  N | Y  N | Y  N | Y  N |
| * 8. Are all the head nurses R.N.'s? | Y  N | Y  N | Y  N | Y  N |
| 9. Do there seem to be enough nurses, nurse's aides, and orderlies on duty? | Y  N | Y  N | Y  N | Y  N |
| 10. Was the staff generally friendly toward you? | Y  N | Y  N | Y  N | Y  N |
| 11. Were they neatly dressed? | Y  N | Y  N | Y  N | Y  N |
| 12. Did the residents seem at ease with the staff? | Y  N | Y  N | Y  N | Y  N |
| 13. Did the staff speak to the residents in respectful, noncondescending terms? | Y  N | Y  N | Y  N | Y  N |
| 14. Did the staff seem to like the residents? | Y  N | Y  N | Y  N | Y  N |
| 15. Did the staff generally have pleasant expressions on their faces? | Y  N | Y  N | Y  N | Y  N |

**Medical/Nursing Care**

| | A: | B: | C: | D: |
|---|---|---|---|---|
| * 1. Is a physician on the premises for a fixed period of time each day? | Y  N | Y  N | Y  N | Y  N |
| * 2. Is a physician on call in case of emergency? | Y  N | Y  N | Y  N | Y  N |
| * 3. Is a registered nurse on duty during the day, seven days a week? | Y  N | Y  N | Y  N | Y  N |
| * 4. Is at least one R.N. or one L.P.N. on duty day and night? | Y  N | Y  N | Y  N | Y  N |
| * 5. Are dental services provided in the home itself? | Y  N | Y  N | Y  N | Y  N |
| * 6. Are there facilities outside of the residents' rooms for physical examinations? | Y  N | Y  N | Y  N | Y  N |
| * 7. May the resident select his or her own physician? | Y  N | Y  N | Y  N | Y  N |
| * 8. May the resident select his or her own hospital? | Y  N | Y  N | Y  N | Y  N |
| * 9. Does the home have a contract with an ambulance service? | Y  N | Y  N | Y  N | Y  N |
| *10. Does the home have access to a pharmacist who maintains records on each resident and reviews them when new medications are ordered? | Y  N | Y  N | Y  N | Y  N |
| *11. Is the family allowed to make alternative arrangements for purchasing prescription drugs? | Y  N | Y  N | Y  N | Y  N |
| *12. Are arrangements made for patients who wish to use alternative professional services such as podiatrists or chiropractors? | Y  N | Y  N | Y  N | Y  N |
| *13. Does the home make arrangements for private duty nurses when the family thinks one is required? | Y  N | Y  N | Y  N | Y  N |
| *14. Does the home have policies that severely restrict the use of physical restraints? | Y  N | Y  N | Y  N | Y  N |
| *15. Are the majority of the residents free of physical restraints? | Y  N | Y  N | Y  N | Y  N |

| THE BUILDING AND GROUNDS | NURSING HOMES | | | |
|---|---|---|---|---|
| | A: | B: | C: | D: |
| 16. Are the rooms and halls free of any smell of human excrement? | Y   N | Y   N | Y   N | Y   N |
| 17. Do they smell of heavy perfume? | Y   N | Y   N | Y   N | Y   N |
| 18. Does each resident have a call button within easy reach? | Y   N | Y   N | Y   N | Y   N |
| 19. Can it be turned off only at the patient's bed? | Y   N | Y   N | Y   N | Y   N |
| 20. Are there call buttons in the bathrooms and bathing areas? | Y   N | Y   N | Y   N | Y   N |
| 21. Does each resident have a water container and clean glass in his/or her room? | Y   N | Y   N | Y   N | Y   N |
| 22. Are the more inactive residents' fingernails trimmed, and are the men cleanly shaved? | Y   N | Y   N | Y   N | Y   N |
| *23. Does the home keep its own medical records? | Y   N | Y   N | Y   N | Y   N |
| *24. Does the resident (or resident's family) have access to them? | Y   N | Y   N | Y   N | Y   N |

**Recreational/Social Arrangements**

| | | | | |
|---|---|---|---|---|
| * 1. Does the home employ a full-time social director? | Y   N | Y   N | Y   N | Y   N |
| * 2. Are residents permitted to entertain visitors in their rooms? | Y   N | Y   N | Y   N | Y   N |
| * 3. Are visiting hours liberal? | Y   N | Y   N | Y   N | Y   N |
| * 4. Are residents given reasonable leeway in establishing when they go to bed? | Y   N | Y   N | Y   N | Y   N |
| * 5. Are members of the opposite sex permitted to visit one another in their rooms with the doors closed? | Y   N | Y   N | Y   N | Y   N |
| * 6. Is alcohol permitted in the home? | Y   N | Y   N | Y   N | Y   N |
| * 7. Are there no limitations on outgoing or incoming telephone calls? | Y   N | Y   N | Y   N | Y   N |
| * 8. Do the published rules and regulations seem reasonable to you? | Y   N | Y   N | Y   N | Y   N |
| * 9. Are children permitted to visit? | Y   N | Y   N | Y   N | Y   N |
| 10. Is there a quiet, private place where residents can entertain visitors? | Y   N | Y   N | Y   N | Y   N |
| 11. Does there seem to be a wide range of recreational activities? | Y   N | Y   N | Y   N | Y   N |
| *12. Are residents included in this planning in some formal way? | Y   N | Y   N | Y   N | Y   N |
| *13. Is there an actively functioning patient council? | Y   N | Y   N | Y   N | Y   N |
| 14. Is there sufficient room for the residents to engage in recreational/social events? | Y   N | Y   N | Y   N | Y   N |
| 15. Are calendars of such events posted in convenient places? | Y   N | Y   N | Y   N | Y   N |
| 16. Did you observe a substantial number of patients engaging in recreational/social events? | Y   N | Y   N | Y   N | Y   N |

| THE BUILDING AND GROUNDS | NURSING HOMES | | | |
|---|---|---|---|---|
| | A: | B: | C: | D: |
| 17. Is there a newsletter for families of residents? | Y  N | Y  N | Y  N | Y  N |
| *18. Are religious services held on the premises? | Y  N | Y  N | Y  N | Y  N |
| *19. Are arrangements made to allow patients to attend outside religious services if they wish? | Y  N | Y  N | Y  N | Y  N |
| 20. Is there a library with recent magazine issues and a good selection of books? | Y  N | Y  N | Y  N | Y  N |
| 21. Does the home sponsor frequent outings for those residents who are able to go? | Y  N | Y  N | Y  N | Y  N |
| 22. Is there a canteen? | Y  N | Y  N | Y  N | Y  N |
| 23. Do patients appear to socialize with one another? | Y  N | Y  N | Y  N | Y  N |
| *24. Does the home have any special programs with area schools to bring young people in to interact with the resident? | Y  N | Y  N | Y  N | Y  N |
| *25. Does the home subscribe to (and provide you with a copy of) a liberal Patient Bill of Rights? | Y  N | Y  N | Y  N | Y  N |
| *26. Is there a formal health education program for residents? | Y  N | Y  N | Y  N | Y  N |
| *27. Does the home provide frequent continuing education courses for its staff? | Y  N | Y  N | Y  N | Y  N |

**Food**

| | A: | B: | C: | D: |
|---|---|---|---|---|
| 1. Are fresh fruits and vegetables served in season? | Y  N | Y  N | Y  N | Y  N |
| 2. Does the home prepare meals from scratch rather than use frozen or prepackaged meals? | Y  N | Y  N | Y  N | Y  N |
| 3. Do the residents have a choice in the selection of meals? | Y  N | Y  N | Y  N | Y  N |
| * 4. Are provisions for special diets made? | Y  N | Y  N | Y  N | Y  N |
| * 5. Is help available for residents requiring feeding assistance? | Y  N | Y  N | Y  N | Y  N |
| * 6. Is this help available both in the resident's room and in the dining area? | Y  N | Y  N | Y  N | Y  N |
| * 7. Are residents served in their rooms if they prefer? | Y  N | Y  N | Y  N | Y  N |
| * 8. Is there a reasonable amount of flexibility as to when residents can eat? | Y  N | Y  N | Y  N | Y  N |
| * 9. Are dining hours for the convenience of the residents rather than the staff? | Y  N | Y  N | Y  N | Y  N |
| 10. Are residents given sufficient time to eat their meals? | Y  N | Y  N | Y  N | Y  N |
| 11. Does the food appear appetizing to you? | Y  N | Y  N | Y  N | Y  N |
| *12. Can the kitchen accommodate special, nonmedically prescribed diets (e.g., for religious reasons)? | Y  N | Y  N | Y  N | Y  N |
| 13. Is the kitchen basically clean by your standards? | Y  N | Y  N | Y  N | Y  N |
| 14. Does the kitchen staff appear neat and clean? | Y  N | Y  N | Y  N | Y  N |
| 15. Is the menu cycle adequately varied? | Y  N | Y  N | Y  N | Y  N |

| THE BUILDING AND GROUNDS | NURSING HOMES | | | |
| --- | --- | --- | --- | --- |
| | A: | B: | C: | D: |
| 16. Does the meal being served match the one on the menu? | Y N | Y N | Y N | Y N |
| 17. Are the food carts closed for sanitation purposes? | Y N | Y N | Y N | Y N |
| 18. Does the kitchen have a dishwashing machine? | Y N | Y N | Y N | Y N |
| *19. Are snacks available between meals and at bedtime? | Y N | Y N | Y N | Y N |
| *20. Do residents have access to a refrigerator to store their snacks? | Y N | Y N | Y N | Y N |
| 21. Is the dining area clean and attractive? | Y N | Y N | Y N | Y N |
| 22. Are the tables convenient for wheelchair use? | Y N | Y N | Y N | Y N |

*After the Visit*

After you have completed the checklist, it may appear as though you have found out everything there is to know about the homes you have just visited. There is more to choosing a nursing home, however, than just answering questions. Your overall impression of each home is equally as important as its different services. One of the chief purposes of answering all these questions is to get this overall impression. (It is possible to have answered "yes" to all the questions in a particular category and still have a negative overall impression.) Therefore, we suggest that you do the following as soon after your visit as possible:

- Find a quiet place where you can work.
- Review the questions and answers under each of the six categories in the checklist.
- Attempt to rate each of the six categories on a scale of 1 to 5:
  1 Completely unsatisfactory
  2 Poor
  3 Adequate (barely)
  4 Good (improvement possible)
  5 Excellent
- Using these individual ratings, try to come up with an overall rating for each nursing home. Try to answer the following question:

  *Overall, how do you rate this facility as a potential nursing home for the person?*
  1 Completely unsatisfactory
  2 Poor
  3 Adequate
  4 Good
  5 Excellent

There is no magical way to come up with this important rating. In the final analysis, you (possibly with input from the potential resident if he or she is able to provide it) must decide how to weigh the different categories. A single "1", for example, on some categories might be enough to remove a home from serious consideration for most people. For others, the quality of the medical/nursing care provided, or even the recreational/social services provided, may completely overshadow all others.

- Finally, place all the ratings (individual and overall) in the Overall Ratings Chart on page 216. (You may prefer to write in the words instead of the number — for example, "poor" instead of "2".)

*Overall Rating:* This chart should now enable you to choose the best home from among the ones you visit. If it doesn't, go back to the original Nursing Home Checklist in this chapter and compare the homes question by question. If this still doesn't resolve the issue, try this next strategy.

*A Final Strategy*

If you still find it difficult to decide among the homes you visited, examine the reason for the problem. Is it because none is really suitable, and you have to choose among the least of several evils? If so, consider visiting some more homes, possibly making a more systematic effort to get recommendations from acquaintances and health professionals.

In the first strategy, you rated each home "Unsatisfactory" to "Excellent," or you may have used a one (1) to five (5) scale. If this did not produce one home that seemed to stand out from all the others, perhaps you should consider converting your responses into percentages. A score of 90 percent in a particular category, or 90 percent overall, may tell you more about a particular home than a rating of "Adequate."

If you decide to convert your responses into percentages, use the chart entitled Overall Ratings by Percentage of Responses on page 216 along with the following steps:

- Go back to the Nursing Home Checklist and for each category (taking each home separately) count the number of "yes" answers you have recorded (e.g., under Nursing Home A, in the category "Rooms" you have 12 "yes" answers). Place this number above the fraction bar in the appropriate cell in the Overall Ratings by Percentage of Responses Chart.

- Now count the total number of questions you answered (both "yes" and "no") in a particular category (e.g., under Nursing Home A, in the category "Rooms," you answered 15 questions). Put this number below the fraction bar in the appropriate cell. Your numbers should look like this:

$$\frac{12}{15}$$

## OVERALL RATINGS CHART

| | NURSING HOMES | | | |
| --- | --- | --- | --- | --- |
| | A: | B: | C: | D: |
| Name | | | | |
| Address | | | | |
| Telephone | | | | |
| CHECKLIST CATEGORIES Building and grounds | | | | |
| Rooms | | | | |
| Personnel | | | | |
| Medical/nursing care | | | | |
| Recreational/social arrangements | | | | |
| Food | | | | |
| **Overall Rating** | | | | |

## OVERALL RATINGS BY PERCENTAGE OF RESPONSES CHART

| CHECKLIST CATEGORIES | NURSING HOMES | | | |
| --- | --- | --- | --- | --- |
| | A: | B: | C: | D: |
| Building and grounds | ___ ___% | ___ ___% | ___ ___% | ___ ___% |
| Rooms | ___ ___% | ___ ___% | ___ ___% | ___ ___% |
| Personnel | ___ ___% | ___ ___% | ___ ___% | ___ ___% |
| Medical/nursing care | ___ ___% | ___ ___% | ___ ___% | ___ ___% |
| Recreational/social arrangements | ___ ___% | ___ ___% | ___ ___% | ___ ___% |
| Food | ___ ___% | ___ ___% | ___ ___% | ___ ___% |
| **Overall Rating** | ___ ___% | ___ ___% | ___ ___% | ___ ___% |
| | 6 | 6 | 6 | 6 |

- At this point you have a fraction. You should now divide the bottom number into the top number. In our example, when you divide 15 into 12, you get a decimal of 0.8, which is then converted into a percentage by moving the decimal point two places to the right (0.8 = 80., or 80 percent). Or you could multiply the decimal by 100 (0.8 × 100 = 80 percent).

- You have now calculated the percentage response to your answers in one particular category. Now do this for the remaining categories.

- After determining the percentages in the remaining categories (remember, there are six), you can determine the overall percentage rating of a particular home. To do this, simply add the percentages determined in all six categories and divide by six (e.g., percentages 75 + 80 + 70 + 90 + 85 + 80 = 480 ÷ 6 = 80 percent).

## Dealing with Problems that Arise in Nursing Home Care

It is difficult for nursing home residents to be effective advocates for themselves. If they are on Medicaid, they may have surrendered all their assets to obtain funding for their nursing home stay and may, in effect, be trapped in the home. They do not complain simply because they do not want to make a bad situation worse. The same applies, to a lesser degree, to just about everyone else. Even if they are economically able to move, there may be long waiting lists at the homes they want to move to.

On the other hand, some people have completely unrealistic expectations of nursing homes. No patient in a nursing home should expect the attention that a private duty nurse in a hospital can give. No nursing home can afford to provide that much service routinely. Even if the service is excellent, it may not be possible to accommodate all residents' wishes for particular services (such as bathing) when they want it.

But there's a minimum below which no nursing home should fall:

- No resident should be allowed to remain in a soiled bed a moment longer than absolutely necessary.
- It is close to impossible to prevent all pressure sores, but they should be small in size and promptly treated by positioning the patient, special mattresses, and attention by a doctor when needed.
- Food should be hot or cold as appropriate and of better-than-just-acceptable quality.

- Dehydration and malnutrition should *not* develop and should be promptly and vigorously treated if found.
- Medications should be given, and given reasonably close to the prescribed schedule. Drug reactions should be noted in writing and reported to the doctor quickly.

The best way to make sure that a friend or relative is getting the kind of services he or she should is by visiting frequently and randomly. It is good to arrange visits so that promised events can be checked on. If a particular program is scheduled, such as a movie, exercise, a walk, a presentation by a visiting speaker, visit when it is scheduled and make sure that it happens from time to time. Some cancellations are unavoidable due to weather and such, but the general program the home promises should be carried out.

Appendix L contains the Bill of Rights for Nursing Home Patients suggested by the **Health Care Financing Administration,** which runs Medicare and Medicaid. Real, serious violations of these rights should be reported to the state authorities listed in appendix K. You should also contact the state nursing home ombudsman's office; a list is provided in appendix O.

Generally, it is best to deal with problems by pointing them out, politely but firmly, to the appropriate person — the nurse, the administrator, the billing office. The approach of being firm but not antagonistic works best. Keep repeating, in a polite manner, the problem you see and the solution you want.

Example: *You discover that your mother has not had her heart medication for three days. You contact the nurse and tell her this. Ask why the problem occurred. Listen carefully. (If the answer is "She had a drug reaction, so we called Dr. Fanyatz, who said to stop the drug," the right thing, not the wrong thing, has probably been done.) Depending on the response, you may need to suggest that the doctor be called, or that the medicine be obtained from a local pharmacy while the nursing home's pharmacy is awaiting its order, and so on.*

An important point to remember is this: *Don't let the nursing home put the monkey on your back.* You do not have to solve, or even sympathize with, their difficulties. In some situations, the proper answer to "What would you suggest?" is "I don't have to suggest anything. *You* have to find a way to deliver the services you promised, even if the pharmacy order is late."

Finally, it is not useful to threaten to move the patient. Besides the antagonism this may create, it may carry no weight in some areas. Many nursing homes have waiting lists and are well aware of the difficulties that often occur with nursing home placement. If a move is clearly indicated, make the arrangements and carry them out.

## Home Health Services

You may be able to stay out of a nursing home with the assistance of **home health care**. Home health care consists of the following services:

- Part-time or intermittent nursing care, provided by or under the supervision of a registered professional nurse (R.N.)
- Physical, occupational, or speech therapy
- Medical social services provided under the direction of a doctor
- Part-time or intermittent services of a home health aide
- Medical supplies (excluding drugs and biologicals) and **durable medical equipment**
- If the **Home Health Agency (HHA)** is affiliated with or under the control of a hospital, services of interns or residents of the hospital.

Not covered under home health care are transportation, housekeeping services, and those services that are normally not covered if provided in a hospital.

To qualify for home health services, you must be one of the following:

- Confined to your home or to an institution that is not a skilled nursing facility or rehabilitation facility
- Under the care of a doctor who is a medical doctor, an osteopath, or a podiatrist
- In need of intermittent skilled nursing care, physical therapy, or speech therapy
- In need of occupational therapy *after* a period during which skilled nursing care, physical therapy, or speech therapy was needed. (In other words, needing *only* occupational therapy does not qualify you for home care, but needing occupational therapy *plus* another service, or after another service, does.)

You are entitled to an unlimited number of home visits, as long as you need the service. The HHA providing the services must be one that is Medicare-participating.

You can have home health care visits for up to 21 consecutive days. After this, a gap of at least one day must follow before home health care visits can be prescribed again.

It is important to understand that home care under Medicare is composed of some (not all) *medical* services that will allow you to remain at home, rather than in a nursing home, *and these only*. It is not a "total care package" such as the social **health maintenance organization** experiments tried to provide.

*Paying for Services Medicare Doesn't Cover*

What can you do if you need services beyond what Medicare can offer? Many HHAs offer these. They may include services such as delivery of hot meals, homemaker assistance, and companions. Your supplemental insurance may cover some of these services, for a limited time. You will also find that the HHA is almost always willing to bill Medicare for the Medicare-covered services and bill you for the remainder. You may find that the charge for noncovered services, such as homemaker assistance, is affordable.

Many HHAs will help you assess your home to see if modifications will make it more suitable for home care. If what is needed falls under the category of **durable medical equipment** and a doctor prescribes it, Medicare usually will pay for all of the cost if it is provided under Part A and 80 percent of the cost under Part B. Many vendors of durable medical equipment know what Medicare covers and what it doesn't, and can tell you. You can also check with your Social Security district office.

*Some Cautionary Notes About Home Care*

First, when ordering medical equipment and having your home checked for suitability for home care, make sure there is a way for you to terminate the rental or return the item if it turns out that it is not Medicare-covered and you decide you cannot afford it. You may be stuck with large expenses otherwise.

Second — and we regret having to mention this — you should make sure your money and valuables are in a safe place that you control before the home health worker visits. You should treat a visit from the home health worker like any other instance in which a stranger enters your home. There have been many instances of theft. Even very reputable agencies cannot always control the behavior of the people they hire. You should ask the HHA about its policies in case of theft. Are they insured for theft by employees? What do they require in the way of proof? Is it enough to prove that no one other than the HHA worker was in your home?

Because of prejudices against older people, you may be told that a stolen item was not stolen and you simply forgot where you put it. (Of course, you should make sure that the item *was* stolen before you report it.) If something is stolen, report it to the police, to the HHA, and to your insurance agent, if you have homeowner's or renter's insurance.

Third, as with all services, *complain (politely) if you are unsatisfied.* HHAs cannot make up for all the burdens of being old and ill, but they should, at a minimum, provide the medical services that were prescribed and any services that you are paying for, and provide them well. The authorities regulating HHAs in various states are listed in appendix M. Complain to them if your discussion with the HHA does not produce good results.

## Hospice Care

Hospice care is care provided to those who are **terminally ill,** either in their homes or in a hospice facility. It is designed to help those who are dying do so with the greatest possible dignity and comfort, while avoiding treatment that will only prolong suffering. Hospice care is available for a total of 210 days, which consists of two 90-day periods and one 30-day period, provided that a physician or the hospice director certifies that the person is still terminally ill.

Medicare covers hospice care. Your Medicare supplemental insurance may cover any charges that Medicare does not pay. Check with your Medicare supplemental insurer about coverage. We also suggest that you look at chapter 5, which contains information on care for the dying and information on representation.

## Respite Care

Respite care is a part of hospice care. Periodically, the hospice may arrange for inpatient care in either a hospital or skilled nursing home to give temporary relief to the primary caregiver. Inpatient care is limited to no more than five days in a row. You are responsible for 5 percent of the cost up to the Part A deductible.

In this chapter, we'll review: What to do when the system doesn't work ▪ How to appeal decisions involving your doctor ▪ How to protect your assets ▪ What to look for when purchasing insurance ▪ How to clarify problems when Medicare rejects a claim ▪ When to request a refund from a doctor for a service that wasn't medically necessary ▪ When and how to use the appeal process ▪ How to protect your rights

# 8. If It Can Go Wrong, It Will

The purpose of this chapter is to provide troubleshooting advice for dealing with the various things that can go wrong with the Medicare program. Medicare is so complicated that there are literally hundreds of reasons why a particular bill might not be paid.

The number of people and agencies who have a hand somewhere in the process is enormous. They include Congress, the Health Care Financing Administration, the various federal district courts, the Medicare carriers and intermediaries, your various doctors, the hospital utilization review committee, the peer review organizations, your employer's or former employer's health care insurer, the employer's review agent, home health agencies, nursing homes, and suppliers of medical equipment. Every one of them can do something, somewhere along the way, that can result in a medical expense you thought would be covered not being covered. It's a safe bet that in the vast majority of cases, you won't be told about it until you're informed that the bill isn't paid. And not having bills paid is just part of what can go wrong.

This chapter covers the most common problems under the following headings:

▪ Eligibility and Enrollment
▪ Hospitals
▪ Nursing Homes and Home Care
▪ Insurance

- Getting Bills Paid/Filing Claims
- Appeals
- Coordination with employers' health insurance and retirement plans

Most of the chapter is in question-and-answer format, but we depart from this when the information can best be presented in some other way. Most of the questions are ones that **People's Medical Society (PMS)** members have asked us over the years.

## Three Important Points, Again

We'd like to emphasize three points that we raised earlier in this book but that are important enough to bear repeating:

- You are not responsible for any medical bill you could not reasonably have been expected to know was not covered. But *you* have to make the case that you did not know that the service or expense was not covered.

- Increasingly, rejections of claims and termination or denial of services under Medicare are being based on *medical necessity*. If payment is denied, you usually have nothing to worry about — see the section on claims below. For denials of admission to hospitals, inpatient surgery, and notices of noncoverage of further hospital or nursing home stays, you should work closely with your doctor — after all, it's *your doctor's* medical judgement that is being questioned.

- It is vitally important to *keep records* of your dealings with Medicare. We believe that the Claims Log, in appendix B, is the best way of doing this for routine bills. But for requests for reconsideration of denials, appeals, and the like, it is important to *keep copies* of correspondence. When the correspondence has to be sent by a certain date, we recommend that you send it *certified mail, return receipt requested,* so that you will have proof of mailing and proof of receipt. This is inexpensive, and the window clerks at any post office can show you how to do it.

You should also remember to *ask questions* of your local Social Security office if you have them. If the people there don't know the answer, they can refer you to someone who does. Keep asking until you get an answer, and until you're satisfied it's the right answer. Your local Social Security office *is* your Medicare office for many issues. You can always call them and receive help or be directed to the right place.

## Eligibility and Enrollment

**1. I've applied for Medicare and have been told that I'm ineligible. What should I do?**

Find out exactly why you are ineligible. (If you filed an application, you should receive a letter telling you the reason.) If you do not meet one of the *categorical* requirements of the program — for example, you are not yet 65, or are under 65 and not disabled, or are not an alien admitted for permanent residence — you should try to alter your status. (There's no way to be 65 faster, but you can consult a lawyer who specializes in disability cases, apply for citizenship or alien resident status, and — if you were found ineligible because you had not worked enough — check your earnings record.)

If you feel that a clear error has been made and that it is not being corrected, you can appeal the finding of ineligibility.

You should also check to see if you are entitled on the basis of someone else's earnings. See chapter 2, which offers several examples. You may be eligible as the wife, widow, divorced woman, husband, widower, divorced man, child, or parent of someone else.

**2. I don't know when I should apply for Medicare.**

To be safe, you should apply for both Part A (hospital insurance) and Part B (doctor insurance) three months before you turn 65. This will allow you time to gather the proofs of earnings, date of birth, and so on that you need, and for cleaning up of any errors in your earnings record. It will also avoid increases in your Part B premium due to late enrollment. Medicare and Social Security have been changing their procedures on automatic enrollment, and they may change them again. *If you want Medicare, apply for it.* Call your Social Security office for forms and procedures.

It is *very important* to remember that if you do not have 40 quarters of coverage (are not "fully insured"), you may need to continue working until you have earned the required number of quarters. Another option is that you may be eligible on the earnings of someone who is qualified for Social Security. This is especially important to spouses who may qualify on each others' work record or spouses who are now divorced, but were married to each other for at least 10 years.

**3. I suspect my earnings record at Social Security is wrong, but I don't know how to check it.**

Contact the Social Security Administration at 800-772-1213 and request a copy of Form 7004-SM, "Request for Earnings and Benefits

Estimate Statement," or see chapter 2 for a sample letter.

**4. I applied on the basis of disability, and have been turned down. I want to appeal. What can I do?**

Realistically, you have to hire a lawyer. Disability law is complicated, is affected variously by different precedents in different judicial districts, and changes constantly due to court decisions. Beware of lawyers who promise to get you disability benefits. No one can promise that; it depends on the facts of your case. Also, be aware that the federal regulations governing disability limit the fees the attorney may charge you for representation before the **Social Security Administration (SSA)**. The fee is limited to the smallest of the following:

- Twenty-five percent of past-due benefits

- The fee you and the attorney agreed on

- The fee set by the Social Security Administration

If the case goes to a federal court, the court may award a fee higher than any of the above, but the amount the SSA will pay out of past-due benefits awarded is limited to the smallest of the three amounts. You are responsible for any fees above that amount that are awarded by the court. The SSA does not pay any fees if you lose, because in that case there are no past-due benefits from which to pay. In other words, you always have to pay the attorney, but the fee is paid from past-due benefits if you win.

Before paying for an attorney, contact senior citizens' centers, area agencies on aging, and welfare rights projects that are listed in the phone book. No-cost or reduced-cost legal services may be available from them.

**5. I now know that I am definitely not eligible for Medicare. What can I do?**

Persons who are age 65 and do not otherwise qualify for Medicare can purchase Medicare coverage just like private insurance. This is expensive, running $311 a month for Part A hospital insurance and $43.80 a month for Part B doctor insurance, for a monthly total of $354.80. If you purchase Medicare coverage, you will still have to purchase supplemental insurance to have a package that really protects you against the financial effects of illness. You may find that it is cheaper to purchase individual coverage from a **health maintenance organization (HMO)**, which offers very comprehensive benefits for one fixed price, if an HMO is available where you live. See chapter 4.

You are permitted to purchase Part B of Medicare (insurance for doctor bills) if you are a resident of the United States, are 65 or over, and are either a citizen or an alien lawfully admitted for permanent residence who has resided in the United States for the last five years. (It is under this rule that *everyone* enrolls in Part B.) If you are not eligible for Part A of Medicare, enrolling for Part B entitles you to purchase it. So you have to buy Part B to get Part A.

### 6. How do I apply?

The first step is to telephone your local Social Security Office. These offices are commonly listed under the federal government section in the blue pages of your local telephone directory, and under "U. S. Government" in the white pages. If you can't find a listing, call the information operator and ask for any Social Security office. Calling one will enable you to find out which one you should go to.

Call that office. Tell them that you want to apply for Medicare (and Social Security if you are not already receiving it.) The SSA is making a determined effort to carry out as much business as possible over the phone. This is generally more efficient, and it saves you a visit to the Social Security office. At the same time, if you have trouble dealing with matters like this over the phone (if, for example, you have trouble hearing and don't have an amplified phone), you can insist on a face-to-face visit. (For more on this, see chapter 2.)

Whichever way you apply, the Social Security office representative will fill out most of the forms for you. This is done to ensure that the type of answers SSA needs to make a decision get answered on the forms involved. After the representative has filled out the forms, you should read them — and insist on the correction of any errors — before signing them. If you need special assistance — if, for example, you are blind, deaf, or illiterate — special help will be made available to you. You may have to go to another Social Security office to find the right person to help you. The representative at the first Social Security office you go to will give you instructions. If you think you will need special help, you should mention this when you first call.

The representative will ask you to bring certain documents when you come to the Social Security office, usually the following:

- Proof of age
- Records of earnings, such as W-2 forms (or tax returns for the self-employed) for the past two years
- Your Social Security card

If you are applying because you think you are disabled, you will be asked to bring some documents relating to your medical problems. The Social Security office representative will tell you what they are.

*Keep your originals. Keep your originals. Keep your originals.* More on the application process can be found in chapter 2.

### 7. I've lost my Social Security card and don't think I can remember the number. What can I do?

You need not worry if you have lost your Social Security card. If you can remember the number, you can apply for a duplicate. If you can't remember the number, it is likely to be on other documents around your house, such as payroll stubs, credit card bills, and insurance policies. If all else fails, the Social Security office can access its computer system, which will retrieve your name or any that sound like it. This considerably narrows the search for your number.

## Hospitals

### 1. I want to visit my sister in Canada this summer and have some surgery done while we are together so she can take care of me. Will Medicare pay for a hospital stay outside the United States?

No. People think that Medicare pays for care anywhere in the world. It doesn't. Only care in hospitals in the fifty states and the District of Columbia, Puerto Rico, and the last two U.S. territories — Guam and the Virgin Islands — is paid for. Care you receive in Europe, Canada, Mexico, and the rest of the world is *not* covered. The only exceptions are situations in which you are close to the Mexican or Canadian borders and need emergency care, and the nearest hospital is a Mexican or Canadian one, or if the Mexican or Canadian hospital is much closer to your home than any American hospital and is accredited by the Joint Commission on Accreditation of Healthcare Organizations or a comparable body in the foreign country. In these situations, Medicare will pay for services in a Mexican or Canadian hospital.

Please note that doctors' services outside the United States are covered only if they are provided during an inpatient hospitalization that is paid for under the circumstances described above. *No other doctors' services outside the United States are paid for by Medicare.*

**2. I am worried that I will have to leave the hospital when my DRG runs out, even if I'm not well.**

Don't be. It's illegal for the hospital even to suggest it. During the early days of the **diagnosis-related groups (DRG) system**, there were a number of instances of abuse. Patients were told that they had to leave the hospital "because your DRG has run out" or something similar. Discharging any patient who still needs hospital care because of financial considerations is a total violation of the hospital's contract with Medicare. The hospital has agreed to provide services to you as long as they are medically necessary.

Because of abuses observed, the **People's Medical Society (PMS)** and the **American Association for Retired Persons (AARP)** joined forces to ask Medicare to require hospitals to "mirandize" Medicare patients: just as persons being arrested are told of their constitutional rights. Medicare now requires *all* hospitals to provide Medicare beneficiaries with an *Important Message from Medicare* upon admission for *any* patient care. It appears on pages 229–231.

To sum up: the only reasons you can be discharged from a hospital under Medicare are *medical* ones. Even if Medicare is no longer paying, you should not be discharged for lack of ability to pay. The hospital's social service staff should explore your eligibility for **Medicaid** and see what alternative sources of care are available. State law in many states is rapidly evolving to the position that no patient who needs hospital care for *medical* reasons should ever be discharged or transferred for lack of ability to pay.

**3. The hospital tells me that I have to leave because "my DRG has run out."**

Telling you this is (a) untrue, and (b) a violation of the hospital's contract with Medicare. You are entitled to hospital services as long as they are medically necessary. The hospital can always apply for additional payment.

We suggest that you, or someone helping you, first write down the name and presumptive title of anyone who told you this. Then call the administrator's office. Tell them that you are aware that the hospital will be paid the full DRG for your admission. Tell them that you are aware that they can apply for **outlier** payments. Ask them if they have done so. Then tell them the only reason that you can be discharged is because you no longer need hospital care. Tell them that hospitals don't discharge people, doctors do. Ask which doctor made the deter-

## AN IMPORTANT MESSAGE FROM MEDICARE

### YOUR RIGHTS WHILE YOU ARE A MEDICARE HOSPITAL PATIENT

- You have the right to receive all the hospital care that is necessary for the proper diagnosis and treatment of your illness or injury. According to Federal law, **your discharge date must be determined solely by your medical needs,** not by "DRGs" or Medicare payments.

- You have the right to be fully informed about decisions affecting your Medicare coverage and payment for your hospital stay and for any post-hospital services.

- You have the right to request a review by a Peer Review Organization of any written Notice of Noncoverage that you receive from the hospital stating that Medicare will no longer pay for your hospital care. Peer Review Organizations (PROs) are groups of doctors who are paid by the Federal Government to review medical necessity, appropriateness and quality of hospital treatment furnished to Medicare patients. The phone number and address of the PRO for your area are:

_____

_____

_____

### TALK TO YOUR DOCTOR ABOUT YOUR STAY IN THE HOSPITAL

You and your doctor know more about your condition and your health needs than anyone else. Decisions about your medical treatment should be made between you and your doctor. **If you have any questions about your medical treatment, your need for continued hospital care, your discharge, or your need for possible post-hospital care, don't hesitate to ask your doctor.** The hospital's patient representative or social worker will also help you with your questions and concerns about hospital services.

### IF YOU THINK YOU ARE BEING ASKED TO LEAVE THE HOSPITAL TOO SOON

- Ask a hospital representative for a written notice of explanation immediately, if you have not already received one. This notice is called a "Notice of Noncoverage." You must have this Notice of Noncoverage if you wish to exercise your right to request a review by the PRO.

- The Notice of Noncoverage will state either that your doctor or the PRO agrees with the hospital's decision that Medicare will no longer pay for your hospital care.

  + If the hospital and your doctor agree, the PRO does not review your case before a Notice of Noncoverage is issued. But the PRO will respond to your request for a review of your Notice of Noncoverage and seek your opinion. You cannot be made to pay for your hospital care until the PRO makes its decision, if you request the review by noon of the first work day after you receive the Notice of Noncoverage.

+ If the hospital and your doctor disagree, the hospital may request the PRO to review your case. If it does make such a request, the hospital is required to send you a notice to that effect. In this situation the PRO must agree with the hospital or the hospital cannot issue a Notice of Noncoverage. You may request that the PRO reconsider your case after you receive a Notice of Noncoverage but since the PRO has already reviewed your case once, you may have to pay for **at least one day of hospital care** before the PRO completes this reconsideration.

IF YOU **DO NOT** REQUEST A REVIEW, **THE HOSPITAL MAY BILL YOU** FOR ALL THE COSTS OF YOUR STAY BEGINNING WITH THE THIRD DAY AFTER YOU RECEIVE THE NOTICE OF NONCOVERAGE. THE HOSPITAL, HOWEVER, CANNOT CHARGE YOU FOR CARE UNLESS IT PROVIDES YOU WITH A NOTICE OF NONCOVERAGE.

## HOW TO REQUEST A REVIEW OF THE NOTICE OF NONCOVERAGE

• If the Notice of Noncoverage states that your **physician agrees** with the hospital's decision:
  + You must make your request for review to the PRO by **noon of the first work day** after you receive the Notice of Noncoverage by contacting the PRO by phone or in writing.
  + The PRO must ask for your views about your case before making its decision. The PRO will inform you by phone and in writing of its decision on the review.
  + If the PRO agrees with the Notice of Noncoverage, you may be billed for all costs of your stay beginning at noon of the day **after** you receive the PRO's decision.
  + Thus, you will **not** be responsible for the cost of hospital care before you receive the PRO's decision.

• If the Notice of Noncoverage states that the PRO agrees with the hospital's decision:
  + You should make your request for reconsideration to the PRO **immediately** upon receipt of the Notice of Noncoverage by contacting the PRO by phone or in writing.
  + The PRO can take up to three working days from receipt of your request to complete the review. The PRO will inform you in writing of its decision on the review.
  + Since the PRO has already reviewed your case once, prior to the issuance of the Notice of Noncoverage, the hospital is permitted to begin billing you for the cost of your stay beginning with the third calendar day after you receive your Notice of Noncoverage even **if the PRO has not completed its review.**
  + Thus, if the PRO continues to agree with the Notice of Noncoverage, **you may have to pay for at least one day of hospital care.**

NOTE: The process described above is called "immediate review." If you miss the deadline for this immediate review while you are in the hospital, you may still request a review of Medicare's decision to no longer pay for your care at any point during your hospital stay or after you have left the hospital. The Notice of Noncoverage will tell you how to request this review.

## POST-HOSPITAL CARE

When your doctor determines that you no longer need all the specialized services provided in a hospital, but you still require medical care, he or she may discharge you to a skilled nursing facility or home care. The discharge planner at the hospital will help arrange for the services you may need after your discharge. Medicare and supplemental insurance policies have limited coverage for skilled nursing facility care and home health care. Therefore, you should find out which services will or will not be covered and how payment will be made. Consult with your doctor, hospital discharge planner, patient representative and your family in making preparations for care after you leave the hospital. **Don't hesitate to ask questions.**

ACKNOWLEDGEMENT OF RECEIPT — My signature only acknowledges my receipt of this Message from (name of hospital) on (date) and does not waive any of my rights to request a review or make me liable for any payment.

_____

Signature of beneficiary or
person acting on behalf of beneficiary.

mination that you no longer needed hospital care. Write down all the answers you get from every person you talk to. Then call the Office of the Inspector General at Health and Human Services, 1-800-447-8477. Say that you want to report a case of abuse of the Medicare program. They'll take it from there.

**4. I want to have an operation in the hospital, and Medicare has denied me, saying that I have to have it done in an outpatient facility. What can I do?**

You can appeal, even though there is generally no problem with outpatient surgery and you may be at less risk than you would be in the hospital. Your proposed admission was turned down because the **peer review organization (PRO)**, or the hospital's **utilization review committee (URC)** acting for the PRO, did not find it medically necessary. You can request a reconsideration of this decision, just as you can any other PRO decision. The procedure is given below. Please note that this is a generic procedure for the filing of requests for reconsideration and appeals. These are two different stages of the same process; we'll refer to them all as "appeals" except where that might be confusing.

*How to Appeal (Request a Reconsideration) of a Peer Review Organization Decision*

You can appeal the PRO decision by filing a request for reconsideration with the PRO itself, at the address for the PRO shown on the notice you received; at any Social Security office, or at a Railroad Retirement Board office, if you are a railroad retirement beneficiary.

Your doctor and the hospital also have the right to file an appeal. They *do not* have the right to an "expedited reconsideration" that you have.

*Time to File the Request for Reconsideration*

You must file your request for reconsideration within 60 days of the date you received the Notice of Noncoverage. Unless you can prove otherwise, the notice is deemed to have been received by you five days after the date on it. (Example: The notice is dated January 5. You are deemed to have received it on January 10, unless you can prove you received it later. Your 60-day period for appeal started on January 10. The last day you can file an appeal is March 10, the sixtieth day after the deemed receipt of the notice.)

*"Good Cause" for Late Filing*

Generally, you will be allowed to file late if there is what the PRO considers to be "good cause" for it. The regulations are very broad, and it is hard to see what exactly might count. The regulations give examples such as serious illness, a death in the family, failure to receive information you had requested before the sixty-day limit, a misunderstanding of what the PRO notice told you, and so on.

*Obtaining Information*

Both you and your doctor have a right to see the information on which the PRO based its decision. You should ask for this when you file your request for reconsideration. You may add to the information anything you or your doctor want to add.

*Expedited Reconsideration and Time Limits*

You can request that the PRO make an expedited reconsideration of the denial. How fast "expedited" has to be depends on the circumstances:

- Within three working days if you are still a patient in the hospital (this doesn't really apply here, of course, since you're trying to get in);
- Within three days if the initial determination was a denial of hospital admission and you are still in the hospital;
- Within ten working days if you are in a skilled nursing facility;
- Within thirty working days in all other situations, and in every situation where someone other than you files the appeal. Having expedited redetermination available is a very important reason for *you* to file the appeal and have the doctor or hospital submit information as part of an appeal.

*What to Include*

You should file your claim using HCFA Form 2649, which is shown on page 234. You can request an appeal with just a letter, but using the form will ensure that you include everything that is needed. You should ask your doctor to provide medical documentation. It is important for both you and your doctor to focus on the issue at hand and not to editorialize. The general issue you will be dealing with in PRO denials of admission is the *medical necessity* for you to be hospitalized at all, or to have a procedure done in the hospital or done at all. Keep the focus on these issues. They will boil down to appropriate medical judgment. Your doctor will probably want to submit information regarding your condition, plus evidence from the medical literature indicating that what the PRO wants done is unwise.

*Notices and Appeals*

When the PRO provides you with its reconsidered decision, it must do so *in writing* and inform you of the following:

- The decision
- The reasons for it

DEPARTMENT OF HEALTH, EDUCATION, AND WELFARE
HEALTH CARE FINANCING ADMINISTRATION

Form Approved.
OMB No. 066-R-0067

# REQUEST FOR RECONSIDERATION OF PART A HEALTH INSURANCE BENEFITS

INSTRUCTIONS: *Please type or print firmly.* Leave the block empty if you cannot answer it. Take or mail the WHOLE form to your Social Security office which will be glad to help you. Please read the statement on the reverse side of page 2.

1. BENEFICIARY'S NAME

2. HEALTH INSURANCE CLAIM NUMBER

3. REPRESENTATIVE'S NAME, IF APPLICABLE

(☐ RELATIVE   ☐ ATTORNEY   ☐ OTHER PERSON)   ☐ PROVIDER FILING

## 4. PLEASE ATTACH A COPY OF THE NOTICE(S) YOU RECEIVED ABOUT YOUR CLAIM TO THIS FORM.

5. THIS CLAIM IS FOR
☐ INPATIENT HOSPITAL   ☐ SKILLED NURSING FACILITY (SNF)   ☐ HEALTH MAINTENANCE ORGANIZATION (HMO)
☐ EMERGENCY HOSPITAL   ☐ HOME HEALTH AGENCY (HHA)

6. NAME AND ADDRESS OF PROVIDER *(Hospital, SNF, HHA, HMO)*   |   CITY AND STATE   |   PROVIDER NUMBER

7. NAME OF INTERMEDIARY   |   CITY AND STATE   |   INTERMEDIARY NUMBER

8. DATE OF ADMISSION OR START OF SERVICES   |   9. DATE(S) OF THE NOTICE(S) YOU RECEIVED

10. I DO NOT AGREE WITH THE DETERMINATION ON MY CLAIM. PLEASE RECONSIDER MY CLAIM BECAUSE

11. YOU MUST OBTAIN ANY EVIDENCE *(For example, a letter from a doctor)* YOU WISH TO SUBMIT.

☐ I HAVE ATTACHED THE FOLLOWING EVIDENCE:

☐ I WILL SEND THIS EVIDENCE WITHIN 10 DAYS:

☐ I HAVE NO ADDITIONAL EVIDENCE OR OTHER INFORMATION TO SUBMIT WITH MY CLAIM.

12. IS THIS REQUEST FILED WITHIN 60 DAYS OF THE DATE OF YOUR NOTICE?
☐ YES   ☐ NO
IF YOU CHECKED "NO" ATTACH AN EXPLANATION OF THE REASON FOR THE DELAY TO THIS FORM.

13. ONLY ONE SIGNATURE IS NEEDED. THIS FORM IS SIGNED BY:
☐ BENEFICIARY   ☐ REPRESENTATIVE   ☐ PROVIDER REP.

SIGN HERE ▶

14. STREET ADDRESS

CITY, STATE, ZIP CODE

TELEPHONE   |   DATE

15. If this request is signed by mark (X), TWO WITNESSES who know the person requesting reconsideration must sign in the space provided on the reverse side of this page of the form.

## DO NOT FILL IN BELOW THIS LINE — FOR SOCIAL SECURITY USE — THANK YOU

16. ROUTING
☐ INTERMEDIARY
☐ HCFA, RO-MEDICARE
☐ BSS, ODR

18. SSA OR INTERMEDIARY DATE STAMP

17. ADDITIONAL INFORMATION

FORM **HCFA-2649** (8-79   FORMERLY SSA-2649)
DESTROY PRIOR EDITIONS

INTERMEDIARY

Page 1 of 4

- A statement of the effect the decision has on what Medicare will pay for or has paid for
- A statement of your appeal rights, with complete instructions for filing the appeal

When you receive a notice of a reconsidered decision that is not in your favor, consider whether you want to request a hearing. A hearing is more formal than a reconsideration, and entitles you to appear before an **administrative law judge (ALJ)**. If you do request a hearing, it is wise to have a lawyer involved. Hearings can involve subpoenaing witnesses and other legal steps. It is less formal than a court case, but far more formal than a request for reconsideration.

Only you, not your doctor or the hospital, have this right. The rules for filing an appeal are exactly the same as for filing for reconsideration with the PRO — sixty days, counted from five days after the date of the notice, and all that. You should file your appeal on HCFA HA-501-US, unless the information you received with the PRO's Notice of Reconsideration tells you to do something else.

The first thing the ALJ will attempt to determine is whether or not the controversy involves at least $200 (with the price of health care these days, it almost surely will). If the ALJ determines that the amount is less than $200, he will notify you and any other concerned parties that he has determined this and that they have fifteen days to show why he is wrong. If no evidence is submitted within fifteen days, the request for a hearing is dismissed. (You will not have to worry about this if you don't receive such a notice.)

You will be notified by the ALJ of the date of the hearing at least ten days before it is filed.

If the ALJ's decision is unfavorable, you can appeal to the Social Security Appeals Council. Your attorney can tell you how to do this. The Appeals Council does not take all the appeals addressed to it. If $2,000 or more is involved, you can appeal an Appeals Council determination (or the ALJ's decision if the Appeals Council refused a hearing) to the federal courts. This must be done within sixty days of the date of the Appeals Council determination, or its decision not to hear your case.

**5. My doctor wants to do my operation in the hospital, but the PRO says no. What can I do?**

See the answer to the preceding question.

## Nursing Homes and Home Care

**1. I need to go to a nursing home, but I'm not sure Medicare will pay for it. How can I tell?**

Medicare does not cover what people usually think of as "nursing home care." There are three levels of nursing home care:

- **Skilled nursing facilities (SNFs)** offer care delivered by registered and licensed practical nurses on the orders of an attending physician. They offer services such as oxygen therapy, intravenous and tube feedings, care of catheters and wound drains, and physical, occupational, and speech therapy.

- **Intermediate care facilities (ICFs)** provide less intensive care than do SNFs. Patients are generally more mobile, and rehabilitation therapies are stressed.

- **Sheltered, or custodial, care** is nonmedical. Residents do not require constant attention from nurses and aides, but need assistance with one or more daily activities or no longer want to be bothered with keeping up a house. The social needs of residents are met in a secure environment free of as many anxieties as possible.

Medicare covers nursing home care at the SNF level only. This coverage is intended for basically one situation: if you need more care to recuperate, but care that is less intense than that provided in a hospital. Medicare covers the first 20 days in full. From the 21st day through the 100th, you are responsible for a copayment of $95 per day. Medicare picks up any amount over the $95 for these days. Beginning on the 101st day Medicare pays nothing, and you are responsible for all costs. You are once again eligible for another 100 days of SNF care in the next benefit period.

**2. There should be no question that I need a nursing home and that Medicare will pay for it. After all, I can't do for myself a lot of the things that I used to. That's a health problem, and Medicare covers those — correct?**

Not really. Nursing home care is covered only for a short time, and only if it will improve physical or mental functioning to a degree that makes the nursing home stay *medically* "reasonable and necessary." **Medical necessity** is *the* key issue in payment for SNF services. The SNF regulations go to great lengths to define what is and is not SNF.

The key is that care that is complex enough to require the services of a nurse or skilled rehabilitation personnel is covered; care that you could do yourself is not. But complications may require SNF-level care, even for situations that would normally not be covered. Basically, SNF care is rehabilitation; if your condition cannot be expected to improve as a result of SNF care *and* you do not need observation by skilled personnel, your care will not be covered. Obviously, what your doctor writes in the chart makes a big difference in what gets covered. If you are worried about coverage of SNF services, discuss this with her.

**3. Is there anything I can do to stay out of a nursing home?**

Yes. There are many alternatives that may enable you to stay out, depending on your level of functioning and the exact services you may need. Use the Health Status checklist in Chapter 7 to assess your needs.

For those who are not bedridden, adult day care, home health care, homemaker services, sharing a home with other elderly people, Meals on Wheels, shopping services, and adult foster care may be alternatives that will avoid a nursing home stay. For the availability of these services, you can check with your local agency on aging, the medical social services office of the hospital (if the person is in the hospital awaiting discharge), and departments of social services. Many are listed in the telephone book under the names we've used, for example, "shopping services."

**4. What about home health care? What does Medicare cover?**

Home health care consists of the following services:

- Part-time or intermittent nursing care provided by or under the supervision of a registered professional nurse (R.N.)
- Physical, occupational, or speech therapy
- Medical social services provided under the direction of a doctor
- Part-time or intermittent services of a home health aide
- Medical supplies (excluding drugs and biologicals) and **durable medical equipment**
- If the **Home Health Agency (HHA)** is affiliated with or under the control of a hospital, services of interns or residents of the hospital

Not covered under home health care are transportation, housekeeping services, and those services that are normally not covered if provided in a hospital.

To qualify for home health services, you must be one of the following:

- Confined to your home or to an institution that is not a SNF or rehabilitation facility

- Under the care of a doctor who is a medical doctor, an osteopath, or a podiatrist
- In need of intermittent skilled nursing care, physical therapy, or speech therapy
- In need of occupational therapy *after* a period during which skilled nursing care, physical therapy, or speech therapy were needed. (In other words, needing *only* occupational therapy does not qualify you for home care, but needing occupational therapy *plus* another service, or after another service, does.)

You are entitled to an unlimited number of home visits, as long as you need the service, but for no more than 21 consecutive days. After that, a gap of at least one day must occur before you can receive home health services again. The HHA providing the services must be one that is Medicare-participating.

It is important to understand that home care under Medicare is composed of some (not all) *medical* services that will allow you to remain at home, rather than in a nursing home, *and these only*. It is not a "total care package."

**5. Are there some things I should watch out for in regard to home care?**

First, ordering medical equipment and when having your home checked for suitability for home care, make sure there is a way for you to terminate the rental or return the item if it turns out that it is not Medicare-covered and you decide you cannot afford it. You may be stuck with large expenses otherwise.

Second — and we regret having to mention this — you should make sure your money and valuables are in a safe place that you control before the home health worker visits. You should treat a visit from the home health worker like any other instance in which a stranger enters your home. There have been many instances of theft. Even very reputable agencies cannot always control the behavior of the people they hire. You should ask the HHA about its policies in case of theft. Are they insured for theft by employees? What do they require in the way of proof? Is it enough to prove that no one other than the HHA worker was in your home?

Because of prejudices against older people, you may be told that a stolen item was not stolen and you simply forgot where you put it. (Of course, you should make sure that the item *was* stolen before you report it.) If something is stolen, report it to the police, to the HHA, and to your insurance agent, if you have homeowner's or renter's insurance.

Third, as with all services, *complain (politely) if you are unsatisfied.* HHAs cannot make up for all the burdens of being old and ill, but they should, at a minimum, provide the medical services that were prescribed and any services that you are paying for, and provide them well. The authorities regulating HHAs in the various states are listed in appendix M. Complain to them if your discussion with the HHA does not produce good results.

**6. I've considered every alternative to care in a nursing home that you listed in chapter 7, and I still find I need nursing home care. Medicare won't pay for it. What can I do?**

The Medicaid programs covers nursing home care. Medicaid is intended for the *very* poor who have nowhere else to turn, but not all of the very poor are covered. It is a state-run program that receives federal funds. States make most of the rules, and the trend in recent years has been to make Medicaid requirements more stringent. The old law virtually guaranteed that the spouse who stayed at home would have to impoverish him- or herself to pay for the care of the spouse in the nursing home.

Legislation passed in 1988 greatly reduces the burden but can still lead to substantial loss of assets.

- In any month in which a married person is in a nursing home, no income of the at-home spouse is to be considered available to the spouse in the nursing home.

- Income is considered the property of the person to whom it is paid. Income paid to both spouses is attributed 50 percent to each.

- The home, household goods, and personal effects of both spouses are not counted in considering Medicaid eligibility.

- All assets other than these will be counted and divided in two. If the at-home spouse has less than $15,000, the spouse in the nursing home may transfer assets to him or her to make up to $15,000 available to the at-home spouse. (States may, at their option, raise this figure to any amount less than $76,000. The $15,000 amount will be indexed to inflation.)

- The assets that remain in the name of the spouse in the nursing home are considered available to pay for his or her nursing home care. All assets in excess of $76,000 are attributed to the spouse in the nursing home and are considered available to pay for nursing home care.

- States must allow nursing home residents to retain certain sums for medical expenses not covered by Medicare or Medicaid before contributing to the expense of their nursing home care. The states may place "reasonable limits" on the amounts spent.

- States must allow the at-home spouse sufficient income from the other spouse to bring total household income of the at-home spouse to at least 150 percent of the federal poverty level for a two-person household. States will not be required to allow more than $1,918 per month, except by court order or change in regulation.

These requirements dramatically reduce the economic stress on the spouse who remains at home, but they still may require him or her to part with large amounts of income and assets. Your spouse and, in rare cases, your parents do not *actually* have to give anything toward the cost of your care, but your *eligibility* is determined as though they do. The exact requirements, as well as the amount of assets and income you may retain and still be eligible, vary from state to state. Check the list of state Medicaid offices in appendix N to find out where to call to determine the exact eligibility requirements for your state.

You are automatically eligible for Medicaid if you are eligible for, or receiving, *Supplemental Security Income (SSI)* payments for the aged, blind, and disabled, but you must apply at a state welfare office. If you meet the requirements for SSI, there is little chance that you would have to give up additional income or assets to qualify for Medicaid.

If your income, less certain deductions and medical bills, is within certain (low) limits, you may be eligible for Medicaid as medically needy. You must "spend down" to pay medical bills to the point at which you are eligible; after that, Medicaid pays for all medical bills as long as you are eligible.

**7. But I don't have the money to pay my medical bills *now*. You're telling me that I have to pay them all off in order to get Medicaid to pay for future ones?**

No. This is a common misunderstanding. The requirements for the medically needy spend-down is that you have *incurred* enough medical bills so that your income, less allowances and the medical bills, is less than the income limit for eligibility. Medicaid pays all of the bills, both current and future, if you meet this test, have assets under the asset limit, and meet other requirements, such as age and residency, your particular state may impose.

**8.  I don't want to give up my home. Can't I transfer it and my other assets over the limit to my children, and continue to keep it?**

You no longer have to give up your home to become eligible for Medicaid. Legislation passed in 1988 greatly reduces the burden but can still lead to substantial loss of assets.

- In any month in which a married person is in a nursing home, no income of the at-home spouse is to be considered available to the spouse in the nursing home.

- Income is considered the property of the person to whom it is paid. Income paid to both spouses is attributed 50 percent to each.

- The home, household goods, and personal effects of both spouses are not counted in considering Medicaid eligibility.

- All assets other than these will be counted and divided in two. If the at-home spouse has less than $15,000, the spouse in the nursing home may transfer assets to him or her to make up to $15,000 available to the at-home spouse. (States may, at their option, raise this figure to any amount less than $76,000. The $15,000 amount will be indexed to inflation.)

- The assets that remain in the name of the spouse in the nursing home are considered available to pay for his or her nursing home care. All assets in excess of $76,000 are attributed to the spouse in the nursing home and are considered available to pay for nursing home care.

- States must allow nursing home residents to retain certain sums for medical expenses not covered by Medicare or Medicaid before contributing to the expense of their nursing home care. The states may place "reasonable limits" on the amounts spent.

- States must allow the at-home spouse sufficient income from the other spouse to bring total household income of the at-home spouse to at least 150 percent of the federal poverty level for a two-person household. States will not be required to allow more than $1,918 per month, except by court order or change in regulation.

You can transfer your assets to someone *other* than your spouse (for example, to a child) in order to become eligible for Medicaid, but you must have done so before you become eligible for Medicaid (time frames vary by state). If you want to transfer your assets in order to become eligible for nursing home coverage under Medicaid, *you should do so only with the services of a lawyer who understands the Medicaid program.* This is both to protect you and to ensure that you actually will be found eligible for Medicaid based on the action you took. There is no point in transferring assets only to find that you are still not eligible.

### 9. How do I apply for Medicaid?

Medicaid applications are taken at welfare offices, but many states also take them at senior citizens' centers, agencies on aging, and other locations. Call the Medicaid office for your state (listed in appendix N) to find out where you can apply in your area. When you call the office in your area, find out what you need to bring with you for the application process.

Generally, you should bring proof of age, financial status, and any disability you may have. The proof of financial status should include the last six months' bank statements for checking and savings accounts, rent or mortgage payment receipts, loan papers for your car or the title to it, any documents relating to stock or bond ownership, and check stubs for any regular payments you receive. You should also have the amount of your Social Security check, if you are currently receiving Social Security payments. You should always have your Social Security number. Bring your medical bills, or copies of them, for the last year.

### 10. How can I select a good nursing home?

You can begin the process of selecting a nursing home by eliminating those you know you don't want to use. Don't consider nursing homes that are as follows:

- Too far away to allow visiting by relatives and friends
- Too expensive
- Not properly certified or licensed
- Not offering the medical or other services needed
- Unsuitable for some other reason, such as being owned by a religious denomination with which you do not want to associate

You can find out whether or not a home is properly certified or licensed by contacting the state agencies regulating nursing homes that are listed in appendix K at the back of this book.

Chapter 7 contains a checklist, on pages 209–214, and several more suggestions for selecting a nursing home.

**11. Now that I'm in the nursing home, I'm shocked by the conditions. What can I do about it?**

It is difficult for nursing home residents to be effective advocates for themselves. If they are on Medicaid, they may have surrendered all their assets to obtain funding for their nursing home stay and may, in effect, be trapped in the home. They do not complain simply because they do not want to make a bad situation worse. The same applies, to a lesser degree, to just about everyone else. Even if they are economically able to move, there may be long waiting lists at the homes they want to move to.

On the other hand, some people have completely unrealistic expectations of nursing homes. No patient in a nursing home should expect the attention that a private duty nurse in a hospital can give. No nursing home can afford to provide that much service routinely. Even if the service is excellent, it may not be possible to accommodate all residents' wishes for particular services (such as bathing) exactly when they want it.

But there's a minimum below which no nursing home should fall:

- No resident should be allowed to remain in a soiled bed a moment longer than absolutely necessary.
- It is close to impossible to prevent all pressure sores for totally bedridden people, but they should be small in size and promptly treated by positioning the patient, special mattresses, and immediate attention by a doctor when needed.
- Food should be hot or cold as appropriate and of better-than-just-acceptable quality.
- Dehydration and malnutrition should *not* develop and should be promptly and vigorously treated if found.

- Medications should be given, and given reasonably close to the pre-scribed schedule. Drug reactions should be noted in writing and re-ported to the doctor quickly.

The best way to make sure that a friend or relative is getting the kind of services he or she should is by visiting frequently and ran-domly. It is good to arrange visits so that promised events can be checked on. If a particular program is scheduled, such as a movie, exercise, a walk, a presentation by a visiting speaker, visit when it is scheduled and make sure that it happens from time to time. Some cancellations are unavoidable due to weather and such, but the general program the home promises should be carried out.

Appendix L contains the Bill of Rights for Nursing Home Patients suggested by the **Health Care Financing Administration**, which runs Medicare and Medicaid. Real, serious violations of these rights should be reported to the state authorities listed in appendix K. You should also contact the state nursing home ombudsman's office; a list is pro-vided in appendix O.

Generally, it is best to deal with problems by pointing them out, politely but firmly, to the appropriate person — the nurse, the admin-istrator, the billing office. The approach of being firm but not antag-onistic works best. Keep repeating, in a polite manner, the problem you see and the solution you want.

An important point to remember is this: *Don't let the nursing home put the monkey on your back.* You do not have to solve, or even sympathize with, their difficulties. In some situations, the proper an-swer to "What would you suggest?" is "I don't have to suggest any-thing. *You* have to find a way to deliver the services you promised and are being paid for."

Finally, it is not useful to threaten to move a resident. Besides the antagonism this may create, it may carry no weight at all in some areas. Many nursing homes have waiting lists and are well aware of the difficulties that often occur with nursing home placement. If a move is clearly indicated, make the arrangements and carry them out.

## Insurance

**1. I want to buy insurance to supplement my Medicare. What should I look for?**

We suggest that, at a minimum, you should purchase a policy that covers *all* the deductibles and copayments for hospital and doctor bills. This means that you will have to pay only what Medicare does not reimburse, which limits your expense to relatively minor items (with the exception of nursing home care). You should also look for policies that cover physician charges in excess of the Medicare–approved charge. Policies that cover these expenses should pay at least 80 percent of the excess fee up to the full balance billing limit. The policy should also cover the SNF copayment for days 21 through 100.

Here are some other features to look for:

- Guaranteed renewable
- No more than a six-month exclusion for preexisting conditions
- No limitations to single diseases, such as cancer, etc.
- No waiting periods for coverage

Chapter 4 provides more information about supplemental insurance and gives you a means of comparing policies.

## Getting Bills Paid/Filing Claims

### 1. How do I file a Medicare claim?

You don't! Thanks to a change in Medicare regulations, physicians and medical suppliers must prepare and submit your Medicare claims for any Part B services you receive. More precisely:

- Your doctor or medical supply company (medical equipment or supplies) must send in the claim even if they do not agree to accept Medicare assignment.

- They cannot charge you extra for filing the claim.

- If they do not agree to accept Medicare assignment, you are responsible for paying the whole bill; the Medicare payment will be sent to you.

- If they refuse to prepare and submit your Medicare claim, contact your Medicare carrier.

That's the long and short of filing a Medicare claim.

### 2. My doctor filled out my claim form and I filed a claim with my supplemental carrier, yet here I sit with a pile of rejection notices in front of me and no check. What went wrong?

Well ...... what should be a simple, effective process offering maximum speed of payment for providers and minimum worry for beneficiaries doesn't always work out that way. A large part of the problem is the number of hands spoiling the broth: your doctor, the Part B carrier, your supplemental insurance carrier, the peer review organization, Medicare itself and so on (and on, and on). Even with doctors and suppliers filing Part B claims for you, sometimes things can go wrong. Here are some suggestions for the situation you face. First, you need to find out why the claim was rejected. Check the message found on the **Explanation of Medicare Benefits (EOMB)** or the notice you received from your supplemental carrier. It may well be some variation of "claim already paid," "duplicate claim," "provider has not submitted claim," "no EOMB submitted," or some such message. What happens is this:

- Your doctor completes the claim form, as required by law, but has not yet submitted it to the carrier. In this case you don't have an EOMB to file with your supplemental insurer, and therefore, cannot recover your 20 percent copayment. Check with your doctor to find out when he/she is going to submit the claim.

- You paid in full for the service because your doctor does not accept assignment (he/she is required to file the claim), but you never received your reimbursement from Medicare. The doctor has not submitted the claim to the carrier and legally doesn't need to for up to one year. However, Medicare has warned that doctors and suppliers who willfully and repeatedly fail to submit assigned or nonassigned claims within one year will be subject to sanctions.

- He's a doctor who *does* take assignment (and therefore bills Medicare directly for 80 percent of the approved charge); his billing agency sent in a duplicate claim. Same situation, although here you don't even know that someone else's sending in a duplicate claim caused the rejection.

- Medicare has already paid its 80 percent of the approved fee on an assigned claim. You send Medicare a claim for the 20 percent copayment (which you must pay) instead of sending it to your Medicare supplemental insurer. Many carriers' computers often can't distinguish this situation from other duplicate claims, so you're told it's being rejected as duplicate, rather than being told that you're filing a claim for something that you or your insurer must pay.

- You pay the doctor in full for the service you received because he/she does not accept assignment. The doctor files the Medicare claim and you receive a check for 80 percent of the approved amount, as well as an EOMB. You now submit a second claim to Medicare to collect for the difference between the approved amount and what you paid the doctor. You receive a rejection notice from Medicare stating that the claim has been paid. Your claim should have been sent to your supplemental carrier for the 20 percent copayment. Some supplemental insurance policies may also cover charges above the Medicare-approved amount.

Second, check for these other common reasons for claims rejection:

- Medicare had paid for the maximum number of services you can have. For example, Part A of Medicare pays for home health visits for twenty-one consecutive days, but after that a gap of at least one day must elapse before more visits can be paid for.

- You sent Medicare a claim for a service that *is* covered under your Medicare supplemental policy but *not* under Medicare. Your Medicare supplemental insurer may maintain a help line (perhaps a toll-free number) that can help you determine where to file for what services. Also check your policy: it may provide a chart, or a simple English explanation, of what should be filed with it and what with Medicare.

- The claim, or part of it, was not paid because the money was needed to meet the Part A or Part B deductible.

- For psychiatric services, you have already received the lifetime maximum number (190) of inpatient days.

**3. But my claim was rejected because the peer review organization (or the carrier, or the intermediary) found that it was not medically necessary. What should I do now?**

You don't need to do anything unless the doctor (or some other Medicare provider) demands payment. Rejection of claims because the services the doctor rendered were not "reasonable and necessary" — which translates into *medically necessary* in the eyes of the PRO — is becoming more common. As we've noted repeatedly: *You are not required to pay for any service which you could not reasonably have been expected to know was not covered by Medicare. The only circumstance in which you are required to pay is one in which you were informed that no Medicare payment would be made for the specific service and you agreed to have the service performed in spite of this.* That a service (a course of treatment, a single treatment, a hospital stay) was not medically necessary is a judgment that the PRO is in most cases making after the fact. Hence, you're not required to pay: you cannot reasonably have been expected to know that the PRO, three months down the line, would find that the service you received wasn't needed. Does the PRO function of judging medical necessity mean that what Medicare routinely pays for on one side of some state or county line will be routinely rejected on the other? The answer is *yes*. This is, however, the nature of medical peer review. Groups of doctors in one part of the country don't necessarily always agree with groups of doctors in another.

How do you make use of this protection? Remember that in the vast majority of cases, you owe the doctor nothing. (You will probably get at least one bill, if the doctor's billing service is at all efficient, before you get the Explanation of Medicare Benefits [EOMB] with the rejection notice.) If you get a bill, send the doctor a *copy* of the EOMB (keep your original) together with the appropriate letter from pages 248–254.

Exactly how you make sure you don't have to pay, or get a refund if you have paid, is a bit complicated. The following letters cover all the situations you will encounter. The essence is this:

- For a participating or nonparticipating doctor whom you have not paid, you should pay nothing; just send the letter if the doctor bills you.

- For a participating or nonparticipating doctor whom you *have* paid, you are owed a refund within thirty days unless the doctor appeals, in which he must pay the refund within fifteen days after he receives the notice of the decision. If the decision is to pay him, you will receive a revised Explanation of Medicare Benefits.

**For a Doctor Who Is a Medicare Participant or Who Accepted Assignment on the Rejected Claim, to Whom You *Have Not Paid* the 20 percent Copayment**

Your name
Your street address
Your city, state, and ZIP code

The date [*Important!*]

Your doctor's name
His street address
His city, state, and ZIP code

Dear Doctor [*insert your doctor's name*]:

I recently received your bill for $ [*insert amount*] for [*insert name of service, such as "fulguration of warts," from bill or*

*Explanation of Medicare Benefits*] rendered on [*insert date*].

As you can see from the enclosed copy of my Explanation of Medicare Benefits, Medicare has rejected this claim because the services were found not to be medically necessary. A notice to this effect should have been sent to you by Medicare.

I am sure that you always try to give me the best care you can, and that doctors may differ from time to time. It is important that you know that I am not required to pay the 20 percent Medicare copayment under these circumstances. Depending on the circumstances, you may or may not be paid by Medicare for the other 80 percent of the Medicare approved charge.

Please correct your records to show that I do not owe you anything for this service.

Thank you for your attention to this request.

> Sincerely yours,
> Your signature

---

**For a Doctor Who is a Medicare Participant or Who Accepted Assignment on the Rejected Claim, to Whom You *Have Paid* the 20 percent Copayment**

Your name
Your street address
Your city, state and ZIP code

The date [*Important!*]

Your doctor's name
His street address
His city, state, and ZIP code

Dear Doctor [*insert your doctor's name*]:

I recently received your bill for $[*insert amount*] for [*insert name of service, such as "fulguration of warts," from bill or Explanation of Medicare Benefits*] rendered on [*insert date*].

As you can see from the enclosed copy of my Explanation of Medicare Benefits, Medicare has rejected this claim because the services were found not to be medically necessary. A notice to this effect should have been sent to you by Medicare.

I am sure that you always try to give me the best care you can, and that doctors may differ from time to time. It is important that you know that I am not required to pay the 20 percent Medicare copayment under these circumstances. Depending on the circumstances, you may or may not be paid by Medicare for the other 80 percent of the Medicare-approved charge.

I would appreciate your refunding me the amount of $[*insert amount*], which I paid [*insert "by check number" and number if you paid by check, "by money order" and number if you paid by money order*] on [*insert date*].

Thank you for your attention to this request.

Sincerely yours,
Your signature

---

**For a Doctor Who Is Not a Medicare Participant or Who Did Not Accept Assignment on the Rejected Claim, to Whom You *Have Not Paid* the 20 percent Copayment and Any Additional Amount**

Your name
Your street address
Your city, state and ZIP code

The date [*Important!*]

Your doctor's name
His street address
His city, state, and ZIP code

Dear Doctor [*insert your doctor's name*]:

I recently received your bill for $[*insert amount*] for [*insert name of service, such as "fulguration of warts," from bill or Explanation of Medicare Benefits*] rendered on [*insert date*].

As you can see from the enclosed copy of my Explanation of Medicare Benefits, Medicare has rejected this claim because the services were found not to be medically necessary. A notice to this effect should have been sent to you by Medicare.

I am sure that you always try to give me the best care you can, and that doctors may differ from time to time. It is important that you know that I am not required to pay any of your bill under these circumstances. Depending on the circumstances, you may or may not be paid by Medicare for the other 80 percent of the Medicare approved charge.

Thank you for your attention to this request.

Sincerely yours,
Your signature

**For a Doctor Who Is Not a Medicare Participant or Who Did Not Accept Assignment on The Rejected Claim, to Whom You *Have Paid* the 20 percent Copayment and Any Additional Amounts**

Your name
Your street address
Your city, state and ZIP code

The date [*Important!*]

Your doctor's name
His street address
His city, state, and ZIP code

Dear Doctor [*insert your doctor's name*]:

I recently received your bill for $[*insert amount*] for [*insert name of service, such as "fulguration of warts," from bill or Explanation of Medicare Benefits*] rendered on [*insert date*].

As you can see from the enclosed copy of my Explanation of Medicare Benefits, Medicare has rejected this claim because the services were found not to be medically necessary. A notice to this effect should have been sent to you by Medicare.

I am sure that you always try to give me the best care you can, and that doctors may differ from time to time. It is important that you know that I am not required to pay the 20 percent Medicare copayment under these circumstances. Depending on the circumstances, you may or may not be paid by Medicare for the other 80 percent of the Medicare approved charge.

I would appreciate your refunding me the amount of $ [*insert amount*], which I paid [*insert "by check number" and number if you paid by check, "by money order" and number if you paid by money order*] on [*insert date*].

Thank you for your attention to this request.

Sincerely yours,
Your signature

**4. My claim wasn't rejected totally, but I got a notice that it was reduced because of a judgment of medical necessity. What does that mean?**

Essentially, the situation is exactly the same as for a rejected claim, but the PRO found that some other procedure, logically part of what the doctor did, *was* medically justified. For example, a charge for a lengthy office visit was changed to a charge for a brief office visit, and the doctor was paid 80 percent of the approved charge for that. You can use letters similar to the ones cited. Samples with the appropriate changes follow.

**For a Doctor Who Is a Medicare Participant or Who Accepted Assignment on the Rejected Claim, to Whom You *Have Not Paid* the 20 percent Copayment**

Your name
Your street address
Your city, state and ZIP code

The date [*Important!*]

Your doctor's name
His street address
His city, state, and ZIP code

Dear Doctor [*insert your doctor's name*]:

I recently received your bill for $[*insert amount*] for [*insert name of service, such as "fulguration of warts," from bill or Explanation of Medicare Benefits*] rendered on [*insert date*].

As you can see from the enclosed copy of my Explanation of Medicare benefits, Medicare has reduced the charge for this claim because the services were found not to be medically necessary. A notice to this effect should have been sent to you by Medicare.

I am sure that you always try to give me the best care you can, and that doctors may differ from time to time. It is important that you know that I am not required to pay more than 20 percent Medicare copayment for the reduced claim under these circumstances.

Please correct your records to show that I do not owe you any more than this amount for this service.

Thank you for your attention to this request.

Sincerely yours,
Your signature

---

**For a Doctor Who Is a Medicare Participant or Who Accepted Assignment on the Rejected Claim, to Whom You *Have Paid* the 20 percent Copayment**

Your name
Your street address
Your city, state and ZIP code

The date [*Important!*]

Your doctor's name
His street address
His city, state, and ZIP code

Dear Doctor [*insert your doctor's name*]:

I recently received your bill for $[*insert amount*] for [*insert name of service, such as "fulguration of warts," from bill or*

*Explanation of Medicare Benefits*] rendered on [*insert date*].

As you can see from the enclosed copy of my Explanation of Medicare Benefits, Medicare has reduced the charge for this claim because some of the services were found not to be medically necessary. A notice to this effect should have been sent to you by Medicare.

I am sure that you always try to give me the best care you can, and that doctors may differ from time to time. It is important that you know that I am not required to pay the 20 percent Medicare copayment for the reduced claim under these circumstances. Depending on the circumstances, you may or may not be paid by Medicare for the other 80 percent of the Medicare-approved charge.

I would appreciate your refunding me the amount of $[*insert amount*], which I paid [*insert "by check number" and number if you paid by check, "by money order" and number if you paid by money order*] on [*insert date*].

Thank you for your attention to this request.

Sincerely yours,
Your signature

---

**For a Doctor Who Is Not a Medicare Participant or Who Did Not Accept Assignment on the Rejected Claim, to Whom You *Have Not Paid* 20 percent Copayment and Any Additional Amount**

Your name
Your street address
Your city, state and ZIP code

The date [*Important!*]

Your doctor's name
His street address
His city, state, and ZIP code

Dear Doctor [*insert your doctor's name*]:

I recently received your bill for $[*insert amount*] for [*insert name of service, such as "fulguration of warts," from bill or Explanation of Medicare Benefits*] rendered on [*insert date*].

As you can see from the enclosed copy of my Explanation of Medicare Benefits, Medicare has reduced this claim because some of the services were found not to be medically necessary. A notice to this effect should have been sent to you by Medicare.

I am sure that you always try to give me the best care you can, and that doctors may differ from time to time. It is important that you know that I am not required to pay more than the balance billing limit, less 80 percent of the Medicare-approved charges, under these circumstances.

Please correct your records to show that I do not owe you any more than this amount for this service.

Thank you for your attention to this request.

Sincerely yours,
Your signature

---

**For a Doctor Who Is Not a Medicare Participant or Who Did Not Accept Assignment on the Rejected Claim, to Whom You *Have Paid* the 20 percent Copayment and Any Additional Amounts**

Your name
Your street address
Your city, state and ZIP code

The date [*Important!*]

Your doctor's name
His street address
His city, state, and ZIP code

Dear Doctor [*insert your doctor's name*]:

I recently received your bill for $[*insert amount*] for [*insert name of service, such as "fulguration of warts," from bill or Explanation of Medicare Benefits*] rendered on [*insert date*].

As you can see from the enclosed copy of my Explanation of Medicare Benefits, Medicare has rejected this claim because the services were found not to be medically necessary. A notice to this effect should have been sent to you by Medicare.

I am sure that you always try to give me the best care you can, and that doctors may differ from time to time. It is important that you know that I am not required to pay more than the balance billing limit, less 80 percent of the Medicare-approved charges, under these circumstances.

I would appreciate your refunding me the amount of $[*insert amount*], which I paid [*insert "by check number" and number if you paid by check, "by money order" and number if you paid by money order*] on [*insert date*].

Thank you for your attention to this request.

Sincerely yours,
Your signature

**5. My doctor says she doesn't have to correct the bill, or pay the refund, because she has a sign in her waiting room that says that Medicare may not cover some services. Is she right?**

No. Medicare has specifically ruled that the display of such a sign does *not* excuse the doctor from correcting bills, reducing charges, or paying refunds.

**6. I've sent the letters you suggested, but my doctor is dunning me and I don't want my credit rating ruined. What should I do?**

Review the situation to make sure that you are facing a claim that you don't have to pay. If you are reasonably certain, ask for assistance from the Medicare carrier or intermediary. If you have asked for assistance and have received none, call the Department of Health and Human Services Office of the Inspector General at 1-800-447-8477.

## Appeals

There are basically three circumstance in which you will want to appeal. The first is that in which you are about to be admitted to a hospital or nursing home, or to have an inpatient or outpatient operation, and the PRO finds it medically unnecessary. The second is the one in which you are a patient, and the PRO or a review body, such as the hospital's utilization review committee (URC), determines that your stay is no longer medically necessary and determines that Medicare will no longer pay. The third is one in which a claim you have submitted for a service already received is denied.

We covered the first two circumstances in chapter 6. That material is repeated below. The procedure is generic for both hospitals and nursing homes. Before you decide to appeal a decision not to pay a claim, check the discussion about claims above to make sure that you do, in fact, have to pay something. If the claim is covered under Medicare's **waiver of liability** rules, your doctor usually has the right to appeal nonpayment and you don't have to pay anything. Appeal procedures for Part A and Part B bills follow.

*Procedure for Appeals of Peer Review Organization Decisions*

The procedure that follows is *generic*. It applies to *all* actions by the PRO. Only the evidence submitted would differ.

*Notices:* Your denial is called a Notice of Noncoverage, and it will explain why something is being denied.

*How to Appeal (Request a Reconsideration) of a Peer Review Organization Decision:* You can appeal the PRO decision by filing a request for reconsideration with the PRO itself, at the address for the PRO shown on the notice you received; at any Social Security office, or at a Railroad Retirement Board office, if you are a railroad retirement beneficiary.

Your doctor and the hospital also have the right to file an appeal. They do *not* have the right to an "expedited reconsideration" that you have.

*Time to File the Request for Reconsideration:* You must file your request for reconsideration within sixty days of the date you receive the Notice of Noncoverage. Unless you can prove otherwise, the notice is deemed to have been received by you five days after the date on it. (Example: The notice is dated January 5. You are deemed to have received it on January 10, unless you can prove you received it later. Your sixty-day period for appeal started on January 10. The last day you can file an appeal is March 10, the sixtieth day after the deemed receipt of the notice.)

*"Good Cause" for Late Filing:* Generally, you will be allowed to file late if there is what the PRO considers to be "good cause" for it. The regulations are very broad, and it is hard to see what exactly might count. The regulations give examples such as serious illness, a death in the family, failure to receive information you had requested before the sixty-day limit, a misunderstanding of what the PRO notice told you, and so on.

*Obtaining Information:* Both you and your doctor have a right to see the information on which the PRO based its decision. You should ask for this when you file your request for reconsideration. You may add to the information anything you or your doctor want to add.

*Expedited Reconsideration and Time Limits:* You can request that the PRO make an expedited reconsideration of the denial. How fast "expedited" has to be depends on the circumstances.

DEPARTMENT OF HEALTH, EDUCATION, AND WELFARE
HEALTH CARE FINANCING ADMINISTRATION

Form Approved.
OMB No. 066-R-0067

# REQUEST FOR RECONSIDERATION OF PART A HEALTH INSURANCE BENEFITS

INSTRUCTIONS: *Please type or print firmly.* Leave the block empty if you cannot answer it. Take or mail the WHOLE form to your Social Security office which will be glad to help you. Please read the statement on the reverse side of page 2.

| 1. BENEFICIARY'S NAME | 2. HEALTH INSURANCE CLAIM NUMBER |
|---|---|

3. REPRESENTATIVE'S NAME, IF APPLICABLE

(☐ RELATIVE  ☐ ATTORNEY  ☐ OTHER PERSON)  ☐ PROVIDER FILING

## 4. PLEASE ATTACH A COPY OF THE NOTICE(S) YOU RECEIVED ABOUT YOUR CLAIM TO THIS FORM.

5. THIS CLAIM IS FOR
☐ INPATIENT HOSPITAL  ☐ SKILLED NURSING FACILITY (SNF)  ☐ HEALTH MAINTENANCE ORGANIZATION (HMO)
☐ EMERGENCY HOSPITAL  ☐ HOME HEALTH AGENCY (HHA)

| 6. NAME AND ADDRESS OF PROVIDER *(Hospital, SNF, HHA, HMO)* | CITY AND STATE | PROVIDER NUMBER |
|---|---|---|

| 7. NAME OF INTERMEDIARY | CITY AND STATE | INTERMEDIARY NUMBER |
|---|---|---|

| 8. DATE OF ADMISSION OR START OF SERVICES | 9. DATE(S) OF THE NOTICE(S) YOU RECEIVED |
|---|---|

10. I DO NOT AGREE WITH THE DETERMINATION ON MY CLAIM. PLEASE RECONSIDER MY CLAIM BECAUSE

11. YOU MUST OBTAIN ANY EVIDENCE *(For example, a letter from a doctor)* YOU WISH TO SUBMIT.

☐ I HAVE ATTACHED THE FOLLOWING EVIDENCE:

☐ I WILL SEND THIS EVIDENCE WITHIN 10 DAYS:

☐ I HAVE NO ADDITIONAL EVIDENCE OR OTHER INFORMATION TO SUBMIT WITH MY CLAIM.

13. ONLY ONE SIGNATURE IS NEEDED. THIS FORM IS SIGNED BY:
☐ BENEFICIARY  ☐ REPRESENTATIVE  ☐ PROVIDER REP.

SIGN HERE ▶

14. STREET ADDRESS

12. IS THIS REQUEST FILED WITHIN 60 DAYS OF THE DATE OF YOUR NOTICE?

☐ YES  ☐ NO

IF YOU CHECKED "NO" ATTACH AN EXPLANATION OF THE REASON FOR THE DELAY TO THIS FORM.

CITY, STATE, ZIP CODE

| TELEPHONE | DATE |
|---|---|

15. If this request is signed by mark (X), TWO WITNESSES who know the person requesting reconsideration must sign in the space provided on the reverse side of this page of the form.

## DO NOT FILL IN BELOW THIS LINE — FOR SOCIAL SECURITY USE — THANK YOU

16. ROUTING
☐ INTERMEDIARY
☐ HCFA, RO-MEDICARE
☐ BSS, ODR

18. SSA OR INTERMEDIARY DATE STAMP

17. ADDITIONAL INFORMATION

FORM **HCFA-2649** (8-79  FORMERLY SSA-2649)
DESTROY PRIOR EDITIONS

INTERMEDIARY

Page 1 of 4

- Within three working days if you are still a patient in the hospital (this doesn't really apply here, of course, since you're trying to get in)
- Within three days if the initial determination was a denial of hospital admission and you are still in the hospital
- Within ten working days if you are in a skilled nursing facility
- Within thirty working days in all other situations, and in every situation where someone other than you files the appeal. Having expedited redetermination available is a very important reason for *you* to file the appeal and have the doctor or hospital submit information as part of an appeal.

***What to Include:*** You should file your claim using HCFA Form 2649, which is shown on page 257.

You can request an appeal with just a letter, but using the form will ensure that you include everything that is needed. You should ask your doctor to provide medical documentation. It is important for both you and your doctor to focus on the issue at hand, and not editorialize. The general issue you will be dealing with in PRO denials of admission is the *medical necessity* for you to be hospitalized at all, or to have a procedure done in the hospital or done at all. Keep the focus on these issues. They will boil down to appropriate medical judgment. Your doctor will probably want to submit information regarding your condition, plus evidence from the medical literature indicating that what the PRO wants done is unwise.

***Notices and Appeals:*** When the PRO provides you with its reconsidered decision, it must do so *in writing* and inform you of the following:

- The decision
- The reasons for it
- A statement of the effect the decision has on what Medicare will pay for or has paid for
- A statement of your appeal rights, with complete instructions for filing the appeal
- When you receive a notice of a reconsidered decision that is not in your favor, you should consider whether you want to request a hearing. A hearing is more formal than a reconsideration, and it entitles you to appear before an **administrative law judge (ALJ)**. If you do request a hearing, it is wise to have a lawyer involved. Hearings can

involve subpoenaing witnesses and other legal steps. It is less formal than a court case, but far more formal than a request for reconsideration. Medicare is emphasizing doing all business possible, including hearings, over the phone. Although a hearing can be conducted over the phone, you should carefully consider appearing in person. It is sometimes easier to make your case in person, depending on the circumstances.

- Only you, not your doctor or the hospital, have this right. The rules for filing an appeal are exactly the same as for filing for reconsideration with the PRO — sixty days, counted from five days after the date of the notice, and all that. You should file your appeal on HCFA HA-501-US, unless the information you received with the PRO's Notice of Reconsideration tells you to do something else.

- The first thing the ALJ will attempt to determine is whether or not the controversy involves at least $200 (with the price of health care these days, it almost surely will). If the ALJ determines that the amount is less than $200, he will notify you and any other concerned parties that he has determined this and that they have fifteen days to show why he is wrong. If no evidence is submitted within fifteen days, the request for a hearing is dismissed. (You will not have to worry about this if you don't receive such a notice.)

- You will be notified by the ALJ of the date of the hearing at least ten days before it is filed.

- If the ALJ's decision is unfavorable, you can appeal to the Social Security Appeals Council. Your attorney can tell you how to do this. The Appeals Council does not take all the appeals addressed to it. If $2,000 or more is at issue, you can appeal an Appeals Council decision, or the ALJ's decision if the Appeals Council refused a hearing, to the federal courts. This must be done within sixty days of the date of the Appeals Council decision on your case, or its decision not to hear it.

*Requesting Reconsiderations (Appealing Decisions) on Payment of Claims*

The procedures in this section apply to denial of payment for all services, other than doctors' services, after you have left the hospital. They also apply to notices regarding hospital care that you receive from the Medicare intermediary while you are in the hospital.

*Notices:* Your Notice of Noncoverage will come either in the form of an **Explanation of Medicare Benefits (EOMB)** or in the form of a letter. In any case, it must be in writing. It will explain the reason that something is being denied. A typical EOMB is shown on page 260.

# Explanation of Your Medicare Part B Benefits

Name of Beneficiary

Iphigenia Smith
4321 Edgar Allen Poe Drive
San Diego, CA 99110

Your Medicare number:   120-99-6789

A summary about this notice dated December 30, 1996.

| | |
|---|---|
| Total charges: | $1,755.00 |
| Total Medicare approved: | $1,339.00 |
| Medicare paid your provider: | $1,071.20 |
| You are responsible for: | $ 367.80 |

---

**Details about this claim (See the back of this notice for more information.)**

You received these services from your provider;
Dr. Sherman T. Potter, claim-#9876-1234-2468

Midway Medical Clinic, 2552 Baskerville Rd.,
San Diego, CA 99110

This indicates amount billed and approved.

| Services and Service Codes | Dates | Charge | Medicare approved | Notes |
|---|---|---|---|---|
| 65850 surgery, incision of eye | Nov 15, 1996 | $975.00 | $780.00 | a |
| 90040 brief office visit | Nov 19, 1996 | $100.00 | $ 0 | b |
| 90070 extended office visits | Nov 17–29, 1996 | $600.00 | $516.00 | a |
| 90040 brief office visit | Nov 30, 1996 | $ 40.00 | $ 21.50 | a |
| 90040 brief office visit | Dec 15, 1996 | $ 40.00 | $ 21.50 | a |
| | Total | $1,755.00 | $1,339.00 | |

This indicates the service and date provided.

Notes:

a  We based the approved amount on the fee schedule for this service.

b  Medicare did not pay for this test. Medicare pays for this only when the laboratory is certified for this type of test.

This tells you if assignment was taken and the dollar amount billed.

Here's an explanation of this claim:

| | | |
|---|---|---|
| Of the total charges, Medicare approved | $1,339.00 | The provider accepted this amount. See #4 on the back of this notice. |
| The deductible you still owe | $ 0 | You have met the $100 deductible for 1996. |
| | $1,339.00 × .80 | Medicare pays 80 percent of this total. |
| We are paying the provider | $1,071.20 | Your copayment is 20 percent or $267.80. |
| Of the amount approved | $1,339.00 | |
| Subtract what we pay the provider | $1,071.20 | |
| You are responsible for | $ 267.80 | |
| plus charges not covered by Medicare | $ 100.00 | |
| The total you are responsible for: | $ 367.80 | The provider may bill you for this amount. If you have other insurance, the other insurance may pay this amount. |

This indicates whether or not you have met the $100 deductible this year.

This explains what you pay.

---

If you have questions about this notice, call Blue Cross Blue Shield of Maryland at 410-861-2273 or toll free at 800-662-5170 or visit us at 1946 Greenspring Drive, Timonium, Maryland.
You'll need this notice when you call or visit us about this claim.
If you want to appeal this claim, see #5 on the other side. You must write us by June 30, 1997.

This gives you the time frame to file any appeal.

This is your Part B carrier. If you suspect a mistake, contact this office.

# Important Information You Should Know About Your Medicare Part B Benefits

**This part of the notice answers some common questions that people ask about collecting Medicare benefits. If you have other questions, see your copy of *The Medicare Handbook* or call us for more information.**

**1. What should I do if I have questions about this notice?**

If you have questions about this notice, call, write, or visit us and we will tell you the facts that we used to decide what and how much to pay. Turn to the front of this notice: our address and phone number are on the bottom of the page.

**2. Can I appeal how much Medicare paid for these services?**

If you do not agree with what Medicare approved for these services, you may appeal our decision. To make sure that we are fair to you, we will not allow the same people who originally processed these services to conduct this review.

However, in order to be eligible for a review, you **must** write to us within **6 months** of the date of this notice, unless you have a good reason for being late (for example, if you had an extended illness which kept you from being able to file on time).

Turn to the front of this notice: the deadline date and our address are on the bottom of the page. It may help your case if you include a note from your doctor or supplier (provider) that tells us what was done and why.

If you want help with your appeal, you can have a friend, lawyer, or someone else help you. Some lawyers do not charge unless you win your appeal. There are groups, such as lawyer referral services, that can help you find a lawyer. There are also groups, such as legal aid services, who will give you free legal services if you qualify.

**3. How much does Medicare pay?**

The details on the front of this notice explain how much Medicare paid for these services. See your copy of *The Medicare Handbook* for more information about the benefits you are entitled to as a beneficiary in the Medicare Part B program. If you need another copy of the handbook, call or visit your local Social Security office.

Medicare may make adjustments to your payment. We may reduce the amount we pay for services by a certain percentage (Balanced Budget Law). If your provider accepted assignment, you are not liable to pay the amount of this reduction. We pay interest on some claims not paid within the required time.

All Medicare payments are made on the condition that you will pay Medicare back if benefits are also paid under insurance that is primary to Medicare. Examples of other insurance are employer group health plans, automobile medical, liability, no fault, or workers' compensation. Notify us immediately if you have filed or could file a claim with insurance that is primary to Medicare.

**4. How can I reduce my medical costs?**

Many providers have agreed to be part of **Medicare's participation program.** That means that they will always accept the amount that Medicare approves as their full payment. Write or call us for the name of a participating provider or for a free list of participating providers.

A provider who accepts assignment can charge you only for the part of the annual deductible you have not met and the copayment which is the remaining 20 percent of the approved amount.

If you are treated by one of these doctors you can save money. See *The Medicare Handbook* for more information about how you can reduce your medical costs.

**5. How can I use this notice?**

You can use this notice to:

- Contact us immediately if you think Medicare paid for a service you did not receive

- Show your provider how much of your deductible you have met

- Claim benefits with another insurance company. If you send this notice to them, make a copy of it for your records.

---

**Keep this notice for your records.**
*Health Care Financing Administration*

*How to Appeal (Request a Reconsideration) of a Payment Denial or Intermediary Determination that Care is Not Medically Necessary:* You can appeal the PRO decision by filing a request for reconsideration with the intermediary itself, at the address shown on the EOMB, at any Social Security office, or a Railroad Retirement Board office, if you are a railroad retirement beneficiary, or at any office of the Health Care Financing Administration.

Your doctor and the hospital have the right to file an appeal only if you do not plan to do so and you certify this in writing on a form they will provide. They do *not* have the right to an "expedited reconsideration" that you have.

*Time to File the Request for Reconsideration:* You must file your request for reconsideration within sixty days of the date you receive the notice of denial. Unless you can prove otherwise, the notice is deemed to have been received by you five days after the date on it. (Example: The notice is dated January 5. You are deemed to have received it on January 10. The last day you can file an appeal is March 10, the sixtieth day after the deemed receipt of the notice.)

*Request for Extension of Time to File:* If you need more than sixty days to file your appeal, you can request more time at any Social Security office, Medicare office, or the Railroad Retirement Board. You cannot file an extension request with an intermediary. You will be notified in writing of the time granted you.

*"Good Cause" for Granting a Time Extension:* Generally, you will be allowed to file late if there is what PRO considers to be "good cause" for it. The regulations are very broad and it is hard to see what exactly might count. The regulations give examples such as serious illness, a death in the family, failure to receive information you had requested before the sixty-day limit, a misunderstanding of what the PRO notice told you, and so on.

*Obtaining Information:* Both you and your doctor have a right to see the information on which the PRO based its decision. You should ask for this when you file your request for reconsideration. You may add to the information anything you or your doctor want to add.

*Expedited Reconsideration:* There is a procedure for expedited appeals under Part A (hospital insurance), but it may be used only if both the person appealing and the secretary of Health and Human Services (HHS) agree that the only issue is a constitutional one. This is a rare situation.

*What to Include:* You should file your claim using HCFA Form 2649. You can request an appeal with just a letter, but using the form will ensure that you include everything that is needed. You should ask your doctor to provide medical documentation. It is important for both you and your doctor to focus on the issue at hand, and not editorialize. The general issues you will be dealing with are as follows:

- The medical necessity of the service
- Whether or not Medicare covers it
- Whether or not you are entitled to it
- Whether or not the amount paid is what ought to have been paid

Medical necessity issues will boil down to appropriate medical judgment. Your doctor will probably want to submit information regarding your condition, plus evidence from the medical literature that indicates that the decision is unwise.

*Time Limits:* The regulations provide no time limit for a decision on a Part A request for reconsideration.

*Notices and Appeals:* When you are provided with the reconsidered decision, it will include, in writing, the following:

- The decision
- The reasons for it
- A statement of the effect the decision has on what Medicare will pay for, or has paid for
- A statement of your appeal rights, with complete instructions for filing the appeal

When you receive a notice of a reconsidered decision that is not in your favor, consider whether you want to request a hearing. A hearing is more formal than a reconsideration, and entitles you to appear before an ALJ. If you do request a hearing, it is wise to have a lawyer involved. Hearings can involve subpoenaing witnesses and other legal steps. It is less formal than a court case, but far more formal than a request for reconsideration.

Only you, not your doctor or the hospital, have this right. The rules for filing an appeal are exactly the same as for filing for reconsideration — sixty days, counted from five days after the date of the notice, and all that. You should file your appeal on HCFA HA-501-US, unless the information you received with the Notice of Reconsideration tells you to do something else.

You may request a hearing only if the amount in controversy is $100 or more.

You should also note that your request for a hearing will be deemed received *five days* after the date on it, unless you can show that it was received earlier. If you are within five days of the sixty-day limit, send it *certified mail, return receipt requested,* so you will have proof of the date it was actually received.

The first thing the ALJ will attempt to determine is whether or not the controversy involves at least $100 (with the price of health care these days, it almost surely will). If the ALJ determines that the amount is less than $100, he will notify you and any other concerned parties that he has determined this and that they have fifteen days to show why he is wrong. If no evidence is submitted within fifteen days, the request for a hearing is dismissed. (You will not have to worry about this if you don't receive such a notice.)

You will be notified by the ALJ of the date of the hearing at least ten days before it is filed.

If the ALJ's decision is unfavorable, you can appeal to the Social Security Appeals Council. Your attorney can tell you how to do this. The Appeals Council does not take all the appeals addressed to it. If $1,000 or more is at issue, you can appeal an Appeals Council decision, or the ALJ's decision if the Appeals Council refused a hearing, to the federal courts. This must be done within sixty days of the date of the Appeals Council decision on your case, or its decision not to hear it.

If you receive a favorable determination, Medicare will pay its usual amounts for the services rendered. If you do not receive a favorable determination, you pay.

*Appeals of Health Maintenance Organization Decisions*

As a member of a health maintenance organization, you have all the appeal rights that Medicare beneficiaries have. In addition, Medicare requires that the HMO have a written appeals procedure for all members for matters within the HMO. Which one you should use depends on the circumstances. We suggest using the HMO appeals process for matters that can be resolved within the HMO (for example, you want a treatment and your doctor does not think it is medically indicated) and the Medicare process for matters that you cannot resolve using the

HMO procedure. Just keep in mind the time limits for Medicare appeals. Do not fail to file a Medicare appeal of a Notice of Non-coverage, for example, just because you are trying to work matters out with the HMO.

## Coordination with Employers' Health Insurance and Retirement Plans

Plans are so varied, and changes so rapid, that it is hard to give specific advice. Keep in mind that employer-provided health insurance for persons over 65 who continue to work is now the *secondary* payer, with Medicare picking up the difference between what the plan doesn't pay and what Medicare does — *not* the difference between what the plan pays and what you are charged. Look carefully at the list of Medicare-covered items in chapter 3, and if you think Medicare covers something that the employer plan does not cover (the most common example is likely to be skilled nursing facility services), make sure you file a claim with Medicare.

Also remember that many employer health plans are, in fact, health insurance policies purchased from a carrier for a group of employees and are regulated by the insurance commission or equivalent body in your state. Contact the insurance commission if you suspect you are not receiving fair treatment or the benefits to which you are entitled.

# Appendix A: Medicare Intermediaries and Carriers

Carriers can answer questions about Medical Insurance (Part B).

Note: Funding for the toll-free, or 800, numbers listed may be discontinued. Medicare will advise you of any changes in telephone numbers.

**Alabama**
Medicare/Blue Cross-Blue Shield
  of Alabama
450 Riverchase Parkway, E.
Birmingham, AL 35298
205-988-2100
800-292-8855

**Alaska**
Medicare/Aetna Life Insurance Co.
P.O. Box 1997
Portland, OR 97207-1997
503-243-5351
800-547-6333

**Arizona**
Medicare/Aetna Life Insurance Co.
P.O. Box 37200
7600 N. 16th Street, Suite 100
Phoenix, AZ 85020
602-870-6203
800-352-0411

**Arkansas**
Medicare/Arkansas Blue Cross
  and Blue Shield
601 S. Gaines Street
Little Rock, AR 72201-4041
501-378-2000
800-482-5525

**California**
*(North)*
Medicare/California Physician's Service
(d/b/a Blue Shield of California)
P.O. Box 7013
San Francisco, CA 94130-7013
415-445-5971
800-675-2266

*(South)*
Medicare/Transamerica Occidental
  Life Insurance Co.
P.O. Box 54905
Los Angeles, CA 90054-0905
213-748-2311

**Colorado**
Medicare/Blue Cross and Blue Shield
  of North Dakota
711 Second Avenue, N.
Fargo, ND 58102
701-282-1100

**Connecticut**
Medicare/The Travelers Insurance Co.
P.O. Box 9000
538 Preston Avenue
Meriden, CT 06454-9000
203-639-3000
800-982-6819

**Delaware**
Medicare/Medical Services
  of Pennsylvania
(d/b/a Xact Medicare Services)
P.O. Box 890065
Camp Hill, PA 17089-0065
717-763-3151
800-851-3535

**District of Columbia**
Medicare/Pennsylvania Blue Shield
P.O. Box 890065
Camp Hill, PA 17089-0065
717-763-3151
800-233-1124

**Florida**
Medicare/Blue Shield of Florida, Inc.
P.O. Box 2078
532 Riverside Avenue
Jacksonville, FL 32231-0019
904-791-6111
800-333-7586
For fast service on simple inquiries
    including requests for copies of
    explanation of Medicare benefits
    notices, requests for Medpard
    directories, brief claims inquiries
    (status or verification of receipt),
    and address changes:
800-666-7586

**Georgia**
Medicare/Aetna Life Insurance Co.
P.O. Box 60010
Savannah, GA 31402-0010
912-921-3010
800-727-0827

**Hawaii**
Medicare/Aetna Life & Casualty
P.O. Box 3947
Honolulu, HI 96812-3947
808-539-5216
800-272-5242

**Idaho**
Medicare/Aetna Life Insurance Co.
Two Vantage Way
Nashville, TN 37228
615-244-5600

**Illinois**
Medicare Claims/Health Care
    Service Corp.
3109 W. DeYoung Street
Marion, IL 62959-5543
618-997-2311
800-642-6930

**Indiana**
Medicare Part B/Associated
    Insurance Co.
8115 Knue Street
Indianapolis, IN 46250-2804
317-842-4425
800-622-4792

**Iowa**
Medicare/IASD Health Services Inc.
636 Grand Avenue, Station 112
Des Moines, IA 50309
515-245-4618
800-532-1285

**Kansas**
Medicare/Blue Cross and Blue Shield
    of Kansas
1133 S.W. Topeka Boulevard
Topeka, KS 66629-0001
913-291-7000

**Kentucky**
Medicare Part B/Adminastar of
    Kentucky, Inc.
(d/b/a Blue Cross and Blue Shield
    of Kentucky)
9901 Linn Station Road
Louisville, KY 40223
502-329-8512
800-999-7608

**Louisiana**
Arkansas Blue Cross and Blue Shield
    Medicare Administration
601 Gaines Street
Little Rock, AR 72203
501-378-2000
800-462-9666

**Maine**
Medicare/Blue Shield of
    Massachusetts
100 Summer Street
Boston, MA 02110
617-741-3300
800-492-0919

**Maryland**

*Counties of Prince Georges and*
*Montgomery:*
Medicare/Medical Services Association
of Pennsylvania
(d/b/a Xact Medicare Services)
P.O. Box 890065
Camp Hill, PA 17089-0065
717-763-3151

*Rest of state:*
Medicare/Blue Cross and Blue Shield
of Texas
901 South Central Expressway
Richardson, TX 75080
214-766-6900
800-233-1124

**Massachusetts**

Medicare/Blue Cross and Blue Shield
of Massachusetts
100 Summer Street
Boston, MA 02110
617-741-3300
800-882-1228

**Michigan**

Medicare Claims/Health Care
Service Corp.
3109 W. DeYoung Street
Marion, IL 62959-5543
618-997-2311

**Minnesota**

*Counties of Anoka, Dakota, Fillmore,*
*Goodhue, Hennepin, Houston*
*Olmstead, Ramsey, Wabasha,*
*Washington, and Winona:*
Minnesota Medicare/The Travelers
Insurance Co.
8120 Penn Avenue S.
Bloomington, MN 55431-1394
612-885-2800
800-352-2762

*Rest of state:*
Medicare/Blue Cross and Blue Shield
of Minnesota
P.O. Box 64357
St. Paul, MN 55164-0357
612-456-8000
800-392-0343

**Mississippi**

Medicare/The Travelers Insurance Co.
P.O. Box 22545
Jackson, MS 39225-2545
601-977-5750
800-682-5417 (In Mississippi)
800-227-2349 (Outside Mississippi)

**Missouri**

*Counties of Andrew, Atchison, Bates,*
*Benton, Buchanan, Caldwell,*
*Carroll, Cass, Clay, Clinton,*
*Daviess, DeKalb, Gentry, Grundy,*
*Harrison, Henry, Holt, Jackson,*
*Johnson, Lafayette, Livingston,*
*Mercer, Nodaway, Pettis, Platte,*
*Ray, St. Clair, Saline, Vernon,*
*and Worth:*
Medicare/Blue Cross and Blue Shield
of Kansas
1133 S.W. Topeka Boulevard
Topeka, KS 66629-0001
913-291-7000
800-892-5900

*Rest of state:*
Medicare/General American Life
Insurance Co.
P.O. Box 505
St. Louis, MO 63166
314-525-5441
800-392-3070

**Montana**

Medicare/Blue Cross and Blue Shield
of Montana
P.O. Box 4310
2501 Beltview
Helena, MT 59601
406-444-8350
800-332-6146

**Nebraska**

Medicare/Blue Cross and Blue Shield
of Kansas
1133 S.W. Topeka Boulevard
Topeka, KS 66629-0001
913-291-7000
800-633-1113

**Nevada**
Medicare/Aetna Life & Casualty Co.
1515 E. Tropicana Avenue, Suite 640
Las Vegas, NV 89119
702-736-1790
800-528-0311

**New Hampshire**
Medicare/Blue Cross and Blue Shield
   of Massachusetts, Inc.
100 Summer Street
Boston, MA 02110
617-741-3300
800-447-1142

**New Jersey**
Medicare/Medical Services
   Association of Pennsylvania
(d/b/a Xact Medicare Services)
P.O. Box 890065
Camp Hill, PA 17089-0065
717-763-3151
800-462-9306

**New Mexico**
Medicare/Aetna Life Insurance Co.
Medicare Claims Administration
Northpointe Plaza
5700 Harper Drive, N.E.
Albuquerque, NM 87109
505-821-7350
800-423-2925

**New York**
*Counties of Bronx, Columbia,*
   *Delaware, Duchess, Greene, Kings,*
   *Nassau, New York, Orange,*
   *Putnam, Richmond, Rockland,*
   *Suffolk, Sullivan, Ulster, and*
   *Westchester:*
Medicare/Empire Blue Cross and
   Blue Shield
622 Third Avenue
New York, NY 10017
212-476-1000

*Rest of state:*
Medicare/Blue Cross and Blue Shield
   of Western New York
P.O. Box 80
1901 Main Street
Buffalo, NY 14240-0080
716-887-6900
800-252-6550

**North Carolina**
Medicare/Connecticut General
   Life Insurance
One Triad Center, Suite 240
7736 McCloud Road
Greensboro, NC 27409
910-665-0341

**North Dakota**
Medicare/Blue Cross/Shield of
   North Dakota
711 Second Avenue, N.
Fargo, ND 58102
701-282-1100
800-247-2267

**Ohio**
Medicare/Nationwide Mutual
   Insurance Co.
P.O. Box 16788
Columbus, OH 43216
614-249-7111
800-282-0530

**Oklahoma**
Medicare/Aetna Life Insurance Co.
701 N.W. 63rd Street, 3rd Floor
Oklahoma City, OK 73116-7693
405-848-6257

**Oregon**
Medicare/Aetna Life Insurance Co.
   Medicare Claims Administration
P.O. Box 1997
Portland, OR 97207-1997
503-243-5351
800-452-0125

**Pennsylvania**
Medicare/Medical Services of
   Pennsylvania
(d/b/a Xact Medicare Services)
P.O. Box 890065
Camp Hill, PA 17089-0065
717-763-3151
800-382-1274

**Puerto Rico**
Medicare/Triple-S, Inc.
Box 36328
San Juan, PR 00936-3628
809-749-4080

**Rhode Island**
Medicare/Blue Cross and Blue Shield
   of Rhode Island
444 Westminster Street
Providence, RI 02903-3279
401-459-1000
800-662-5170

**South Carolina**
Medicare/Blue Cross and Blue Shield
   of South Carolina
(d/b/a Palmetto Government Benefits
   Adminstrators)
300 Arbor Lake Drive, Suite 1300
Columbia, SC 29219
803-735-1034
800-868-2522

**South Dakota**
Medicare/Blue Cross and Blue Shield
   of North Dakota
711 Second Avenue, N.
Fargo, ND 58102
701-282-1100
800-437-4762

**Tennessee**
Medicare/Connecticut General
   Life Insurance
Two Vantage Way
Nashville, TN 37228
615-782-4545

**Texas**
Medicare/Blue Cross and Blue Shield
   of Texas
901 S. Central Expressway
Richardson, TX 75080
214-766-6900
800-442-2620

**Utah**
Medicare/Blue Cross and Blue Shield
   of Utah
P.O. Box 30270, Medicare B
2455 Parley's Way
Salt Lake City, UT 84130
801-487-6441
800-426-3477

**Vermont**
Medicare/Blue Cross and Blue Shield
   of Massachusetts
100 Summer Street
Boston, MA 02110
617-741-3300
800-447-1142

**Virgin Islands**
Medicare/Triple-S, Inc.
Box 363628
San Juan, PR 00936-3628
809-749-4949

**Virginia**
Medicare/The Travelers Insurance Co.
P.O. Box 26463
300 Arboretum Place
Richmond, VA 23261
804-330-6100

**Washington**
Medicare/Aetna Life Insurance Co.
1301 Fifth Avenue, Suite 1300
Seattle, WA 91099
206-442-4810

**West Virginia**
Medicare/Nationwide Mutual
   Insurance Co.
P.O. Box 3183
Charleston, WV 25332
304-346-0411
800-848-0106

**Wisconsin**
Medicare/Wisconsin Physicians'
   Services Insurance Corp.
P.O. Box 1787
Madison, WI 53701
608-221-4711
800-362-7221

**Wyoming**
Medicare/Blue Cross/Blue Shield
   of North Dakota
711 Second Avenue, N.
Fargo, ND 58102
701-282-1100
800-442-2371

# Appendix B: Medicare Claims Log

| | | | Medicare Claims Log, Parts A and B | | | | | |
|---|---|---|---|---|---|---|---|---|
| (1) DATE OF SERVICE | (2) NAME OF PROVIDER OR FACILITY | (3) MEDICARE CLAIM NUMBER | (4) CLAIM UNDER | | (5) AMOUNT OF CLAIM | | (6) DEDUCTIBLE MET | |
| | | | PART A | PART B | BILLED | APPROVED | PART A | PART B |
| | | | | | | | | |

| (7) DATE CLAIM SUBMITTED TO CARRIER | (8) BALANCE OR COPAYMENT DUE | (9) AMOUNT CLAIMED | (10) AMOUNT RECEIVED | (11) OUT-OF-POCKET PAYMENT | (12) COMMENTS |
|---|---|---|---|---|---|
|  |  |  |  |  |  |

# Appendix C: State Insurance Offices

**Alabama**
Insurance Department
Retirement Systems Building
P.O. Box 303351
Montgomery, AL 36130-3351
334-269-3550

**Alaska**
Division of Insurance
Department of Commerce and
    Economic Development
State Office Building
P.O. Box 110805
Juneau, AK 99811-0805
907-465-2515

**Arizona**
Insurance Department
2910 N. 44th Street, Suite 210
Phoenix, AZ 85018-7256
602-912-8400

**Arkansas**
Insurance Department
University Tower Building, Room 500
1123 S. University Avenue
Little Rock, AR 72204
501-686-2945

**California**
Department of Insurance
300 S. Spring Street
Los Angeles, CA 90013
213-897-8921

**Colorado**
Division of Insurance
1560 Broadway, Suite 850
Denver, CO 80202
303-894-7499

**Connecticut**
Insurance Department
P.O. Box 816
Hartford, CT 06142-0816
203-297-3800

**Delaware**
Insurance Department
First Federal Plaza
710 N. King Street, Suite 350
Wilmington, DE 19801
302-577-3119

**District of Columbia**
Insurance Administration
Department of Consumer and
    Regulatory Affairs
441 4th Street, N.W.
Washington, DC 20001
202-727-7424

**Florida**
Department of Insurance
Insurance Consumer Services Division
Larson Building
200 E. Gaines Street
Tallahassee, FL 32399-0300
904-922-3100
800-342-2762

**Georgia**
Office of Commissioner of Insurance
Floyd Memorial Building, West Tower,
    7th Floor
2 Martin Luther King, Jr., Drive
Atlanta, GA 30334
404-656-2056

**Hawaii**
Insurance Division
Department of Commerce and
    Consumer Affairs
P.O. Box 3614
Honolulu, HI 96811
808-586-2790

**Idaho**
Department of Insurance
State Office Building
P.O. Box 83720
Boise, ID 83720-0043
208-334-2250

**Illinois**
Department of Insurance
320 W. Washington Street
Springfield, IL 62767
217-782-4515

**Indiana**
Department of Insurance
311 W. Washington Street, Suite 300
Indianapolis, IN 46204
317-232-2385
800-622-4461

**Iowa**
Division of Insurance
Department of Commerce
Lucas State Office Building
Des Moines, IA 50319
515-281-5705

**Kansas**
Insurance Department
State Office Building
420 S.W. 9th Street
Topeka, KS 66612-1678
913-296-3071

**Kentucky**
Department of Insurance
Public Protection and Regulation
  Cabinet
Fitzgerald Building
215 W. Main Street
Frankfort, KY 40601
502-564-3630

**Louisiana**
Insurance Building
P.O. Box 94214
Baton Rouge, LA 70804-9214
504-342-5900

**Maine**
Bureau of Insurance
Department of Professional and
  Financial Regulation
State House Station 35
Augusta, ME 04333
207-624-8475

**Maryland**
Insurance Division
Department of Licensing and
  Regulation
Stanbalt Building
501 St. Paul Place
Baltimore, MD 21202
410-333-6300

**Massachusetts**
Division of Insurance
470 Atlantic Avenue, 6th Floor
Boston, MA 02210
617-521-7794

**Michigan**
Insurance Bureau
P.O. Box 30220
Lansing, MI 48909
517-373-9273

**Minnesota**
Insurance Division
Department of Commerce
133 E. 7th Street
St. Paul, MN 55101
612-296-4026
800-657-3602

**Mississippi**
Insurance Department
P.O. Box 79
Jackson, MS 39205
601-359-3569

**Missouri**
Company Regulations
Division of Insurance
P.O. Box 690
301 W. High Street, Suite 630
Jefferson City, MO 65102
314-751-2640

**Montana**
Commissioner of Insurance
State Auditor Office
P.O. Box 4009
Helena, MT 59604-4009
406-444-2040

**Nebraska**
Department of Insurance
941 O Street, Suite 400
Lincoln, NE 68508
402-471-2201

**Nevada**
Department of Business and Industry
Insurance Division
1665 Hot Springs Road, Room 152
Carson City, NV 89710
702-687-4270

**New Hampshire**
Insurance Department
169 Manchester Street
Concord, NH 03301-5151
603-271-2261

**New Jersey**
Division of Administration
Department of Insurance
CN 325
20 W. State Street
Trenton, NJ 08625
609-292-5360

**New Mexico**
Department of Insurance
State Corporation Commission
Pera Building, P.O. Drawer 1269
Santa Fe, NM 87504-1269
505-827-4500

**New York**
Insurance Department
160 W. Broadway
New York, NY 10013
212-602-0429

**North Carolina**
Department of Insurance
401 Glenwood Avenue
Raleigh, NC 27603
919-733-2205

**North Dakota**
Insurance Department
State Capitol, 5th Floor
600 E. Boulevard Avenue
Bismarck, ND 58505-0320
701-328-2440

**Ohio**
Department of Insurance
2100 Stella Court
Columbus, OH 43215-1067
614-644-2658

**Oklahoma**
Insurance Department
State Insurance Building
P.O. Box 53408
Oklahoma City, OK 73152-3408
405-521-2828

**Oregon**
Insurance and Finance Division
350 Winter Street, N.E., Room 440-2
Consumer Services and Enforcement
Salem, OR 97310
503-378-4474
503-378-4636

**Pennsylvania**
Department of Insurance
1321 Strawberry Square
Harrisburg, PA 17120
717-787-2317

**Puerto Rico**
Office of the Insurance Commissioner
P.O. Box 8330
Fernandez Juncos Station
Santurce, PR 00910
809-722-8686

**Rhode Island**
Office of the Commissioner
233 Richmond Street, Suite 233
Providence, RI 02903-4233
401-277-2223
401-277-2246

**South Carolina**
Office of the Commissioner
Department of Insurance
P.O. Box 100105
Columbia, SC 29202-3105
803-737-6160
803-737-6268

**South Dakota**
Division of Insurance
Department of Commerce and
   Regulation
500 E. Capitol
Pierre, SD 57501-5070
605-773-4104

**Tennessee**
Department of Commerce & Insurance
500 James Robertson Parkway
4th Floor
Nashville, TN 37243-0565
615-741-2241
800-342-8385

**Texas**
State Board of Insurance
Consumer Protection Division
State Insurance Building
333 Guadalupe Street, Room 111-1A
P.O. Box 149091
Austin, TX 78714-9091
512-463-6464

**Utah**
Insurance Department
State Office Building, Room 3110
Salt Lake City, UT 84114
801-538-3800

**Vermont**
Banking, Insurance and Securities
89 Main Street, Drawer 20
Montpelier, VT 05620-3101
802-828-3301

**Virgin Islands**
Office of the Lieutenant Governor
Lieutenant Governor's Office Building
18 Kongens Gade
St. Thomas, VI 00802
809-774-2991

**Virginia**
Bureau of Insurance
P.O. Box 1157
Richmond, VA 23219
804-371-9741

**Washington**
Office of the Insurance Commissioner
Insurance Building
P.O. Box 40255
Olympia, WA 98504
360-664-4095

**West Virginia**
Department of Insurance
2100 Washington Street, E.
Charleston, WV 25305
304-348-3354

**Wisconsin**
Office of the Commissioner
   of Insurance
Loraine Building
P.O. Box 7873
Madison, WI 53707
608-266-3585

**Wyoming**
Insurance Department
Herschler Building, 3rd Floor E.
122 W. 25th Street
Cheyenne, WY 82002
307-777-7401

# Appendix D: NAIC Medicare Supplemental Insurance Standard Policies

| NATIONAL ASSOCIATION OF INSURANCE COMMISSIONERS STANDARD MEDICARE SUPPLEMENTAL INSURANCE POLICIES** | | | | | | | | | | |
|---|---|---|---|---|---|---|---|---|---|---|
| **BENEFITS ↓** PACKAGE PLANS → | **A** | **B** | **C** | **D** | **E** | **F** | **G** | **H** | **I** | **J** |
| *Core Coverage* | | | | | | | | | | |
| Part A Copayment Days 61–90 | | | | | | | | | | |
| Part A Copayment Reserve Days 91–150 | | | | | | | | | | |
| Parts A & B Blood Deductible | ● | ● | ● | ● | ● | ● | ● | ● | ● | ● |
| Part B 20% Copayment | | | | | | | | | | |
| 365 Lifetime Hospital Days 100% | | | | | | | | | | |
| *Additional Coverage* | | | | | | | | | | |
| Part A Hospital Deductible | | ● | ● | ● | ● | ● | ● | ● | ● | ● |
| Part B Doctor Deductible | | | ● | | | ● | | | | ● |
| SNF Copayment Days 21–100 | | | ● | ● | ● | ● | ● | ● | ● | ● |
| At-Home Recovery | | | | ● | | | ● | | ● | ● |
| Excess Doctor Charges | | | | | | 100% | 80% | | 100% | 100% |
| Foreign Travel (Emergency Care) | | | ● | ● | ● | ● | ● | ● | ● | ● |
| Prescription Drugs | | | | | | | | Basic[1] | Basic[1] | Extend[2] |
| Preventive Services | | | | | ● | | | | | ● |

[1]Basic prescription plan includes: $250 deductible; 50% copayment; and $1,250 maximum benefit.
[2]Extended prescription plan includes: $250 deductible; 50% copayment; and $3,000 maximum benefit.

**Only policies meeting these standards may be sold as supplements to Medicare.

*NAIC Standard Medicare Supplemental Insurance Policies*

The chart on the opposite page lists the ten standard Medicare supplemental insurance packages that have been designed by the National Association of Insurance Commissioners. When fully implemented, they will make it much easier to shop for supplemental insurance because you will be able to compare like coverage and premiums.

The heart of the new insurance plans is a core of basic coverage that must be included in all plans. This is labeled as Plan A and includes: Part A copayment for hospital days 61–90, the lifetime reserve copayment for hospital days 91–150, Parts A & B blood deductible, Part B 20 percent copayment, and additional hospital days beyond Medicare coverage.

The other nine plans, labeled B through J contain the core coverage plus variations of coverage. Nine plans cover the Part A hospital deductible, while only two plans, E and J, cover preventive health care services. Excess doctor charges above the Medicare-approved amounts are covered by plans F, G, I, and J. Prescription drugs are covered by plans H, I, and J.

In order to determine if a particular service is included with a specific plan, read across the top of the chart until you find the plan. Read down the chart and note the coverage indicated by the black dots.

If you have any questions concerning a particular plan or insurance company, contact your state's insurance commissioners office (See Appendix C.)

# Appendix E: Explanation of Your Medicare Part B Benefits

Name of Beneficiary

Iphigenia Smith
4321 Edgar Allen Poe Drive
San Diego, CA 99110

Your Medicare number:   120-99-6789

A summary about this notice dated December 30, 1996.

| | |
|---|---|
| Total charges: | $1,755.00 |
| Total Medicare approved: | $1,339.00 |
| Medicare paid your provider: | $1,071.20 |
| You are responsible for: | $ 367.80 |

---

## Details about this claim (See the back of this notice for more information.)

You received these services from your provider;
Dr. Sherman T. Potter, claim-#9876-1234-2468

Midway Medical Clinic, 2552 Baskerville Rd.,
San Diego, CA 99110

This indicates
amount billed
and approved.

| Services and Service Codes | Dates | Charge | Medicare approved | Notes |
|---|---|---|---|---|
| 65850 surgery, incision of eye | Nov 15, 1996 | $975.00 | $780.00 | a |
| 90040 brief office visit | Nov 19, 1996 | $100.00 | $ 0 | b |
| 90070 extended office visits | Nov 17–29, 1996 | $600.00 | $516.00 | a |
| 90040 brief office visit | Nov 30, 1996 | $ 40.00 | $ 21.50 | a |
| 90040 brief office visit | Dec 15, 1996 | $ 40.00 | $ 21.50 | a |
| | Total | $1,755.00 | $1,339.00 | |

This indicates the
service and date
provided.

Notes:

a   We based the approved amount on the fee schedule for this service.

b   Medicare did not pay for this test. Medicare pays for this only when the laboratory is certified for this type of test.

This tells you if
assignment was
taken and the dollar
amount billed.

Here's an explanation of this claim:

| | | |
|---|---|---|
| Of the total charges, Medicare approved | $1,339.00 | The provider accepted this amount. See #4 on the back of this notice. |
| The deductible you still owe | $ 0 | You have met the $100 deductible for 1996. |
| | $1,339.00 | Medicare pays 80 percent of this total. |
| | × .80 | |
| We are paying the provider | $1,071.20 | Your copayment is 20 percent or $267.80. |
| Of the amount approved | $1,339.00 | |
| Subtract what we pay the provider | $1,071.20 | |
| You are responsible for | $ 267.80 | |
| plus charges not covered by Medicare | $ 100.00 | |
| The total you are responsible for: | $ 367.80 | The provider may bill you for this amount. If you have other insurance, the other insurance may pay this amount. |

This indicates
whether or not you
have met the $100
deductible this year.

This explains what
you pay.

---

If you have questions about this notice, call Blue Cross Blue Shield of Maryland at 410-861-2273 or toll free at 800-662-5170 or visit us at 1946 Greenspring Drive, Timonium, Maryland.
You'll need this notice when you call or visit us about this claim.
If you want to appeal this claim, see #5 on the other side. You must write us by June 30, 1997.

This is your Part B
carrier. If you
suspect a mistake,
contact this office.

This gives you the time
frame to file any appeal.

# Important Information You Should Know About Your Medicare Part B Benefits

This part of the notice answers some common questions that people ask about collecting Medicare benefits. If you have other questions, see your copy of *The Medicare Handbook* or call us for more information.

1. **What should I do if I have questions about this notice?**
   If you have questions about this notice, call, write, or visit us and we will tell you the facts that we used to decide what and how much to pay. Turn to the front of this notice: our address and phone number are on the bottom of the page.

2. **Can I appeal how much Medicare paid for these services?**
   If you do not agree with what Medicare approved for these services, you may appeal our decision. To make sure that we are fair to you, we will not allow the same people who originally processed these services to conduct this review.

   However, in order to be eligible for a review, you **must** write to us within **6 months** of the date of this notice, unless you have a good reason for being late (for example, if you had an extended illness which kept you from being able to file on time).

   Turn to the front of this notice: the deadline date and our address are on the bottom of the page. It may help your case if you include a note from your doctor or supplier (provider) that tells us what was done and why.

   If you want help with your appeal, you can have a friend, lawyer, or someone else help you. Some lawyers do not charge unless you win your appeal. There are groups, such as lawyer referral services, that can help you find a lawyer. There are also groups, such as legal aid services, who will give you free legal services if you qualify.

3. **How much does Medicare pay?**
   The details on the front of this notice explain how much Medicare paid for these services. See your copy of *The Medicare Handbook* for more information about the benefits you are entitled to as a beneficiary in the Medicare Part B program. If you need another copy of the handbook, call or visit your local Social Security office.

Medicare may make adjustments to your payment. We may reduce the amount we pay for services by a certain percentage (Balanced Budget Law). If your provider accepted assignment, you are not liable to pay the amount of this reduction. We pay interest on some claims not paid within the required time.

All Medicare payments are made on the condition that you will pay Medicare back if benefits are also paid under insurance that is primary to Medicare. Examples of other insurance are employer group health plans, automobile medical, liability, no fault, or workers' compensation. Notify us immediately if you have filed or could file a claim with insurance that is primary to Medicare.

4. **How can I reduce my medical costs?**
   Many providers have agreed to be part of **Medicare's participation program.** That means that they will always accept the amount that Medicare approves as their full payment. Write or call us for the name of a participating provider or for a free list of participating providers.

   A provider who accepts assignment can charge you only for the part of the annual deductible you have not met and the copayment which is the remaining 20 percent of the approved amount.

   If you are treated by one of these doctors you can save money. See *The Medicare Handbook* for more information about how you can reduce your medical costs.

5. **How can I use this notice?**
   You can use this notice to:
   - Contact us immediately if you think Medicare paid for a service you did not receive

   - Show your provider how much of your deductible you have met

   - Claim benefits with another insurance company. If you send this notice to them, make a copy of it for your records.

---

**Keep this notice for your records.**
*Health Care Financing Administration*

# CODE
## —of—
# PRACTICE

As a PMS Code of Practice practitioner, I will assist you in finding information resources, support groups and health care providers to help you maintain and improve your health. When you seek my care for specific problems, I will abide by the following Code of Practice:

## Office Procedures

1. I will post or provide a printed schedule of my fees for office visits, procedures, testing and surgery, and provide itemized bills.

2. I will provide certain hours each week when I will be available for non-emergency telephone consultation.

3. I will schedule appointments to allow the necessary time to see you with minimal waiting. I will promptly report test results to you and return phone calls.

4. I will allow and encourage you to bring a friend or relative into the examining room with you.

5. I will facilitate your getting your medical and hospital records, and will provide you with copies of your test results.

## Choice in Diagnosis and Treatment

6. I will let you know your prognosis, including whether your condition is terminal or will cause disability or pain, and will explain why I believe further diagnostic activity or treatment is necessary.

7. I will discuss diagnostic, treatment and medication options for your particular problem with you (including the option of no treatment) and describe in understandable terms the risk of each alternative, the chances of success, the possibility of pain, the effect on your functioning, the number of visits each would entail, and the cost of each alternative.

8. I will describe my qualifications to perform the proposed diagnostic measures or treatments.

9. I will let you know of organizations, support groups, and medical and lay publications that can assist you in understanding, monitoring and treating your problem.

10. I will not proceed until you are satisfied that you understand the benefits and risks of each alternative and I have your agreement on a particular course of action.

## People's Medical Society.
462 Walnut Street • Allentown, PA 18102

# Appendix G: Books for a People's Medical Library

This list is a suggestion of what a basic People's Medical Library might contain.

*Alternative Medicine: The Definitive Guide.* Fife, WA: Future Medicine Publishing, 1994.

*Alzheimer's & Dementia: Questions You Have . . . Answers You Need,* by Jennifer Hay. Allentown, PA: People's Medical Society, 1996.

*America's Best Hospitals/U.S. News & World Report,* edited by Avery Comarow. New York: Joseph Wiley & Sons, Inc., 1996.

*American Medical Association Directory of Physicians in the U.S.,* 34th edition. Chicago: American Medical Association, 1995.

*Arthritis: Questions You Have . . . Answers You Need,* by Ellen Moyer. Allentown, PA: People's Medical Society, 1997.

*Asthma: Questions You Have . . . Answers You Need,* by Paula Brisco. Allentown, PA: People's Medical Society, 1994.

*Back Pain: Questions You Have . . . Answers You Need,* by Sandra Salmans. Allentown, PA: People's Medical Society, 1995.

*Blood Pressure: Questions You Have . . . Answers You Need.* Allentown, PA: People's Medical Society, 1996.

*Cancer,* by Robert McAllister, M.D., Sylvia Teich Horowitz, Ph.D., and Raymond V. Gilden, Ph.D. New York: Basic Books, 1993.

*Cancer Prevention and Nutritional Therapies,* revised and updated, by Richard A. Passwater, Ph.D. New Canaan, CT: Keats Publishing, Inc., 1994.

*Cecil Textbook of Medicine,* 20th edition, edited by J. Claude Bennett, M.D., and Fred Plum, M.D. Philadelphia: W. B. Saunders, 1996.

*Current Medical Diagnosis and Treatment,* 22nd edition, by Marcus Krupp and Milton L. Chatton. Los Altos, CA: Appleton-Lange, 1993.

*DHEA: A Practical Guide,* by Ray Sahelian, M.D. Garden City Park, NY: Avery Publishing Group, 1996.

*Diabetes: Questions You Have . . . Answers You Need,* by Paula Brisco. Allentown, PA: People's Medical Society, 1997.

*Dial 800 For Health.* New York: Wings Books, 1993.

*Directory of Medical Specialists,* 25th edition. Chicago: Marquis Who's Who, 1991.

*Doctor in the House: Your Best Guide to Effective Medical Self-Care,* by John C. Harbert, M.D. Totowa, NJ: Hummana Press, 1994.

*Dorland's Illustrated Medical Dictionary,* 28th edition. Philadelphia: W. B. Saunders, 1994.

*Every Parent's Nightmare,* by Daniel R. Tomal and Annette Tomal. Grand Rapids, MI: Zondervan Publishing House, 1993.

*Every Woman's Body,* by Diana Korte. New York: Fawcett Columbine, 1994.

*Examining Your Doctor: A Patient's Guide to Avoiding Harmful Medical Care,* by Timothy B. McCall, M.D. New York: Birch Press, 1995.

*Fifty Plus: The Graedons' People's Pharmacy for Older Adults,* by Joe and Teresa Graedon. New York: Bantam Books, 1988.

*First Aid Handbook,* by Alton L. Thygerson. Boston: Jones and Bartlett Publishers, 1995.

*Getting the Most for Your Medical Dollar,* by Charles B. Inlander and Karla Morales. New York: Wings Books, 1993.

*Good Operations — Bad Operations,* by Charles B. Inlander and the staff of the People's Medical Society. New York: Viking, 1993.

*Handbook of Nonprescription Drugs,* 10th edition, edited by Timothy R. Covington. Washington, DC: American Pharmaceutical Association, 1993.

*Harrison's Principles of Internal Medicine,* 12th edition, edited by Eugene Braunwald, M.D., et al. New York: McGraw-Hill, 1991.

*Heart Disease: A Textbook of Cardiovascular Medicine,* 5th edition, edited by Eugene Braunwald, M.D. Philadelphia: W. B. Saunders, 1996.

*How to Avoid a Hysterectomy,* by Lynn Payer. New York: Pantheon Books, 1987.

*How to Keep Your Child Fit from Birth to Six,* by Bonnie Prudden. New York: Ballantine Books, 1986.

*Let Me Die Before I Wake,* by Derek Humphry. Los Angeles: Hemlock Society, 1984.

*Mastering Pain: A Twelve Step Program for Coping with Chronic Pain,* by Richard A. Sternbach. New York: Putnam Publishing Group, 1987.

*Mayo Clinic Family Health Book,* edited by David E. Larson, M.D. New York: William Morrow and Co., Inc., 1990.

*Medicine on Trial,* by Charles B. Inlander, Lowell Levin, and Ed Weiner. New York: Prentice Hall, 1988.

*Medicine and Culture: Varieties of Treatments in the United States, England, West Germany and France,* by Lynn Payer. New York: Henry Holt & Co., 1988.

*Medicine for the Outdoors: A Guide to Emergency Medical Procedures and First Aid,* by Paul S. Auerback, M.D. Boston: Little, Brown and Company, 1991.

*Merck Manual of Diagnosis and Treatment,* 16th edition, edited by Robert Berkow, M.D., et al. Rahway, NJ: Merck, Sharp and Dohme, 1995.

*New Our Bodies, Ourselves: A Book by and for Women,* updated and enlarged, by the Boston Women's Healthbook Collective. New York: Simon & Schuster, 1992.

*No Housecalls: Irreverent Notes on the Practice of Medicine,* by Peter Gott, M.D. New York: Poseidon Press, 1986.

*Nursing a Loved One at Home,* by Susan Golden, R.N. Philadelphia: Running Press, 1988.

*On Your Own Terms: The Seniors' Guide to an Independent Life,* by Linda D. Cirino. New York: Hearst Books, 1995.

*Ourselves Growing Older: Women Aging with Knowledge and Power,* by the Boston Women's Healthbook Collective. New York: Simon & Schuster, 1994.

*PDR Medical Dictionary.* Montvale, NJ: Medical Economics Co., Inc., 1995.

*Peace, Love and Healing,* by Bernie S. Siegel, M.D. New York: Harper & Row, 1989.

*Physicians' Desk Reference,* 50th edition. Montvale, NJ: Medical Economics Co., Inc., 1996.

*Playing God: The New World of Medical Choices,* by Thomas and Colin Scully. New York: Simon & Schuster, 1988.

*Smart Patient, Good Medicine,* by Richard L. Sribnick, M.D., and Wayne B. Sribnick, M.D. New York: Walker and Company, 1994.

*Take Care of Yourself: A Consumer's Guide to Medical Care,* 5th edition, by Donald M. Vickery, M.D., and James F. Fries, M.D. Reading, MA: Addison-Wesley, 1993.

*Take This Book to the Hospital With You,* revised and updated edition, by Charles B. Inlander and Ed Weiner. Allentown, PA: People's Medical Society, 1997.

*The American Medical Association Family Medical Guide,* revised edition, edited by Jeffery R. Kuntz, M.D., and Asher J. Finkel, M.D. New York: Random House, 1987.

*The American Medical Association Home Medical Adviser,* edited by Charles Clayman, M.D., et al. New York: Random House, 1988.

*The Clay Pedestal: A Re-Examination of the Doctor-Patient Relationship,* by Thomas Preston, M.D. Seattle: Madrona Publishers, 1981.

*The Columbia University College of Physicians and Surgeons Complete Home Medical Guide,* revised edition, edited by Donald F. Tapley, M.D., et al. New York: Crown Publishers, 1989.

*The Complete Book of Water Therapy,* by Dian Dincin Buchman. New Canaan, CT: Keats Publishing, Inc., 1994.

*The Compete Drug Reference.* Rockville, MD: United States Pharmacopeial Convention, 1991.

*The Complete Guide to Sensible Eating,* by Gary Null. New York: Four Walls Eight Windows, 1990.

*The Endometriosis Answer Book: New Hope, New Help,* by Niels H. Lauerson, M.D., Ph.D., and Constance DeSwaan. New York: Macmillan Publishing Co., 1988.

*The Essential Guide to Prescription Drugs,* 12th edition, by James W. Long. New York: Macmillan Publishing Co., 1993.

*The Home Medical Handbook,* by Jack I. Stern, M.D., and David L. Carroll. New York: William Morrow and Co., Inc., 1987.

*The Layman's Guide to Acupuncture,* by Y. Manaka and I. Urguahart. New York: Weatherhill Press, 1986.

*The Mosby Medical Encyclopedia,* revised edition. New York: Plume, 1992.

*The New Good Housekeeping Family Health and Medical Guide.* New York: Hearst Books, 1989.

*The PDR Family Guide to Prescription Drugs.* Montvale, NJ: Medical Economics Data, Inc., 1993.

*The Patient's Guide to Medical Tests,* 3rd revised and expanded edition, by Cathey and Edward Pinckney. New York: Facts on File, 1987.

*The People's Medical Society Health Desk Reference: Information Your Doctor Won't or Can't Tell You,* by Charles Inlander and the staff of the People's Medical Society. New York: Hyperion, 1995.

*The Right to Die: Understanding Euthanasia,* by Derek Humphry and Ann Wickett. New York: Harper & Row, 1986.

*The Rights of Patients: The Basic ACLU Guide to Patient Rights,* 2nd edition, by George J. Annas. Carbondale, IL: Southern Illinois University Press, 1989.

*The Safe Shopper's Bible: A Consumer's Guide to Nontoxic Household Products, Cosmetics, and Food,* by David Steinman and Samuel S. Epstein, M.D. New York: Macmillan, 1995.

*The Social Transformation of American Medicine,* by Paul Starr. New York: Basic Books, 1982.

*What Your Doctor Didn't Learn in Medical School,* by Stuart M. Berger, M.D. New York: William Morrow and Co., Inc., 1988.

*Worst Pills, Best Pills II,* by Sidney Wolfe, M.D., et al. Washington, DC: Public Citizen Health Research Group, 1993.

*Your Child's Symptoms: A Parent's Guide to Understanding Pediatric Medicine,* by Bruce Taubman, M.D. New York: Fireside, 1992.

*Your Complete Medical Record,* by the staff of the People's Medical Society. Allentown, PA: People's Medical Society, 1993.

*Your Medical Rights,* by Charles B. Inlander and Eugene Pavalon. Allentown, PA: People's Medical Society, 1994.

# Appendix H: Durable Power of Attorney Forms and Living Wills

## California Durable Power of Attorney for Health Care
## Warning To Persons Executing This Document

This is an important legal document which is authorized by the Keene Health Care Agent Act. Before executing this document, you should know these important facts:

This document gives the person you designate as your agent (the attorney in fact) the power to make health care decisions for you. Your agent must act consistently with your desires stated in this document or otherwise made known.

Except as you otherwise specify in this document, this document gives your agent the power to consent to your doctor not giving treatment or stopping necessary treatment to keep you alive.

Notwithstanding this document, you have the right to make medical and other health care decisions for yourself so long as you can give informed consent with respect to the particular decision. In addition, no treatment may be given to you over your objection at the time, and health care necessary to keep you alive may not be stopped or withheld if you object at the time.

This document gives your agent authority to consent, to refuse to consent, or to withdraw consent to any care, treatment, service, or procedure to maintain, diagnose, or treat a physical or mental condition. This power is subject to any statement of your desires and any limitations that you include in this document. You may state in this document any types of treatment that you do not desire. In addition, a court can take away the power of your agent to make health care decisions for you if your agent (1) authorizes anything that is illegal, (2) acts contrary to your desires, or (3) where your desires are not known, does anything that is clearly contrary to your best interests.

The powers given by this document will exist for an indefinite period of time unless you limit their duration in this document. You have the right to revoke the authority of your agent by notifying your agent or your treating doctor, hospital, or other health care provider orally or in writing of the revocation. Your agent has the right to examine your medical records and to consent to their disclosure unless you limit this right in the document.

Unless you otherwise specify in this document, this document gives your agent the power after you die to (1) authorize an autopsy, (2) donate your body or parts thereof for transplant or therapeutic or educational or scientific purposes, and (3) direct the disposition of your remains.

This document revokes any prior durable power of attorney for health care. You should carefully read and follow the witnessing procedure described at the end of this form. This document will not be valid unless you comply with the witnessing procedure.

If there is anything in this document that you do not understand, you should ask a lawyer to explain it to you. Your agent may need this document immediately in case of an emergency that requires a decision concerning your health care. Either keep this document where it is immediately available to your agent and alternate agents or give each of them an executed copy of this document. You may also want to give your doctor an executed copy of this document.

Do not use this form if you are a conservatee under the Lanterman-Petris-Short Act and you want to appoint your conservator as your agent. You can do that only if the appointment document includes a certificate of your attorney.

# CALIFORNIA DURABLE POWER OF ATTORNEY FOR HEALTH CARE

**INSTRUCTIONS**

**PRINT YOUR NAME AND ADDRESS**

**PRINT NAME AND ADDRESS OF YOUR AGENT**

### 1. Designation of Health Care Agent.

I, _____
(name)

_____
(address)

do hereby designate and appoint _____
(name of agent)

_____
(address and telephone number of agent)

as my attorney in fact (agent) to make health care decisions for me as authorized in this document. For the purposes of this document, "health care decision" means consent, refusal of consent, or withdrawal of consent to any care, treatment, service, or procedure to maintain, diagnose, or treat an individual's physical or mental condition.

### 2. Creation of Durable Power of Attorney for Health Care.

By this document I intend to create a durable power of attorney for health care under Sections 2430 to 2443, inclusive, of the California Civil Code. This power of attorney shall not be affected by my subsequent incapacity.

### 3. General Statement of Authority Granted.

Subject to any limitations in this document, I hereby grant to my agent full power and authority to make health care decisions for me to the same extent that I could make such decisions for myself if I had the capacity to do so. In exercising this authority, my agent shall make health care decisions that are consistent with my desires as stated in this document or otherwise made known to my agent, including, but not limited to, my desires concerning obtaining or refusing or withdrawing life-prolonging care, treatment, services, and procedures.

**ADD PERSONAL
INSTRUCTIONS
CONCERNING
LIFE SUPPORT
(IF ANY)**



**ADD OTHER
PERSONAL
INSTRUCTIONS
(IF ANY)**

### 4. Statement of Desires, Special Provisions, and Limitations.

In exercising the authority under this durable power of attorney for health care, my agent shall act consistently with my desires as stated below and is subject to the special provisions and limitations stated below:

(a) Statement of desires concerning life-prolonging care, treatment, services, and procedures:

(b) Additional statement of desires, special provisions, and limitations:

*(You may attach additional pages if you need more space to complete your statement. If you attach additional pages, you must date and sign EACH of the additional pages at the same time you date and sign this document.)*

### 5. Inspection and Disclosure of Information Relating to My Physical or Mental Health.

Subject to any limitations in this document, my agent has the power and authority to do all of the following:

(a) Request, review, and receive any information, verbal or written, regarding my physical or mental health, including, but not limited to, medical and hospital records.

(b) Execute on my behalf any releases or other documents that may be required in order to obtain this information.

(c) Consent to the disclosure of this information.

*(If you want to limit the authority of your agent to receive and disclose information relating to your health, you must state the limitations in paragraph 4 ["Statement of Desires, Special Provisions, and Limitations"] above.)*

### 6. Signing Documents, Waivers, and Releases.

Where necessary to implement the health care decisions that my agent is authorized by this document to make, my agent has the power and authority to execute on my behalf all of the following:

(a) Documents titled or purporting to be a "Refusal to Permit

Treatment" and "Leaving Hospital Against Medical Advice."

(b) Any necessary waiver or release from liability required by a hospital or physician.

### 7. Autopsy; Anatomical Gifts; Disposition of Remains.

Subject to any limitations in this document, my agent has the power and authority to do all of the following:

(a) Authorize an autopsy under Section 7113 of the Health and Safety Code.

(b) Make a disposition of a part or parts of my body under the Uniform Anatomical Gift Act (Chapter 3.5 [commencing with Section 7150] of Part 1 of Division 7 of the Health and Safety Code).

(c) Direct the disposition of my remains under Section 7100 of the Health and Safety Code.

*(If you want to limit the authority of your agent to consent to an autopsy, make an anatomical gift, or direct the disposition of your remains, you must state the limitations in paragraph 4 ["Statement of Desires, Special Provisions, and Limitations"] above.)*

**SPECIFY A DURATION (IF ANY)**

### 8. Duration.

This durable power of attorney for health care expires on _____

_____

*(Fill in this space ONLY if you want to limit the duration of this power of attorney)*

### 9. Designation of Alternate Agents.

If the person designated as my agent in paragraph 1 is not available or becomes ineligible to act as my agent to make a health care decision for me or loses the mental capacity to make health care decisions for me, or if I revoke that person's appointment or authority to act as my agent to make health care decisions for me, then I designate and appoint the following persons to serve as my agent to make health care decisions for me as authorized in this document, such persons to serve in the order listed below:

**PRINT THE NAMES, ADDRESSES AND TELEPHONE NUMBERS OF YOUR ALTERNATE AGENTS**

A. First Alternate Agent: _____
                                              *(name of first alternate agent)*

_____
                        *(address and telephone number of first alternate agent)*

B. Second Alternate Agent: _____
                                               *(name of second alternate agent)*

_____
                     *(address and telephone number of second alternate agent)*

### 10. Nomination of Conservator of Person.

*(A conservator of the person may be appointed for you if a court decides that one should be appointed. The conservator is responsible for your physical care, which under some circumstances includes making health care decisions for you. You are not required to nominate a conservator but you may do so. The court will appoint the person you nominate unless that would be contrary to your best interests. You may, but are not required to, nominate as your conservator the same person you named in paragraph 1 as your health care agent. You can nominate an individual as your conservator by completing the space below.)*

If a conservator of the person is to be appointed for me, I nominate the following individual to serve as conservator of the person:

_____
*(name of person nominated as conservator)*

_____
*(address of person nominated as conservator)*

### 11. Prior Designations Revoked.

I revoke any prior durable power of attorney for health care.

### DATE AND SIGNATURE OF PRINCIPAL
### (YOU MUST DATE AND SIGN THIS POWER OF ATTORNEY)

I sign my name to this Durable Power of Attorney for Health Care on

_____ at _____, _____.
*(date)*                         *(city)*                              *(state)*

_____
*(you sign here)*

(THIS POWER OF ATTORNEY WILL NOT BE VALID UNLESS IT IS SIGNED BY EITHER A NOTARY PUBLIC OR TWO QUALIFIED WITNESSES WHO ARE PRESENT WHEN YOU SIGN OR ACKNOWLEDGE YOUR SIGNATURE. IF YOU HAVE ATTACHED ANY ADDITIONAL PAGES TO THIS FORM, YOU MUST DATE AND SIGN EACH OF THE ADDITIONAL PAGES AT THE SAME TIME YOU DATE AND SIGN THIS POWER OF ATTORNEY.)

# FLORIDA LIVING WILL

**INSTRUCTIONS**

**PRINT THE DATE**

**PRINT YOUR NAME**

**PRINT THE NAME, HOME ADDRESS AND TELEPHONE NUMBER OF YOUR SURROGATE**

Declaration made this _____ day of _____, 19\_\_\_\_\_.

I, _____, willfully and voluntarily make known my desire that my dying not be artificially prolonged under the circumstances set forth below, and I do hereby declare:

If at any time I have a terminal condition and if my attending or treating physician and another consulting physician have determined that there is no medical probability of my recovery from such condition, I direct that life-prolonging procedures be withheld or withdrawn when the application of such procedures would serve only to prolong artificially the process of dying, and that I be permitted to die naturally with only the administration of medication or the performance of any medical procedure deemed necessary to provide me with comfort care or to alleviate pain.

It is my intention that this declaration be honored by my family and physician as the final expression of my legal right to refuse medical or surgical treatment and to accept the consequences for such refusal.

In the event that I have been determined to be unable to provide express and informed consent regarding the withholding, withdrawal, or continuation of life-prolonging procedures, I wish to designate, as my surrogate to carry out the provisions of this declaration:

Name: _____

Address: _____

_____ Zip Code: _____

Phone: _____

**PRINT NAME, HOME ADDRESS AND TELEPHONE NUMBER OF YOUR ALTERNATE SURROGATE**

I wish to designate the following person as my alternate surrogate, to carry out the provisions of this declaration should my surrogate be unwilling or unable to act on my behalf:

Name: _____

Address: _____

_____ Zip Code: _____

Phone: _____

**ADD PERSONAL INSTRUCTIONS (IF ANY)**

Additional instructions (optional):

I understand the full import of this declaration, and I am emotionally and mentally competent to make this declaration.

**SIGN THE DOCUMENT**

Signed: _____

**WITNESSING PROCEDURE**

**TWO WITNESSES MUST SIGN AND PRINT THEIR ADDRESSES**

Witness 1:

    Signed: _____

    Address: _____

Witness 2:

    Signed: _____

    Address: _____

*Courtesy of Choice In Dying*    11/93
200 Varick Street, New York, NY  10014  1-800-989-WILL

# NEW YORK LIVING WILL

*This Living Will has been prepared to conform to the law in the State of New York, as set forth in the case <u>In re Westchester County Medical Center</u>, 72 N.Y.2d 517 (1988). In that case the Court established the need for "clear and convincing" evidence of a patient's wishes and stated that the "ideal situation is one in which the patient's wishes were expressed in some form of writing, perhaps a 'living will.'"*

**PRINT YOUR NAME**

I, _____, being of sound mind, make this statement as a directive to be followed if I become permanently unable to participate in decisions regarding my medical care. These instructions reflect my firm and settled commitment to decline medical treatment under the circumstances indicated below:

I direct my attending physician to withhold or withdraw treatment that merely prolongs my dying, if I should be in an **incurable or irreversible mental or physical condition with no reasonable expectation of recovery.**

These instructions apply if I am (a) **in a terminal condition;** (b) **permanently unconscious;** or (c) **if I am minimally conscious but have irreversible brain damage and will never regain the ability to make decisions and express my wishes.**

I direct that my treatment be limited to measures to keep me comfortable and to relieve pain, including any pain that might occur by withholding or withdrawing treatment.

While I understand that I am not legally required to be specific about future treatments **if I am in the condition(s)** described above I feel especially strongly about the following forms of treatment:

    I do not want cardiac resuscitation.
    I do not want mechanical respiration.
    I do not want artificial nutrition and hydration.
    I do not want antibiotics.

**CROSS OUT ANY STATEMENTS WITH WHICH YOU DO NOT AGREE**

    However, I **do want** maximum pain relief, even if it may hasten my death.

Other directions:

These directions express my legal right to refuse treatment, under the law of New York. I intend my instructions to be carried out, unless I have rescinded them in a new writing or by clearly indicating that I have changed my mind.

Signed _____ Date _____

Address _____

I declare that the person who signed this document is personally known to me and appears to be of sound mind and acting of his or her own free will. He or she signed (or asked another to sign for him or her) this document in my presence.

Witness 1 _____

Address _____

Witness 2 _____

Address _____

*Courtesy of Choice In Dying*   11/93
200 Varick Street, New York, NY 10014 1-800-989-WILL

# Appendix I: Hospital Patient's Bill of Rights

The American Hospital Association presents *A Patient's Bill of Rights* with the expectation that observance of these rights will contribute to more effective patient care and greater satisfaction for the patient, his physician, and the hospital organization. Further, the Association presents these rights in the expectation that they will be supported by the hospital on behalf of its patients as an integral part of the healing process. It is recognized that a personal relationship between the physician and the patient is essential for the provision of proper medical care.

The traditional physician-patient relationship takes on a new dimension when care is rendered within an organizational structure. Legal precedent has established that the institution itself also has a responsibility to the patient. It is in recognition of these factors that these rights are affirmed.

**1.** The patient has the right to considerate and respectful care.

**2.** The patient has the right to obtain from his physician complete current information concerning his diagnosis, treatment, and prognosis in terms the patient can be reasonably expected to understand. When it is not medically advisable to give such information to the patient, the information should be made available to an appropriate person in his behalf. He has the right to know, by name, the physician responsible for coordinating his care.

**3.** The patient has the right to receive from his physician information necessary to give informed consent prior to the start of any procedure and/or treatment. Except in emergencies, such information for informed consent should include, but not necessarily be limited to, the specific procedure and/or treatment, the medically significant risks involved, and the probable duration of incapacitation. Where medically significant alternatives for care or treatment exist, or when the patient requests information concerning medical alternatives, the patient has the right to such information. The patient also has the right to know the name of the person responsible for the procedures and/or treatment.

**4.** The patient has the right to refuse treatment to the extent permitted by law and to be informed of the medical consequences of his action.

**5.** The patient has the right to every consideration of his privacy concerning his own medical care program. Case discussion, consultation, examination, and treatment are confidential and should be conducted discreetly. Those not directly involved in his care must have the permission of the patient to be present.

**6.** The patient has the right to expect that all communications and records pertaining to his care should be treated as confidential.

**7.** The patient has the right to expect that within its capacity a hospital must make reasonable response to the request of a patient for services. The hospital must provide evaluation, service, and/or referral as indicated by the urgency of the case. When medically permissible, a patient may be transferred to another facility only after he has received complete information and explanation concerning the needs for and alternatives to such a transfer. The institution to which the patient is to be transferred must first have accepted the patient for transfer.

**8.** The patient has the right to obtain information as to any relationship of his hospital to other health care and educational institutions insofar as his care is concerned. The patient has the right to obtain information as to the existence of any professional relationships among individuals, by name, who are treating him.

9. The patient has the right to be advised if the hospital proposes to engage in or perform human experimentation affecting his care or treatment. The patient has the right to refuse to participate in such research projects.

10. The patient has the right to expect reasonable continuity of care. He has the right to know in advance what appointment times and physicians are available and where. The patient has the right to expect that the hospital will provide a mechanism whereby he is informed by his physician or a delegate of the physician of the patient's continuing health care requirements following discharge.

11. The patient has the right to examine and receive an explanation of his bill, regardless of source of payment.

12. The patient has the right to know what hospital rules and regulations apply to his conduct as a patient.

No catalog of rights can guarantee for the patient the kind of treatment he has a right to expect. A hospital has many functions to perform, including the prevention and treatment of disease, the education of both health professionals and patients, and the conduct of clinical research. All these activities must be conducted with an overriding concern for the patient, and, above all, the recognition of his dignity as a human being. Success in achieving this recognition ensures success in the defense of the rights of the patient.

# Appendix J: State Peer Review Organizations (PROs)

Note: PROs can answer questions about the quality of care and access to care in a Medicare-certified facility. PROs cannot answer questions about your bill or about what Medicare covers. For Part A or Part B billing or coverage questions, call your Part B carrier or your Part A intermediary.

**Alabama**
Alabama Quality Assurance
  Foundation, Inc.
1 Perimeter Park, S., Suite 200N
Birmingham, AL 35243-2327
800-760-3540

**Alaska**
PRO-WEST
(PRO for Alaska)
10700 Meridian Avenue, N.,
  Suite 100
Seattle, WA 98133-9075
907-562-2252 (In Anchorage)
800-445-6941

**Arizona**
Health Services Advisory Group, Inc.
301 E. Bethany Home Road, B-157
Phoenix, AZ 85012
800-626-1577
800-359-9909 or 800-223-6693
  (In Arizona)

**Arkansas**
Arkansas Foundation for Medical
  Care, Inc.
P.O. Box 2424
809 Garrison Avenue
Fort Smith, AR 72902
800-824-7586
800-272-5528 (In Arkansas)

**California**
California Medical Review, Inc.
60 Spear Street, Suite 500
San Francisco, CA 94105
415-882-5800*
800-841-1602 (In California)

**Colorado**
Colorado Foundation for Medical Care
2821 S. Parker Road
Aurora, CO 80014
303-695-3333*
800-937-3378 (In Colorado)

**Connecticut**
Connecticut Peer Review
  Organization, Inc.
100 Roscommon Drive, Suite 200
Middletown, CT 06457
203-632-2008*
800-553-7590 (In Connecticut)

**Delaware**
West Virginia Medical Institute, Inc.
(PRO for Delaware)
3001 Chesterfield Place
Charleston, WV 25304
302-655-3077 (In Wilmington)
800-642-8686 ext. 266

**District of Columbia**
Delmarva Foundation for Medical
  Care, Inc.
(PRO for D.C.)
9240 Centreville Road
Easton, MD 21601
800-645-0011
800-492-5811 (In Maryland)

**Florida**
Florida Medical Quality
  Assurance, Inc.
1211 N. Westshore Boulevard,
  Suite 700
Tampa, FL 33607
813-281-9024
800-844-0795 (In Florida)

*PRO will accept collect calls from out of state on this number.

**Georgia**
Georgia Medical Care Foundation
57 Executive Park, S., Suite 200
Atlanta, GA 30329
404-982-0411
800-282-2614 (In Georgia)

**Hawaii**
Hawaii Medical Service Association
(PRO for American Samoa/Guam
   and Hawaii)
818 Keeaumoku Street
P.O. Box 860
Honolulu, HI 96808-0860
808-944-3586*

**Idaho**
PRO-WEST
(PRO for Idaho)
10700 Meridian Avenue, N.,
   Suite 100
Seattle, WA 98133-9075
208-343-4617* (Local Boise)
800-445-6941

**Illinois**
Crescent Counties Foundation for
   Medical Care
1001 Warrenville Road, Suite 500
Lisle, IL 60532-1398
708-769-9600
800-647-8089

**Indiana**
Indiana Medical Review Organization
2901 Ohio Boulevard
P.O. Box 3713
Terre Haute, IN 47803-3713
800-288-1499

**Iowa**
Iowa Foundation for Medical Care
6000 Westown Parkway, Suite 350E
West Des Moines, IA 50266-7771
515-223-2900
800-752-7014

**Kansas**
The Kansas Foundation for Medical
   Care, Inc.
2947 S.W. Wanamaker Drive
Topeka, KS 66614
913-273-2552
800-432-0407 (In Kansas)

**Kentucky**
Kentucky Medical Review
   Organization
P.O. Box 23540
10503 Timberwood Circle,
   Suite 200
Louisville, KY 40223
800-288-1499

**Louisiana**
Louisiana Health Care Review, Inc.
8591 United Plaza Blvd., Suite 270
Baton Rouge, LA 70809
504-926-6353
800-433-4958 (In Louisiana)

**Maine**
Health Care Review, Inc.
(PRO for Maine)
Henry C. Hall Building
345 Blackstone Boulevard
Providence, RI 02906
207-945-0244*
800-541-9888 or 800-528-0700
   (In Maine)

**Maryland**
Delmarva Foundation for Medical
   Care, Inc.
(PRO for Maryland)
9240 Centreville Road
Easton, MD 21601
800-645-0011
800-492-5811 (In Maryland)

**Massachusetts**
Massachusetts Peer Review
   Organization, Inc.
235 Wyman Street
Waltham, MA 02154-1231
617-890-0011*
800-252-5533 (In Massachusetts)

**Michigan**
Michigan Peer Review Organization
40600 Ann Arbor Road, Suite 200
Plymouth, MI 48170-4495
800-365-5899

*PRO will accept collect calls from out of state on this number.

**Minnesota**
Foundation for Health Care
    Evaluation
2901 Metro Drive, Suite 400
Bloomington, MN 55425
800-444-3423

**Mississippi**
Mississippi Foundation for Medical
    Care, Inc.
P.O. Box 4665
735 Riverside Drive
Jackson, MS 39296-4665
601-948-8894
800-844-0600 (In Mississippi)

**Missouri**
Missouri Patient Care Review
    Foundation
505 Hobbs Road, Suite 100
Jefferson City, MO 65109
800-347-1016

**Montana**
Montana-Wyoming Foundation for
    Medical Care
400 N. Park, 2nd Floor
Helena, MT 59601
406-443-4020*
800-497-8232 (In Montana)

**Nebraska**
Iowa Foundation for Medical Care/
    The Sunderbruch Corporation (NE)
6000 Westown Parkway, Suite 350E
West Des Moines, IA 50266
402-474-7471*
800-247-3004 (In Nebraska)

**Nevada**
HealthInsight
675 E. 2100 South, Suite 270
Salt Lake City, UT 84106-1864
702-826-1996 (In Reno)
702-385-9933*
800-558-0829 (In Nevada)

**New Hampshire**
New Hampshire Foundation for
    Medical Care
15 Old Rollinsford Road, Suite 302
Dover, NH 03820
603-749-1641*
800-582-7174 (In New Hampshire)

**New Jersey**
The Peer Review Organization of
    New Jersey, Inc.
Central Division
Brier Hill Court, Building J
East Brunswick, NJ 08816
908-238-5570*
800-624-4557 (In New Jersey)

**New Mexico**
New Mexico Medical Review
    Association
P.O. Box 27449
707 Broadway, N.E., Suite 200
Albuquerque, NM 87125-7449
505-842-6236 (In Albuquerque)
800-432-6824 (In New Mexico)

**New York**
Island Peer Review Organization, Inc.
1979 Marcus Avenue, 1st Floor
Lake Success, NY 11042
516-326-7767*
800-331-7767 (In New York)

**North Carolina**
Medical Review of North Carolina
5625 Dillard Drive, Suite 203
Cary, NC 27511-9227
919-851-2955
800-682-2650 (In North Carolina)

**North Dakota**
North Dakota Health Care Review, Inc.
900 N. Broadway, Suite 301
Minot, ND 58701
701-852-4231*
800-472-2902 (In North Dakota)

**Ohio**
Peer Review Systems, Inc.
P.O. Box 6174
757 Brooksedge Plaza **Drive**
Westerville, OH 43081-6174
800-589-7337 (In Ohio)
800-837-0664

*PRO will accept collect calls from out of state on this number.

**Oklahoma**
Oklahoma Foundation for Peer
    Review, Inc.
5801 Broadway Extension
The Paragon Building, Suite 400
Oklahoma City, OK 73118-7489
405-840-2891
800-522-3414 (In Oklahoma)

**Oregon**
Oregon Medical Professional
    Review Organization
1220 S.W. Morrison, Suite 200
Portland, OR 97205
503-279-0100*
800-344-4354 (In Oregon)

**Pennsylvania**
Keystone Peer Review
    Organization, Inc.
P.O. Box 8310
777 E. Park Drive
Harrisburg, PA 17105-8310
717-564-8288
800-322-1914 (In Pennsylvania)

**Puerto Rico**
Puerto Rico Foundation for
    Medical Care
Mercantile Plaza, Suite 605
Hato Rey, PR 00918
809-753-6705* or 809-753-6708*

**Rhode Island**
Health Care Review, Inc.
Henry C. Hall Building
345 Blackstone Boulevard
Providence, RI 02906
401-331-6661*
800-221-1691 (New England-wide)
800-662-5028 (In Rhode Island)

**South Carolina**
Medical Review of North
    Carolina, Inc.
(PRO for South Carolina)
5625 Dillard Drive, Suite 203
Cary, NC 27511
919-851-2955
800-922-3089 (In South Carolina)

**South Dakota**
South Dakota Foundation for
    Medical Care
1323 S. Minnesota Avenue
Sioux Falls, SD 57105
800-658-2285

**Tennessee**
Mid-South Foundation for
    Medical Care
6401 Poplar Avenue, Suite 400
Memphis, TN 38119
800-489-4633

**Texas**
Texas Medical Foundation
Barton Oaks Plaza 2, Suite 200
901 Mopac Expressway, S.
Austin, TX 78746
512-329-6610
800-725-8315 (In Texas)

**Utah**
HealthInsight
675 E. 2100 South, Suite 270
Salt Lake City, UT 84106-1864
800-274-2290

**Vermont**
New Hampshire Foundation for
    Medical Care
(PRO for Vermont)
15 Old Rollinsford Road, Suite 302
Dover, NH 03820
802-655-6302
800-772-0151 (In Vermont)

**Virgin Islands**
Virgin Islands Medical Institute, Inc.
IAD Estate Diamond Ruby
P.O. Box 1566, Christiansted
St. Croix, VI 00821-1566
809-778-6470* (In St. Croix)

**Virginia**
Medical Society of Virginia
    Review Organization
P.O. Box K70
1606 Santa Rosa Road, Suite 200
Richmond, VA 23288-0070
804-289-5397 (In Richmond)
804-289-5320
800-545-3814 (In DC, MD, and VA)

*PRO will accept collect calls from out of state on this number.

**Washington**
PRO-WEST
10700 Meridian Avenue, N.,
   Suite 100
Seattle, WA 98133-9075
206-368-8272 (In Seattle)
800-445-6941

**West Virginia**
West Virginia Medical Institute, Inc.
3001 Chesterfield Place
Charleston, WV 25304
304-346-9864 (In Charleston)
800-642-8686 ext. 266

**Wisconsin**
Wisconsin Peer Review Organization
2909 Landmark Place
Madison, WI 53713
608-274-1940
800-362-2320 (In Wisconsin)

**Wyoming**
Montana-Wyoming Foundation for
   Medical Care
400 N. Park, 2nd Floor
Helena, MT 59601
406-443-4020*
800-497-8232 (In Wyoming)

*PRO will accept collect calls from out of state on this number.

# Appendix K: State Nursing Home Licensure Offices

State Nursing Home Licensure offices inspect institutions to assure a basic standard of care for the resident. They issue certification for institutions that qualify for federal programs: Medicare and Medicaid. These regulations are standard throughout the country. In addition, they issue state licensure for all long-term-care institutions. These regulations vary from state to state. Copies of all regulations should be available from these offices.

**Alabama**
Nursing Home Licensure Office
Division of Licensure and Certification
Alabama Department of Health
434 Monroe Street
Montgomery, AL 36130-3017
334-240-3503

**Alaska**
Nursing Home Licensure Office
Department of Health and
    Social Services
Health Facilities Certification
    and Licensing
4411 Business Park Boulevard, Suite 46
Anchorage, AK 99503
907-561-2171

**Arizona**
Department of Health Services
Office of Health Care Licensure
1647 E. Morton Avenue, Suite 130
Phoenix, AZ 85020
602-255-1177

**Arkansas**
Department of Health
Certification and Licensure Section
Office of Long-Term Care
P.O. Box 8059, Slot 404
Little Rock, AR 72203-8059
501-682-8430

**California**
Nursing Home Licensure Office
Licensure and Certification Division
Facilities Licensing Section
P.O. Box 942732
1800 3rd Street, Suite 210
Sacramento, CA 94234-7320
916-445-3281

**Colorado**
Nursing Home Licensure Office
Department of Health
Health Facilities Division
Evaluation and Licensure Section
4210 E. 11th Avenue, Room 254
Denver, CO 80220
303-866-5901

**Connecticut**
Nursing Home Licensure Office
Department of Public Health
Division of Regulation
410 Capitol Avenue, MS 512
P.O. Box 340308
Hartford, CT 06134
860-509-7444

**Delaware**
Office of Health Facilities Licensing
    and Certification
Nursing Home Division
Division of Public Health
3000 Newport Gap Pike
Wilmington, DE 19808
302-577-3499

**District of Columbia**
Office of Licensing and Certification
Nursing Home Division
Department of Human Services
614 H Street, N.W., Suite 1003
Washington, DC 20001
202-727-7190

**Florida**
Nursing Home Licensure Office
Licensure and Certification Branch
Division of Health
Department of Rehabilitation Services
2727 Mahan Drive
Tallahassee, FL 32308
904-487-3513

**Georgia**
Nursing Home Licensure Office
Standards and Licensure Unit
Office of Regulatory Services
2 Peachtree Street, N.E., Suite 22-418
Atlanta, GA 30303
404-657-5850

**Hawaii**
Nursing Home Licensure Office
Hospital and Medical Facility Branch
1270 Queen Emma, Suite 1100
Honolulu, HI 96813
808-586-4080

**Idaho**
Nursing Home Licensure Office
Facilities Standards and Development
Idaho Department of Health
 and Welfare
450 W. State Street
2nd Floor, Towers Bldg.
Boise, ID 83720-0036
208-334-6626

**Illinois**
Nursing Home Licensure Office
Department of Public Health
Health Facilities and Quality of Care
525 W. Jefferson Street, 5th Floor
Springfield, IL 62761
217-782-5180

**Indiana**
Nursing Home Licensure Office
Division of Health Facilities
State Board of Health
1330 W. Michigan Street
P.O. Box 1964
Indianapolis, IN 46206-1964
317-383-6442

**Iowa**
Nursing Home Licensure Office
State Department of Health
Division of Health Facilities
Lucas State Office Building, 3rd Floor
Des Moines, IA 50319-0083
515-281-4115
800-523-3213

**Kansas**
Department of Health and
 Environment
Bureau of Adult and Child Homes
900 S.W. Jackson, Suite 1001
Topeka, KS 66612-1290
913-296-1240

**Kentucky**
Division for Licensing and Regulation
Office of the Inspector General
CHR Building, 4th Floor, E.
275 E. Main Street
Frankfort, KY 40621
502-564-2800

**Louisiana**
Nursing Home Licensure Office
Health and Hospitals Department
Division of Licensure and
 Certification
P.O. Box 3767
Baton Rouge, LA 70821-3767
504-342-5774

**Maine**
Division of Licensure and
 Certification
35 Anthony Avenue
State House Station 11
Augusta, ME 04333
207-624-5386

**Maryland**
Office of Licensing and
 Certification Program
Department of Health and
 Mental Hygiene
4201 Patterson Avenue, 4th Floor
Baltimore, MD 21215
410-764-2770

**Massachusetts**
Long-Term-Care Facilities Program
Department of Public Health
10 West Street, 5th Floor
Boston, MA 02111
617-727-5864

**Michigan**
Nursing Home Licensure Office
Bureau of Health Care Services
Department of Public Health
P.O. Box 30195
3423 N. Martin Luther King, Jr.,
    Boulevard
Lansing, MI 48909
517-335-8505

**Minnesota**
Department of Health
Health Resources Division
393 N. Dunlop Street
P.O. Box 64900
St. Paul, MN 55164-0900
612-643-2171

**Mississippi**
Nursing Home Licensure Office
Health Facilities Certification
    and Licensure
Department of Health
P.O. Box 1700
Jackson, MS 39215
601-960-7769

**Missouri**
Department of Social Services
Division of Aging
615 Howerton Court
Jefferson City, MO 65109
573-751-3082

**Montana**
Department of Health and
    Environmental Sciences
Health Facilities Division
P.O. Box 200901
Cogswell Building
1400 Broadway
Helena, MT 59620-0901
406-444-2037

**Nebraska**
Health Facilities Standards Bureau
Department of Health
301 Centennial Mall, S.
Lincoln, NE 68509-5007
402-471-2946

**Nevada**
Human Resources Department
Health Administration
Bureau of Regulatory Health Services
1550 E. College Parkway, #158
Carson City, NV 89710
702-687-4475

**New Hampshire**
Department of Health and
    Human Services
Division of Public Health
Bureau of Health Facilities
    Administration
6 Hazen Drive
Concord, NH 03301
603-271-4592

**New Jersey**
Health Facilities Evaluation and
    Licensing Division
Licensing, Certification and
    Standards
300 Whitehead Road, CN 367
Trenton, NJ 08625-0367
609-588-7726

**New Mexico**
Health and Social Service
    Department
Public Health Division
Harold Runnels Building
525 Camino de los Marquez,
    Suite 2
Santa Fe, NM 87501
505-827-4200

**New York**
Bureau of Long-Term-Care Services
Corning Tower, Empire State Plaza,
    Room 1882
Albany, NY 12237-0732
518-473-1564

**North Carolina**
Nursing Home Licensure Office
Licensure and Certification Section
Health Care Facilities Branch
701 Barbour Drive
Raleigh, NC 27603
919-733-2342

**North Dakota**
Department of Health and
    Consolidated Laboratories
Health Resources Section
Health Facilities Division
600 E. Boulevard Avenue
Bismarck, ND 58505-0200
328-224-2352

**Ohio**
Department of Health
Licensing and Certification Division
246 N. High Street, 3rd Floor
P.O. Box 118
Columbus, OH 43266-0118
614-752-9524

**Oklahoma**
Special Health Services
Licensure and Certification Division
1000 N.E. 10th Street
Oklahoma City, OK 73117-1299
405-271-6868

**Oregon**
Long-Term-Care Licensing
Licensing and Certification
500 Summer Street, N.E.
Salem, OR 97310
800-422-6012 (In Oregon)
800-522-2602

**Pennsylvania**
Nursing Home Licensure Office
Division of Long-Term Care
P.O. Box 2649
Harrisburg, PA 17105
717-783-4854
800-822-2113

**Rhode Island**
Department of Health
Division of Facilities Regulation
3 Capitol Hill
Providence, RI 02908
401-277-2566

**South Carolina**
Health and Environmental
    Control Department
Health Regulation Division
Health Facilities Regulation
2600 Bull Street
Columbia, SC 29201
803-737-7211

**South Dakota**
Department of Health
Division of Licensure and
    Certification
445 E. Capitol Avenue
Pierre, SD 57501
605-773-3364

**Tennessee**
Department of Health
Manpower and Facilities Bureau
283 Plus Park Boulevard
Nashville, TN 37247-0530
615-367-6316

**Texas**
Department of Health
Licensing and Certification Bureau
1100 W. 49th Street
Austin, TX 78756-3199
512-834-6650

**Utah**
Department of Health
Health Care Resources
Health Facilities Licensure Bureau
P.O. Box 16990
288 N. 1460 West
Salt Lake City, UT 84116-0990
801-538-6152

**Vermont**
Aging and Disabilities Department
Licensing and Protection Division
19 Commerce Building
P.O. Box 536
Williston, VT 05495
802-863-7250

**Virginia**
Department of Health
Public Health Programs Office
Health Facilities Regulations Office
3600 W. Broad Street, Suite 216
Richmond, VA 23230
804-367-2102

**Washington**
Department of Health
1300 S.E. Quince Street
Olympia, WA 98504-0935
306-586-5846

**West Virginia**
Health and Human Resources
    Department
Administration and Finance Bureau
Health Facilities and Licensure
    Certification Section
Building 3, Room 550
Charleston, WV 25305
304-558-0050

**Wisconsin**
Health and Social Services Department
Health Division
Bureau of Quality Compliance
P.O. Box 7850
Madison WI 53707
608-267-7185

**Wyoming**
Health Department
Division of Health
Office of Health Quality
First Bank Building, 8th Floor
Cheyenne, WY 82002-0480
307-777-7123

# Appendix L: Nursing Home Patient Bill of Rights

Under federal regulations, nursing homes must have written policies covering the rights of patients. These rights must be posted where residents and visitors can easily see them. A Patient Bill of Rights ensures that each person admitted to a facility will have his or her rights protected. Flagrant violations of these rights should be reported to the proper state authorities.

**A Patient:**

1. is fully informed as evidenced by the resident's written acknowledgment of these rights and of all rules and regulations governing the exercise of these rights.

2. is fully informed of services available in the facility and of related charges for services not covered under Medicare/Medicaid, or not covered by the facility's basic daily rate.

3. is fully informed of his or her medical condition unless the physician notes in the medical record that it is not in the patient's interest to be told, and is afforded the opportunity to participate in the planning of his or her medical treatment and to refuse to participate in experimental research.

4. is transferred or discharged only for medical reasons, or for his or her welfare or that of other residents, and is given reasonable advance notice to ensure orderly transfer or discharge.

5. is encouraged and assisted, through his or her period of stay to exercise his or her rights as a resident and as a free citizen. To this end he or she may voice grievances and recommended changes in policies and services to facility staff and/or outside representatives of his or her choice without fear of coercion, discrimination, or reprisal.

6. may manage his or her personal financial affairs, or is given at least a quarterly accounting of financial transactions made on his or her behalf if the facility accepts the responsibility to safeguard the funds.

7. is free from mental and physical abuse, and free from chemical and physical restraints except as authorized in writing by a physician for a specified and limited period of time or when necessary to protect patients from injury to themselves or others.

8. is assured confidential treatment of his or her personal and medical records and may approve or refuse their release to any individual outside facility.

---

*Source:* Suggested by the Health Care Financing Administration, U.S. Department of Health and Human Services, Washington, D.C.

9. is treated with consideration, respect, and full recognition of his or her dignity and individuality, including privacy in treatment and in care of his or her personal needs.

10. is not required to perform services for the facility that are not included for therapeutic purposes in this plan of care.

11. may associate and communicate privately with persons of his or her choice, and send and receive his or her personal mail unopened.

12. may meet with, and participate in activities of social, religious, and community groups at his or her discretion.

13. may retain and use his or her personal clothing and possessions as space permits, unless to do so would infringe upon rights of other patients, or constitute a hazard of safety.

14. is assured privacy for visits by his or her spouse; if both are inpatients in the facility, they are permitted to share a room.

# Appendix M: State Agencies Regulating Home Health Care

**Alabama**
Department of Public Health
State Office Building
572 E. Patton Avenue
Mail to: 434 Monroe Street
Montgomery, AL 36130-3017
334-613-5300

**Alaska**
Department of Health and
  Social Services
Alaska Office Building
P.O. Box 110601
Juneau, AK 99811-0601
907-465-3030

**Arizona**
Department of Health Services
1647 E. Morten
Phoenix, AZ 85020
602-542-1000

**Arkansas**
Department of Health
State Health Building
4815 W. Markham Street
Little Rock, AR 72204
501-661-2112

**California**
Department of Health Services
714 P Street, Room 1253
Sacramento, CA 95814
916-445-4171

**Colorado**
Attn: Home Health Care
Department of Health Care Policy
  & Financing
1575 Sherman, 5th Floor
Denver, CO 80203-1714
303-866-5920

**Connecticut**
Department of Health Services
410 Capitol Avenue
Hartford, CT 06134
860-509-7101

**Delaware**
Division of Public Health
Department of Health and
  Social Services
2055 Limestone Road, Suite 300
Wilmington, DE 19808
302-995-8630

**District of Columbia**
Department of Human Services
Commission of Public Health
2700 Martin Luther King, Jr.,
  Avenue, S.E.
Washington, DC 20032
202-373-7166

**Florida**
Health Program Office
Department of Health and
  Rehabilitative Services
HSH
1317 Winewood Boulevard
Bldg. 6, Room 308
Tallahassee, FL 32399-0700
904-487-3220

**Georgia**
Division of Public Health
Department of Human Resources
2 Peachtree Street, N.W., Room 7-300
Atlanta, GA 30303
404-657-2700

**Hawaii**
Department of Health
P.O. Box 3378
Honolulu, HI 96801
808-586-4410

**Idaho**
Bureau of Preventive Medicine
Division of Health
Department of Health and Welfare
Towers Building, 4th Floor
P.O. Box 83720
450 W. State Street
Boise, ID 83720-0036
208-334-5930

**Illinois**
Department of Public Health
535 W. Jefferson Street
Springfield, IL 62761
217-782-4977

**Indiana**
State Board of Health
1330 W. Michigan Street
Indianapolis, IN 46202-1964
317-383-6100

**Iowa**
Department of Public Health
SCH
Lucas State Office Building
321 E. 12th Street
Des Moines, IA 50319-0075
515-281-5787

**Kansas**
Division of Health
Department of Health &
   Environment
900 S.W. Jackson Street, Suite 1001
Topeka, KS 66612
913-296-1500

**Kentucky**
Department for Health Services
Cabinet for Human Resources
Health Services Building, 1st Floor
275 E. Main Street
Frankfort, KY 40621
502-564-3970

**Louisiana**
Health and Hospitals, Department
   of Public Health Services
P.O. Box 60630
325 Loyola Avenue
New Orleans, LA 70160
504-568-5050

**Maine**
Bureau of Health
Department of Human Services
State House, Station 1
Augusta, ME 04333-0011
207-287-3201

**Maryland**
Department of Health and
   Mental Hygiene
Deputy Secretary
Herbert R. O'Conor State
   Office Building
201 W. Preston Street, Room 525
Baltimore, MD 21201
410-225-6500

**Massachusetts**
Department of Public Health
250 Washington Street
Boston, MA 02108-4619
617-624-5200

**Michigan**
Department of Public Health
P.O. Box 30195
3423 Martin Luther King, Jr.,
   Boulevard
Lansing, MI 48909
517-334-8420

**Minnesota**
Department of Health
P.O. Box 9441
717 Delaware Street, S.E.
Minneapolis, MN 55440-9441
612-623-5000

**Mississippi**
Department of Health
2423 N. State Street
Jackson, MS 39216
601-960-7400

**Missouri**
Department of Health
1738 E. Elm Street
P.O. Box 570
Jefferson City, MO 65102
573-751-6001

**Montana**
Department of Health and
   Environmental Sciences
P.O. Box 200901
Helena, MT 59620-0901
406-444-2544

**Nebraska**
Department of Health
State Office Building
P.O. Box 95007
301 Centennial Mall, S., 3rd Floor
Lincoln, NE 68509-5007
402-471-2133

**Nevada**
Department of Human Resources
Director's Office, Room 600
505 E. King Street
Carson City, NV 89710
702-687-4400

**New Hampshire**
Division of Public Health Services
Department of Health and
    Human Services
Health and Welfare Services Building
6 Hazen Drive
Concord, NH 03301-6527
603-271-4501

**New Jersey**
Department of Health &
    Elderly Services
Health and Agriculture Building
John Fitch Plaza
CN 360
Trenton, NJ 08625-0360
609-292-7837

**New Mexico**
Health Department
Public Health Division
P.O. Box 26110
1190 St. Francis Drive
Santa Fe, NM 87505
505-827-2389

**New York**
Department of Health
Frear Bldg.
2 Third Street, Suite 401
Troy, NY 12180
518-474-2011

**North Carolina**
Office of the State Health Director
Archdale Building
P.O. Box 27687
512 N. Salisbury Street
Raleigh, NC 27611
919-733-4984

**North Dakota**
Department of Health &
    Consolidated Laboratories
State Capitol, Judicial Wing
600 E. Boulevard Avenue
Bismarck, ND 58505-0200
701-328-2372

**Ohio**
Department of Health
246 N. High Street, 3rd Floor
Columbus, OH 43215
614-466-3543

**Oklahoma**
Department of Health
1000 N.E. 10th Street
Oklahoma City, OK 73117
405-271-4200

**Oregon**
Department of Human Resources
Health Division
800 N.E. Oregon Street, 2nd Floor
Portland, OR 97232
503-731-4000

**Pennsylvania**
Department of Health
Health and Welfare Building
P.O. Box 90
Harrisburg, PA 17108
717-787-6436

**Puerto Rico**
Department of Health
P.O. Box 70184
San Juan, PR 00936
809-766-1616

**Rhode Island**
Health Department
3 Capitol Hill
Providence, RI 02908-5097
401-277-2231

**South Carolina**
Department of Health and
    Environmental Control
2600 Bull Street
Columbia, SC 29201
803-734-4880

**South Dakota**
Health Department
445 E. Capitol Avenue
Pierre, SD 57501-3185
605-773-3361

**Tennessee**
Health Department
Cordell Bldg., 3rd Floor
426 Fifth Avenue
Nashville, TN 37247-0101
615-741-3111

**Texas**
Department of Health
1100 W. 49th Street
Austin, TX 78756-3199
512-458-7375

**Utah**
Department of Health
288 N. 1460 West
Salt Lake City, UT 84116
801-538-6101

**Vermont**
Human Services Agency
Health Department
P.O. Box 70
108 Cherry Street
Burlington, VT 05402
802-863-7280

**Virgin Islands**
Health Department
St. Thomas Hospital
48 Sugar Estate
St. Thomas, VI 00802
809-776-8311

**Virginia**
Office of Health Commissioner
P.O. Box 2448
Richmond, VA 23218
804-786-3561

**Washington**
Health Department
1112 S.E. Quince Street
P.O. Box 47890
Olympia, WA 98504-7890
360-753-5871

**West Virginia**
Health and Human Resources
    Department
Office of the Secretary
State Capitol Complex, Building 3,
    Room 206
Charleston, WV 25305
304-558-0684

**Wisconsin**
Health and Social Services
    Department
Office of the Secretary
P.O. Box 7850
Madison, WI 53707-7850
608-266-9622

**Wyoming**
Health Department
Office of the Director
117 Hathaway Building
2300 Capitol Avenue
Cheyenne, WY 82002
307-777-7656

# Appendix N: State Medicaid Offices

Note: Some telephone numbers may have changed; please consult your local directory.

**Alabama**
Medicaid Agency
P.O. Box 5624
501 Dexter Avenue
Montgomery, AL 36103-5624
334-242-5600

**Alaska**
Department of Health and
    Social Services
Division of Medical Assistance
P.O. Box 110660
Juneau, AK 99811-0660
907-465-3355

**Arizona**
Arizona Health Care Cost
    Containment System
801 E. Jefferson Street
Phoenix, AZ 85034
602-417-4000 ext. 4053

**Arkansas**
Department of Human Services
Division of Medical Services
P.O. Box 1437, Slot 1100
Little Rock, AR 72203-1437
501-682-8292

**California**
Department of Health Services
714 P Street, Room 1253
Sacramento, CA 95814
916-657-1425

**Colorado**
Department of Health Care Policy
    and Financing
1575 Sherman, 4th Floor
Denver, CO 80203-1714
303-866-6092

**Connecticut**
Health Care Financing Administration
Department of Social Services
25 Sigourney Street
Hartford, CT 06106-5033
860-424-5167

**Delaware**
Department of Health and
    Social Services
P.O. Box 906, Lewis Bldg.
New Castle, DE 19720
302-577-4901

**District of Columbia**
Department of Human Services
2100 Martin Luther King, Jr.,
    Avenue, S.E.
Suite 302
Washington, DC 20020
202-727-0735

**Florida**
Agency for Health Care
    Administration
P.O. Box 13000
Tallahassee, FL 32317-3000
904-488-3560

**Georgia**
Department of Medical Assistance
2 Peachtree Street, N.W.
27th Floor, Suite 100
Atlanta, GA 30303-3159
404-656-4479

**Hawaii**
Department of Human Services
Med Quest Division
P.O. Box 339
Honolulu, HI 96809-0339
808-586-5391

**Idaho**
Department of Health and Welfare
P.O. Box 83720
Towers Building, Second Floor
Boise, ID 83720-0036
208-334-5747

**Illinois**
Department of Public Aid
Division of Medical Programs
201 S. Grand Avenue, E., 3rd Floor
Springfield, IL 62763-0001
217-782-2570

**Indiana**
Medicaid Policy and Planning
Family and Social Services
   Administration
100 N. Senate Avenue
P.O. Box 6015
Indianapolis, IN 46206-6015
317-232-4455

**Iowa**
Bureau of Medical Services
Department of Human Services
Division of Medical Services
Hoover State Office Building,
   5th Floor
Des Moines, IA 50319-0114
515-281-8794

**Kansas**
Department of Social and
   Rehabilitative Services
Docking State Office Building,
   Room 628-S
915 Harrison
Topeka, KS 66604
913-296-3981

**Kentucky**
Department of Medicaid Services
275 E. Main Street
CHR Bldg., 3rd Floor East
Frankfort, KY 40621
502-564-4321

**Louisiana**
Department of Health and Hospitals
P.O. Box 91030
Baton Rouge, LA 70821-9030
504-342-3891

**Maine**
Department of Human Services
Bureau of Medical Services
249 Western Avenue
Augusta, ME 04333
207-287-2674

**Maryland**
Department of Health &
   Mental Hygiene
Herber R. O'Conor Building
201 W. Preston Street, Room 525
Baltimore, MD 21201
410-225-6505

**Massachusetts**
Division of Medical Assistance
600 Washington Street, 5th Floor
Boston, MA 02111
617-348-5690

**Michigan**
Medical Services Administration
Department of Social Services
P.O. Box 30479
Lansing, MI 48909
517-335-5001

**Minnesota**
Health Care Administration
Department of Human Services
444 Lafayette Road, 6th Floor
St. Paul, MN 55155-3852
612-297-3374

**Mississippi**
Division of Medicaid
Office of the Governor
Robert E. Lee Building
239 N. Lamar Street, Suite 801
Jackson, MS 39201-1399
601-359-6056

**Missouri**
Department of Social Services
Division of Medical Services
P.O. Box 6500
615 Howerton Court
Jefferson City, MO 65102-6500
573-751-6922

**Montana**
Department of Social and
 Rehabilitation Services
Medicaid Services Division
P.O. Box 202951
Helena, MT 59602
406-444-4540

**Nebraska**
Medical Services Division
Department of Social Services
301 Centennial Mall, S., 5th Floor
P.O. Box 95026
Lincoln, NE 68509-5026
402-471-9718

**Nevada**
Department of Human Resources
Welfare Division
Capitol Complex
2527 N. Carson Street
Carson City, NV 89710
702-687-4867

**New Hampshire**
Health and Human Services
 Department
Human Services Division
Office of Medical Services
6 Hazen Drive
Concord, NH 03301-6521
603-271-4353

**New Jersey**
Human Services Department
Division of Medical Assistance
 and Health Services
7 Quakerbridge Plaza, CN-712
Trenton, NJ 08625
609-588-2600

**New Mexico**
Department of Human Services
Medical Assistance Division
P.O. Box 2348
Santa Fe, NM 87504-2348
505-827-3106

**New York**
State Department of Social Services
Division of Health & Long-Term Care
40 N. Pearl Street
Albany, NY 12243
518-474-9132

**North Carolina**
Department of Human Resources
Division of Medical Assistance
P.O. Box 29529
1985 Umstead Drive
Raleigh, NC 27626-0529
919-733-2060

**North Dakota**
Department of Human Services
Medicaid Programs Division
State Capitol Judicial Wing
600 E. Boulevard Avenue
Bismarck, ND 58505-0261
701-328-2310

**Ohio**
Department of Human Services
Office of Medicaid
30 E. Broad Street, 31st Floor
Columbus, OH 43266-0423
614-644-0140

**Oklahoma**
Health Care Authority
4545 N. Lincoln Boulevard, Suite 124
Oklahoma City, OK 73105
405-530-3374

**Oregon**
Department of Human Resources
Office of Medical Assistance Programs
500 Summer Street, N.E., 3rd Floor
Salem, OR 97310-1014
503-945-5772

**Pennsylvania**
Department of Public Welfare
Medical Assistance Programs
Health and Welfare Building,
 Room 515
7th & Forster Streets
Harrisburg, PA 17120
717-787-1870

**Puerto Rico**
Office of Economic Assistance to
 the Medically Indigent
P.O. Box 70184
San Juan, PR 00936-8184
809-765-1230

**Rhode Island**
Department of Human Services
Division of Medical Services
600 New London Avenue
Cranston, RI 02902
401-464-3575

**South Carolina**
Health and Human Service
  Finance Commission
P.O. Box 8206
Columbia, SC 29202-8206
803-253-6100

**South Dakota**
Department of Social Services
Office of Medical Services
Richard F. Kneip Building
700 Governor's Drive
Pierre, SD 57501-2291
605-773-3495

**Tennessee**
Department of Health
Bureau of Medicaid
729 Church Street
Nashville, TN 37202-2630
615-741-0213

**Texas**
Department of Human Services
Health Care Services Division
P.O. Box 149030
Building 4
Austin, TX 78714-9030
512-438-3011

**Utah**
Department of Health
Health Care Financing
Medicaid Information Unit
P.O. Box 142901
Salt Lake City, UT 84114-2901
801-538-6406

**Vermont**
Human Services Agency
Medicaid Division
103 S. Main Street
Waterbury, VT 05671-1201
802-241-2880

**Virgin Islands**
Bureau of Health Insurance and
  Medical Assistance
Health Department
Frostco Center, Suite 302
210-3A Altona
Charlotte Amalie
St. Thomas, VI 00802
809-774-4624

**Virginia**
Department of Medical Services
Division of Medical Social Services
600 E. Broad Street, Suite 1300
Richmond, VA 23219
804-786-8099

**Washington**
Division of Medical Assistance
Department of Social and
  Health Services
P.O. Box 45080
Olympia, WA 98504-5080
360-753-1777

**West Virginia**
Department of Health and
  Human Services
Bureau for Medical Services
State Capitol Complex, Building 6
Charleston, WV 25304
304-926-1700

**Wisconsin**
Department of Health and
  Social Services
Division of Health
P.O. Box 309
Madison, WI 53701
608-266-2522

**Wyoming**
Department of Health
Division of Health Care Financing
6101 Yellowstone Road, Room 259-B
Cheyenne, WY 82002
307-777-7531

# Appendix O: State Long-Term-Care Ombudsman Offices

**Alabama**
Commission on Aging
P.O. Box 301851
Montgomery, AL 36130
334-261-5743
800-243-5463

**Alaska**
Older Alaskans' Commission
Department of Administration
3601 C Street, Suite 260
Anchorage, AK 99503
907-563-6393

**Arizona**
State Agency on Aging
Aging and Adult Administration
1789 W. Jefferson
Phoenix, AZ 85007
602-542-4446

**Arkansas**
Division of Aging and Adult Services
Department of Human Services
P.O. Box 1437, Slot 1412
Little Rock, AR 72203
501-682-2441

**California**
Department of Aging
Office of the Long-Term-Care
  Ombudsman
1600 K Street
Sacramento, CA 95814
800-231-4024
916-322-5290

**Colorado**
State Care Ombudsman Program
455 Sherman Street, Suite 130
Denver, CO 80203
800-582-7410
303-722-0300

**Connecticut**
Department of Social Services
Division of Elderly Services
25 Sigourney Street
Hartford, CT 06106
860-424-4908
800-842-1508

**Delaware**
Division of Aging (Northern)
Delaware State Hospital
2nd Floor Annex
1901 N. DuPont Highway
New Castle, DE 19720
302-577-4791

Division of Aging (Southern)
Milford State Services Center
18 N. Walnut Street
Milford, DE 19963
302-422-1386

**District of Columbia**
Office on Aging
441 4th Street, N.W.,
  Suite 900-South Side
Washington, DC 20001
202-724-5623

**Florida**
Long-Term-Care Ombudsman Council
Carlton Building
501 S. Calhoun Street
Tallahassee, FL 32399-0001
904-488-6190

**Georgia**
Office of Aging
Department of Human Resources
675 Ponce de Leon Avenue
Atlanta, GA 30308
404-817-6702

**Hawaii**
Executive Office on Aging
Office of the Governor
250 S. Hotel Street, Suite 107
Honolulu, HI 96813-2831
808-586-0100

**Idaho**
Office on Aging
700 W. Jefferson, Room 108
Boise, ID 83720-0007
208-334-3833

**Illinois**
Department on Aging
421 E. Capitol Avenue, Suite 100
Springfield, IL 62701-1789
217-785-3140

**Indiana**
Department of Human Services
P.O. Box 7083
402 W. Washington
Indianapolis, IN 46207-7083
800-722-1213
317-232-3645

**Iowa**
Department of Elder Affairs
Clemmons Bldg., 3rd Floor
200 Tenth Street
Des Moines, IA 50309
515-281-5187

**Kansas**
Department on Aging
Docking State Office Building
915 S.W. Harrison Street, Room 150-S
Topeka, KS 66612-1500
913-296-4986

**Kentucky**
Department of Social Services
Division of Aging Services
CHR Building, 5 W.
275 E. Main Street
Frankfort, KY 40621
502-564-6930

**Louisiana**
Governor's Office of Elderly Affairs
P.O. Box 80374
Baton Rouge, LA 70898-0374
504-925-1700

**Maine**
Long-Term-Care Ombudsman Program
Maine Committee on Aging
State House Station 127
Augusta, ME 04333
207-624-5335

**Maryland**
Office on Aging
301 W. Preston Street
Room 1004
Baltimore, MD 21201
410-225-1100

**Massachusetts**
Elder Affairs Executive Offices
1 Ashburton Place
5th Floor
Boston, MA 02108
617-727-7750

**Michigan**
Citizens for Better Care
David Whitney Building
4750 Woodward, Suite 410
Detroit, MI 48201-1308
313-832-6387

**Minnesota**
Board on Aging
Human Services Building
444 Lafayette Road
St. Paul, MN 55155-3843
612-296-2544

**Mississippi**
Council on Aging
750 N. State Street
Jackson, MS 39302
601-359-4929

**Missouri**
Department of Social Services
Aging Division
P.O. Box 1337
Jefferson City, MO 65102
573-751-3082

**Montana**
Office on Aging
P.O. Box 4210
Helena, MT 59604-4210
406-444-4676

**Nebraska**
Department on Aging
301 Centennial Mall, S.
P.O. Box 95044
Lincoln, NE 68509-5044
402-471-2307

**Nevada**
Aging Services Administration
Human Resources Department
340 N. 11th Street, Suite 203
Las Vegas, NV 89101
702-486-3545

**New Hampshire**
Health and Human Services
    Department
Elderly and Adult Services Division
Annex Building #1
115 Pleasant Street
Concord, NH 03301-3843
603-271-4375

**New Jersey**
Department of Community Affairs
Ombudsman for the Elderly
101 S. Broad Street, CN 807
Trenton, NJ 08625-0807
609-292-8016
800-792-8820

**New Mexico**
State Agency on Aging
La Villa Rivera Building
228 E. Palace Avenue
Santa Fe, NM 87501
505-827-7640
800-432-2080

**New York**
Office for Aging
Empire State Plaza
Agency Building 2
Albany, NY 12223
518-474-5731

**North Carolina**
Division of Aging
101 Blaire Drive
Raleigh, NC 27603
919-733-4534

**North Dakota**
Long-Term-Care Ombudsman
Aging Services Division
P.O. Box 7070
600 S. Second Street, Suite 1-C
Bismarck, ND 58504-5729
701-328-8910

**Ohio**
Department on Aging
State Ombudsman
50 W. Broad Street, 9th Floor
Columbus, OH 43215
800-282-1206
614-466-1220

**Oklahoma**
Office of Client Advocacy
Long-Term-Care Ombudsman
P.O. Box 25352
312 N. 28th Street
Oklahoma City, OK 73125
405-521-2281

**Oregon**
Long-Term-Care Ombudsman
2475 Lancaster Drive, N.E.
Building B, Suite 9
Salem, OR 97310
503-378-6533
800-522-2602

**Pennsylvania**
Department of Aging
Bureau of Field Operations
MSSOB
400 Market Street
P.O. Box 1089
Harrisburg, PA 17101-1089
717-783-7247

**Puerto Rico**
Office of the Ombudsman
P.O. Box 41088
Station Meinillas
San Juan, PR 00940-1088
809-725-1886

**Rhode Island**
Department of Elderly Affairs
160 Pine Street
Providence, RI 02903
401-277-2894

**South Carolina**
Division on Aging
202 Arbor Lake Drive, Suite 301
Columbia, SC 29223
803-737-7500

**South Dakota**
Office of Adult Services and Aging
Social Services Department
700 Governor's Drive
Pierre, SD 57501-2291
605-773-3656

**Tennessee**
Commission on Aging
Andrew Jackson State Office Bldg.
500 Deaderick Street, 9th Floor
Nashville, TN 37243-0860
615-741-2056

**Texas**
Department on Aging
Nursing Home Advocacy and
　Long-Term-Care Ombudsman
P.O. Box 12786
Austin, TX 78711
512-444-2727

**Utah**
Long-Term-Care Ombudsman
120 N. 200 West, Room 401
Salt Lake City, UT 84103
801-538-4171
801-538-3910

**Vermont**
Long-Term-Care Ombudsman
　Program
103 S. Main Street, Osgood 1
Waterbury, VT 05671-2301
802-241-2400
800-642-5119

**Virginia**
Department for Aging
700 E. Franklin Street
700 Centre, 10th Floor
Richmond, VA 23219-2327
804-225-2271
800-552-3402

**Washington**
Long-Term-Care Ombudsman
Aging and Adult Services
　Administration
P.O. Box 45600
Olympia, WA 98504-5600
360-493-2560

**West Virginia**
Office of Aging
State Capitol Complex, Holly Grove
1900 Kanawha Boulevard, E.
Charleston, WV 25305-0160
304-558-3317
304-558-2363

**Wisconsin**
Aging & Long-Term Care Board
214 N. Hamilton Street
Madison, WI 53703
608-266-8944
608-266-8945

**Wyoming**
Long-Term-Care Ombudsman
P.O. Box 94
Wheatlyn, WY 82201
307-322-5553

# Glossary

**Administrative law judge (ALJ)**  An official charged with making decisions in matters of administrative, as opposed to civil or criminal, law.

**Advance directives**  Written documents stating how you want medical decisions made for you if you lose the ability to make decisions for yourself. The two most common advance directives are: Living Wills and Durable Powers of Attorney for Health Care.

**Ambulatory surgery**  A large, although limited, range of procedures using operative and anesthesia techniques that allow the patient to recuperate at home, rather than in the hospital, immediately following the operation.

**American Association of Retired Persons (AARP)**  A service and lobbying group composed of people age 50 and over that has the Medicare program among its concerns.

**American Medical Association (AMA)**  The largest, although not the only, trade association of American doctors.

**Anesthesiologist or anesthetist**  A person who administers anesthetics for surgery and diagnostic procedures. An anesthesiologist is always a holder of the M.D. or D.O. degree; an anesthetist may be a nurse-anesthetist or an anesthesia technician.

**Approved charge**  The amount that Medicare has determined is appropriate for payment to a physician for a service, based on his and his colleagues' histories of charge. See *Usual, customary, and reasonable reimbursement system below.*

**Assignment**  A process in which a Medicare beneficiary agrees to have Medicare's share of the cost of a service paid directly to a doctor or other provider, and the provider agrees to accept the Medicare-approved charge as payment in full. Medicare pays 80 percent of the cost and the beneficiary 20 percent, for most services.

**Attending physician**  A doctor with staff privileges at a hospital who treats patients there. Usually applied to physicians on the staff of a teaching hospital who have a role in teaching and supervising interns and residents.

**Balance billing limit**  A Medicare regulation that limits the maximum fee that a non-participating physician may charge a Medicare beneficiary to 115 percent above the Medicare-approved amount. The physician is prohibited from collecting the difference or balance between his/her regular fee and the balance billing limit.

**Biologicals**  Drugs produced by extraction from plant or animal tissue, rather than chemical synthesis. Examples: gamma globulin (from horse serum); human growth hormone.

**Brain stem**  A portion of the brain involved in controlling basic bodily functions.

**Cancer**  A malignant tumor of potentially unlimited growth that expands locally by invading surrounding normal tissues and systemically by metastasis.

**Cardio-pulmonary resuscitation (CPR)**  A set of treatments and procedures used to restart or stabilize heart and lung function when either one ceases.

**Carriers**  Private organizations, usually insurance companies, that have contracts with the Health Care Financing Administration to process claims under Part B (doctor insurance) of Medicare.

**Case law**  The body of court decisions that establishes binding interpretations of the law passed by legislative bodies.

**Catastrophic illness**   Any unusually expensive or lengthy illness that greatly exceeds an individual's ability to pay.

**Catheters**   Tubes used to drain various hollow cavities of the body.

**Chemotherapy**   Generally, the treatment of any disease by drugs; usually used to mean drug therapy for cancer using powerful agents that are toxic to both cancerous and noncancerous cells, but more so to the former.

**Chiropractor**   A holder of the degree of Doctor of Chiropractic (D.C.). Chiropractors treat disorders of location and relationship of bones and joints. Some hold that this type of treatment has positive effects on organ systems other than the musculoskeletal system, others do not. See *Doctor of Chiropractic.*

**Competitive medical plan (CMP)**   An arrangement for prepaid care that is not as restricted (as a health maintenance organization is) in benefits offered, premium calculation, and the like.

**Congressional Budget Office**   The agency of Congress that prepares analyses of various national budget alternatives and studies budget-related issues for Congress.

**Coordination of benefits**   A process in which insurers cooperate to make sure that they do not, together, pay more than the maximum benefit available from any of them.

**Copayments**   Portions of the cost of care an insured person is required to pay, while the insurance usually, but not always, pays for the major part of the cost.

**Deductibles**   Amounts that must be paid by an insured person before an insurance plan pays for any portion of the cost.

**Dentist**   A holder of the degree of Doctor of Dental Medicine (D.D.M.), or Doctor of Dental Surgery (D.D.S.), concerned with care of the teeth, gums, and associated structures.

**Department of Health and Human Services**   The federal department charged generally with administration of national welfare programs. Formed from the old Department of Health, Education, and Welfare when the Department of Education was split off.

**Diagnosis-Related Groups (DRG) system**   A method of paying hospitals based on the average cost of treating patients with statistically similar conditions.

**Diagnostic workup**   The process of testing and checking various hypotheses about possible conditions a patient may have when this cannot be immediately established from symptoms, history, or routine tests.

**Dialysis**   Use of a machine to remove waste products or toxins from the blood to assist or replace kidney function.

**Doctor of Chiropractic**   A holder of the degree of Doctor of Chiropractic, a school of medicine that places almost exclusive reliance on manipulation for alignment of the skeleton, plus exercise and nutrition.

**Doctor of Medicine (M.D.)**   A holder of the degree of Medical Doctor, the dominant school of medicine in the United States, which is committed to allopathic medicine — that is, treatment agents that produce effects different from the symptoms of the disease they are intended to treat, foreign to the body or by high concentrations of naturally occurring agents, and surgery; conventional American medicine.

**Doctor of Osteopathy (D.O.)**   A holder of the degree of Doctor of Osteopathy, a school of medicine that places emphasis, but not exclusive emphasis, on proper alignment of the skeleton.

**Durable medical equipment**   Medical equipment that is intended to be used over and over again, usually by the patient or a caregiver, rather than being used once or a few times and discarded. Examples include wheelchairs, hospital beds, and oxygen tanks.

**Durable power of attorney**   A delegation of some authority to another, which lasts until revoked. See *power of attorney.*

**Earnings record**   The record of amounts earned by each individual for whom Social Security taxes were paid. Maintained by the Social Security Administration.

**Elective surgery or procedure**   A surgery or procedure that, given the patient's diagnosis and condition, can be performed at any convenient time; contrast with urgent procedure, one that must be done very soon, and emergency procedure, one that must be done immediately.

**Electrocardiogram (EKG)**   A medical test to measure the electrical activity of the heart, for diagnosis and therapy.

**Electrolytes**   Ions of sodium, potassium, and calcium in the blood that are intimately involved in regulating muscle contraction and heartbeat.

**Emergency**   A situation requiring immediate care to prevent death, serious injury, or deformity; contrast with *urgent.*

**End stage renal disease**   Kidney disease that is severe enough to require lifetime dialysis or a kidney transplant. End stage renal disease patients are eligible for Medicare and may be eligible for Social Security payments if found to be disabled.

**Executive departments**   The various entities within the federal government that ultimately report to the President (as opposed to Congress or to the Supreme Court).

**Explanation of Medicare Benefits (EOMB)**   A form sent to a Medicare beneficiary after a claim is paid, indicating what Medicare has paid for and why.

**Face sheet**   The top document in a patient's hospital chart, which the doctor attests is correct as to conditions and procedures to obtain payment from Medicare under the DRG system.

**Family practice/Family practitioner**   Delivery of primary health care to all members of families by a physician trained in general practice plus elements of pediatrics and obstetrics and gynecology; one who delivers such care.

**Federal judicial districts**   Major divisions of the United States that are under the jurisdiction of a single federal appeals court. The federal district courts make laws that establish precedents that the Social Security Administration and Medicare must follow, but these precedents have binding force only within the judicial district unless Congress aligns laws with them or the Supreme Court makes them the law of the land by upholding them when an appeal from the federal district court decision is filed.

**Fee-for-service system**   A system of payment for medical services in which each service rendered is charged for individually after the fact; the classic American way of paying for medical care; opposite of prepayment.

**Food and Drug Administration (FDA)**   A part of the Department of Health and Human Services that is charged with administering the Pure Food and Drug Act and various other laws that relate to prescription and veterinary drug production and sales.

**Freedom of choice options**   Arrangements under which members of a health maintenance organization or other prepaid plan can use physicians who are outside the panel of participating doctors, if they wish to do so. Additional payment is usually involved.

**General enrollment period**   The time from January 1 to March 31 of each year when anyone eligible for Part B of Medicare can enroll in it.

**General medical/surgical floors**   The areas of a hospital in which patients who do not require special treatment are cared for.

**General Practice/General Practitioner**    The delivery of a wide range of primary care services by an M.D. or D.O.; one who delivers them. See *Family Practice.*

**Group model health maintenance organization**    A health maintenance organization that is staffed by the doctors in a group practice, who may or may not have ownership interest or control.

**Group practice**    A situation in which a group of doctors shares facilities and support staff, and often makes an attempt to offer patients of the group a range of specialties.

**Gynecological problems**    Conditions and diseases peculiar to women. There is much current controversy about the best ways to treat many of these conditions and about whether some of them are properly considered diseases at all.

**Health Care Financing Administration (HCFA)**    The part of the Department of Health and Human Services that operates Medicare and, together with the states, Medicaid.

**Health maintenance organizations (HMOs)**    Entities that combine the functions of insurer and provider of care, giving most necessary care for a prepaid fee and placing an emphasis on prevention and careful assessment of medical necessity.

**Home health agency (HHA)**    An agency approved by Medicare for the delivery of home health services to Medicare beneficiaries.

**Home health care**    Care rendered in a patient's residence by employees of a home health agency or other approved providers of home health care.

**Hormones**    Naturally occurring chemicals that regulate functions of the body when carried through the bloodstream.

**Hospital-based physicians**    Term for doctors who treat patients exclusively or almost exclusively in hospitals and so use the hospital as their office, the place of primary contact with patients. Often the hospital bills for their services and pays them a salary.

**House staff**    Doctors in training in a hospital, plus hospital-based physicians, who are the primary physicians for patients who do not have personal physicians and assist in the care of those who do.

**Hydration**    Various treatments used to make sure that the body contains adequate water; also, the body's state of water balance.

**Hyperalimentation**    Total nutrition via a tube placed in a vein. Proteins, fats, electrolytes, and carbohydrates are all provided, in contrast to shorter-term administration of intravenous solutions that contain only electrolytes and sugars. Also called total parenteral nutrition. (TPN).

**Iatrogenesis**    Causation of illness by a doctor in the course of treating another real or putative illness.

**Immigration and naturalization records**    Records maintained by, or issued by, the Departments of State and Interior that show that an alien has legally entered the United States or become a citizen.

**Immunosuppressive drug**    A drug given to control the immune system to keep it from damaging a transplanted organ or causing additional damage to normal tissues in an autoimmune disease.

**Individual enrollment period**    The time, running from three months before one's sixty-fifth birthday to three months after, during which one can enroll in Part B of Medicare without a premium increase for delayed enrollment.

**Individual practice association (IPA) health maintenance organization**    A health maintenance organization that is staffed by physicians in private practice who continue to maintain their own offices and see both HMO and non-HMO patients.

**Inpatient** Someone admitted to a hospital for care; an adjective applying to care given in a hospital.

**Inpatient hospital care** Care that is rendered in a hospital to someone who has been formally admitted and temporarily lives in the hospital while receiving treatment.

**Intensive care unit** A part of a hospital in which people whose life support requires constant monitoring, or who require close and constant observation, are cared for.

**Intermediaries** Private organizations, usually insurance companies, that have contracts with the Health Care Financing Administration to process claims under Part A (hospital insurance) of Medicare.

**Intermediate care facility (ICF)** An institution that provides less intensive care than skilled nursing facilities. Patients are generally more mobile, and rehabilitation therapies are stressed.

**Interns** Doctors in their first year of postgraduate training in a hospital. The term is being replaced by "first-year resident."

**Intravenous lines** Tubes placed within, or connecting to a needle placed within, a vein to administer fluids and drugs.

**Licensed practical nurse (L.P.N.) or licensed vocational nurse (L.V.N.)** A person who has undergone training and been granted a license to provide general care to the sick. Considered less well trained than a registered nurse (R.N.).

**Living Will** A document executed prior to or early in the course of an illness, expressing one's wishes in regard to medical treatment if one becomes unable to direct the course of it personally.

**Medicaid** A federal/state program, established by the Title XIX of the Social Security Act, which provides medical care to the poor.

**Medically needy** Eligible for Medicaid, not because of absolute lack of income, but because income, less accumulated medical bills, is below state income limits for the Medicaid program.

**Medical necessity** The state of being thought to be required by the prevailing medical consensus. What is medically necessary in one period or one area may not be so in another.

**Medical necessity determination** A formal judgment, usually made for purposes of insurance payment, that a treatment was or was not medically necessary.

**Medical technician** An individual with training that allows him or her to carry out some of the functions of holders of the M.D. or D.O. degrees, especially in emergency situations outside of hospitals and during transport to hospitals, when limited but intense life support services must be provided.

**Medicare Choices** A HCFA demonstration project designed to increase Medicare beneficiaries' access to managed care.

**Medicare insured group (MIG)** An experimental approach to providing care to Medicare beneficiaries in which a traditional provider of retiree benefits, such as a corporation or union welfare plan, takes over responsibility for all care to those 65 or over in return for a set payment from Medicare.

**Medicare-participating physician** A doctor who has agreed to accept assignment on all claims from all Medicare beneficiaries in return for certain incentives.

**Medicare SELECT** A type of Medigap insurance policy that only pays full supplemental benefits if covered services are provided by selected providers (except in emergencies). The insurance companies that sell Medicare SELECT are responsible for establishing the network of providers. Medicare SELECT policies conform to all Medigap regulations and must have the approval of the insurance department in the states where they are sold.

**Medigap policy**  An insurance policy sold as a supplement to Medicare, usually but not always having coverage of copayments and deductibles as its main features.

**Metastasis**  A secondary growth, in a location of the body apart from the original site, of a cancer.

**Nasogastric tube**  A tube placed through the nose and into the stomach to drain secretions or deliver food and medications.

**Nonprofit voluntary hospitals**  Entities organized to provide hospital services on a nonprofit and nongovernmental basis, generally with alleged oversight from the community they serve via self-perpetuating boards of trustees; classic American hospitals.

**Notarized affidavit**  A document, signed in the presence of a notary public, in which an individual asserts, under penalty of perjury, that an assertion is true; an informal, written form of testimony.

**Nuclear medicine**  The branch of medicine concerned with the use of radioactive chemicals, as opposed to electromagnetic radiation, for therapy and diagnosis; overlaps with radiology and radiation therapy.

**Nurse practitioner**  A registered nurse (R.N.) who has taken additional training and is certified to handle some of the functions of a holder of the M.D. or D.O. degree.

**Office of Management and Budget (OMB)**  The agency of the executive branch of government which prepares the budget the President submits to Congress each year and supervises spending by government agencies during the year.

**Operating room**  A portion of a hospital, or other facility, specially equipped for surgery.

**Ophthalmologist**  A holder of the M.D. or D.O. degree who specializes in treatment of diseases of the eye with drugs and surgery. May or may not prescribe corrective lenses.

**Optometrist**  A holder of the degree of Doctor of Optometry, who specializes in prescribing corrective lenses and diagnosing, but not treating, conditions of the eye that require surgery or medication.

**Outliers**  Cases that fall outside the statistical norms of the DRG system, either in total cost or in days of hospitalization required. Medicare makes additional payments for outliers if the peer review organization approves.

**Out-of-area care**  Care that is given to a member of a health maintenance organization when the member is outside the service area of the HMO. This is an issue largely because federal laws for HMO certification require the definition of a service area. Depending on the HMO, arranging for out-of-area care can be a problem.

**Out-of-pocket limit**  An amount no more than which an insured individual is required to pay, after which his or her insurance policy pays all costs for the services it covers, regardless of other provisions.

**Outpatient**  Having to do with a person, or treatment given to that person, when he or she is not admitted to the hospital; e.g., "outpatient surgery."

**Outpatient prescription drugs**  Drugs that can be given outside a hospital in some or all cases, usually written on the orders of a physician.

**Outpatient surgery**  Surgery performed without admission to a hospital, even though the surgery may be performed in the hospital.

**Outpatient treatment**  Treatment at a hospital, or in a setting outside a hospital, that does not require admission or temporary residence at the hospital.

**Over-the-counter drugs**  Drugs that may be sold without prescription. Examples: aspirin, some decongestants and antihistamines, antibiotic ointments, low-dose cortisone creams, and some eyedrops.

**Pacemaker**   A medical device, implanted in the body, which sends the heart electrical signals to beat when the normal mechanism for generating such signals is defective.

**Packed red cells**   Blood cells that have been separated from the plasma and are administered separately.

**Participating physician agreement**   An agreement a doctor signs with HCFA to accept assignment on all Medicare claims and to follow certain procedures; renewed annually.

**Pathologist**   A doctor specializing in examining tissues removed from the body and in performing autopsies.

**Peer Review Organizations (PRO)**   Groups of doctors who have contracts with the Health Care Financing Administration to evaluate the medical necessity of care rendered to Medicare beneficiaries under the Medicare program and to investigate the quality of care provided to Medicare beneficiaries.

**People's Medical Society (PMS)**   A large health care consumer organization.

**Permanently and totally disabled**   A term of art under the Social Security Act, applying to those persons who meet the definition of disability in the act and qualify for Social Security payments and Medicare on that basis.

**Permanent vegetative state**   A condition in which higher brain functions are permanently suppressed.

**Perverse incentive**   A motivation provided by a system that defeats the system's purpose. In fee-for-service systems, there is a perverse incentive to overtreat; in prepaid systems, there is a perverse incentive to undertreat.

**Physiatrist**   A doctor who specializes in giving and prescribing physical therapy, primarily for rehabilitation.

**Physicians' assistant**   An individual trained to carry out some of the functions of holders of the M.D. or D.O. degree, usually with more training than a nurse practitioner or a medical technician.

**Physician extenders**   Individuals who are trained to do a part of what a holder of the M.D. or D.O. degree can do. They include nurse practitioners, physicians' assistants, and medical technicians. They are used heavily in health maintenance organizations.

**Podiatrist**   A holder of the degree of Doctor of Podiatric Medicine (D.P.M.), concerned with treatment of diseases of the feet.

**Power of attorney**   A legal document giving a person the power to act as the representative of the other in certain situations, which can be defined in the power-of-attorney document.

**Practice patterns**   Statistically detectable tendencies for individual doctors, or groups of them, to treat certain conditions in a certain way.

**Preferred provider organization (PPO)**   An arrangement in which patients are "locked in" to a group of providers, usually by restrictions on payment for services provided by those not in the group of providers, in return for discounts or expanded services. A wide variety exists; some resemble traditional insurance plans, and some resemble health maintenance organizations.

**Primary care physicians**   Physicians who, by training, preference, or necessity, practice a very broad range of medical services for persons not in need of highly specialized medical services. Usually cited as including general practitioners, family practitioners, general internists, pediatricians, and gynecologists who take care of both their patients' gynecological and general medical needs.

**Primary diagnosis**   The chief medical reason for an encounter with a health care provider or admission to a hospital.

**Private room**   In a hospital or nursing home, a room occupied by only one person, as opposed to the standard two-person room or a ward.

**Private duty nursing**   Care given by a nurse who is hired to care for one individual exclusively in a hospital or nursing home and is paid directly by the individual or his or her family.

**Procedure**   A manipulation of the body to give a treatment or perform a test; more broadly, any distinct service a doctor renders to a patient. All distinct physician services have "procedure codes" in various payment schemes.

**Prognosis**   A medical prediction of the course or probable outcome of an illness or condition.

**Prospective payment**   Payment made before a service is rendered, and accepted as payment in full by the provider; the opposite of fee-for-service payment.

**Protocol**   A written plan for caring for a particular condition, intended as a guideline to physicians, and usually adopted by a medical institution such as a clinic, hospital, or health maintenance organization.

**Provider**   A generic term for any person (a doctor) or entity (a home health agency, a hospital) approved to give care to Medicare beneficiaries and to receive payment from Medicare.

**Pulmonary specialist or pulmonologist**   A doctor specializing in lung diseases.

**Qualified Medicare Beneficiary (QMB)**   A Medicare beneficiary who qualifies for financial assistance based upon income and resources. Federal law requires state Medicaid programs to pay Medicare costs such as deductibles, copayments, and Part B premiums for those who qualify. Information on the QMB program is available from any state welfare office.

**Quarter of coverage**   One-fourth of a calendar year during which a person earns enough, in employment covered by Social Security, to have the quarter counted toward the number needed (usually forty) to ensure entitlement to Social Security and Medicare.

**Radiologist**   A physician specializing in taking diagnostic X rays and administering radiotherapy.

**Radiotherapy**   Treatment for cancer and some other conditions using electromagnetic radiation of several varieties.

**Recovery room**   A place in a hospital where patients are brought after surgery for close observation until they are ready to be taken to their floors or special care units.

**Registered nurse (R.N.)**   Generally, the highest trained of nurses; licensed by a state to provide general nursing services after passing a qualifying examination; may or may not hold collegiate degrees.

**Resident**   A doctor taking postgraduate training in a hospital, often working towards certification in a specialty area. Much of the training involves the care of patients under the supervision of more experienced physicians, both those based in the hospital and those who admit patients there.

**Resources-Based Relative Value Scale (RBRVS)**   A physician fee schedule that takes into account the skills and knowledge required to provide medical services. Each service provided by a physician is assigned a relative value unit based on: work required, practice expenses, and the cost of liability (malpractice) insurance. There is also an adjustment factor based on geographic location. The RBRVS replaces the usual, customary, and reasonable payment method.

**Respirator**   A medical device that takes over breathing functions for patients who are permanently or temporarily unable to breathe on their own (e.g., after open heart surgery).

**Retrospective payment**   Payment to a provider after care is given; fee-for-service payment.

**Rider**   An attachment to a standard form of insurance policy, obtained for an additional premium, that provides benefits not covered by the standard policy.

**Risk pooling**   The fundamental idea behind insurance. A large number of people with a low probability of high-cost events share the cost, reducing their individual risks to the amount of their insurance premium rather than the full cost of the event, such as an accident or illness; the fundamental concept of insurance.

**Secondary diagnosis**   A condition that exists in addition to the one that is the chief reason for an encounter with a health care provider or admission to a hospital.

**Sensitivity**   The ability of a medical test to detect something wrong, even if it cannot distinguish among various diagnoses. Contrast with *specificity.*

**Serum**   Biological material remaining after an animal or plant fluid is coagulated or centrifuged.

**Service area**   The geographical region in which a health maintenance organization or other prepaid health care plan has agreed to provide services.

**Sheltered, or custodial, care**   Care that is primarily nonmedical. Residents of sheltered or custodial care facilities do not require constant attention from nurses and aides, but need assistance with one or more daily activities or no longer want to be bothered with keeping up a house. The social needs of residents are met in a secure environment free of as many anxieties as possible.

**Skilled nursing facility (SNF)**   An institution that offers nursing services similar to those given in a hospital, to aid recuperation of those who are seriously ill. Distinguished from intermediate care and custodial care, which may meet some minor medical needs but are intended primarily to support elderly and disabled individuals in the tasks of daily living.

**Social health maintenance organizations (SHMO)**   Experimental programs that try to provide for the medical and social needs of the elderly and disabled in one, prepaid package. These, so far, have not been too successful because they were more expensive than was hoped.

**Social Security Administration (SSA)**   The part of the Department of Health and Human Services that operates the various programs funded under the Social Security Act and determines eligibility for Medicare.

**Social Security office**   Local offices of the Social Security Administration, found throughout the country, which take applications for Social Security and Medicare and handle processing of Medicare requests for reconsideration and appeals.

**Social Security number (SSN)**   A unique number assigned to each individual by the Social Security Administration for tax and benefits purposes. Also used as a unique personal identifier by many other government programs and private enterprises.

**Somatize**   To involuntarily express emotional concerns as physical symptoms.

**Special care units**   Portions of a hospital organized and staffed to take care of one kind of (usually serious) problem; e.g., cardiac care unit, intensive care unit, burn unit.

**Specialist**   A physician who has elected to practice, and usually has special training in, some branch of medicine other than primary care, such as surgery, or an exclusive focus in one area of primary care, such as allergy, gastroenterology, ear-nose-and-throat care, and so on. Especially in urban areas, specialists are expected to have certification (from specialty societies or boards) that they have had adequate training in the specialty.

**Specificity**   The ability of a medical test to identify a specific diagnosis or condition. Contrast with *sensitivity.*

**Specified Low-Income Medicare Beneficiary (SLMB)**   A Medicare beneficiary who is not eligible for the Qualified Medicare Beneficiary program but may still be eligible for financial assistance. The SLMB program is designed for beneficiaries whose income is slightly higher than the national poverty level, but not more than 10 percent higher. The SLMB program pays the monthly Part B premium; however, it does not cover the deductible, copayments, or services not covered by Medicare.

**Staff model health maintenance organization**   A health maintenance organization staffed by doctors who are its employees and are not in individual or group practice.

**Stop-loss provision**   See *out-of-pocket limit.*

**Streptokinase**   A drug, produced by bacteria of the beta-hemolytic streptococcal strains, used to abort heart attacks by dissolving clots that block the arteries of the heart.

**Subluxation of the spine**   A partial dislocation of one of the bones of the spinal column.

**Supplemental Security Income (SSI)**   A program that provides small stipends to the elderly, blind, and disabled who for one reason or another are not eligible for other, more generous welfare programs.

**Swing beds**   Hospital beds approved by Medicare for use as hospital or skilled nursing facility beds, depending on demand.

**Terminally ill**   Having an illness that is expected to end in death.

**Thrombophlebitis**   Irritation of a vein caused by a blood clot.

**Tissue plasminogen activator**   A drug, naturally occurring in small amounts in the human body and produced in quantity by genetically engineered bacteria, used to abort heart attacks by dissolving clots that block the arteries of the heart.

**Tumor**   An abnormal growth of a component of the body that is not inflammatory and possesses no physiological function.

**Urgent**   A situation, less grave than an emergency, in which care is required in the near future to prevent death, serious injury, or deformity. Contrast with *emergency.*

**Usual, customary, and reasonable reimbursement system**   A means of determining payments to doctors based on statistical profiles of their, and their colleagues', history of charges.

**Utilization review committee (URC)**   A group of doctors in a hospital who review lengths of hospital stays and treatments to make sure that they are medically necessary.

**Vaccines**   Biologically produced drugs designed to provide or enhance immunity to specific diseases or disease families.

**Waiver of liability**   A legal removal of an individual's responsibility to pay for a treatment in an instance where Medicare or Medicaid does not pay for it.

**X rays**   Electromagnetic radiation capable of penetrating soft tissue and producing pictures of the inside of the body; also, pictures taken with such radiation.

# Index

Join the People's Medical Society now. **Only $20 a year.** (That's less than the cost of just one office visit with your doctor.) And your contribution is 100 percent tax deductible.

---

*People's Medical Society*
## MEMBERSHIP FORM

☐  **Yes,** I want to join. Start my subscription to the PMS *Newsletter.* My $20 annual membership dues are enclosed.

☐  Send me more information about membership in the People's Medical Society.

Name _____

Address _____

City/State/Zip _____

Please make your check payable to
*People's Medical Society.*

People's Medical Society
462 Walnut Street
Allentown, PA 18102
(610) 770-1670

MME

---

The *PEOPLE'S MEDICAL SOCIETY* is a nonprofit citizens' action group committed to the principles of better, more responsive and less expensive medical care, and dedicated to the belief that people, as individuals or in groups, can make a difference. To this end, the *PEOPLE'S MEDICAL SOCIETY* is involved in the organizing of community efforts around local health-care issues, and in the national debate over the future of the medical care system.